CRASH COURSE
History and
Examination
SECOND EDITION

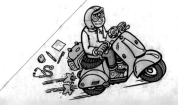

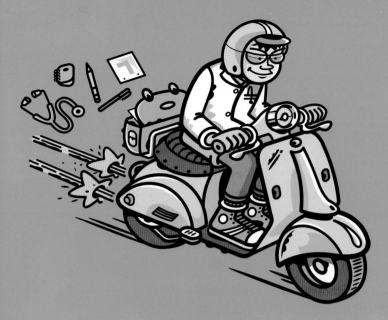

Series editor
Daniel Horton-Szar
BSc(Hons), MBBS(Hons)
GP Registrar
Northgate Medical Practice
Canterbury
Kent

Faculty advisor
Prof John Spencer
Medical Education and Primary
  Health Care
School of Medical Education
  Development
University of Newcastle upon Tyne
Newcastle upon Tyne

History and Examination

SECOND EDITION

Maxwell A. Allan

MBBS, BMedSci(Hons)
Anaesthetics Department
Sunderland Royal Hospital
Sunderland

First Edition Author
James Marsh

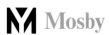

Edinburgh • London • New York • Oxford • Philadelphia • St Louis • Sydney • Toronto 2004

MOSBY
An imprint of Elsevier Limited

Commissioning Editor	Alex Stibbe
Project Development Manager	Duncan Fraser
Project Manager	Frances Affleck
Designer	Andy Chapman
Cover Design	Kevin Faerber
Illustration Manager	Mick Ruddy

First edition 1999
This edition 2004

ISBN 0723433321

British Library Cataloguing in Publication Data
A catalogue record for this book is available from the British Library

Library of Congress Cataloging in Publication Data
A catalog record for this book is available from the Library of Congress

Notice
Medical knowledge is constantly changing. Standard safety precautions must be followed, but as new research and clinical experience broaden our knowledge, changes in treatment and drug therapy may become necessary or appropriate. Readers are advised to check the most current product information provided by the manufacturer of each drug to be administered to verify the recommended dose, the method and duration of administration, and contraindications. It is the responsibility of the practitioner, relying on experience and knowledge of the patient, to determine dosages and the best treatment for each individual patient. Neither the Publisher nor the authors assume any liability for any injury and/or damage to persons or property arising from this publication.

Typeset by Kolam, Pondicherry, India
Printed in China

The Publisher's policy is to use **paper manufactured from sustainable forests**

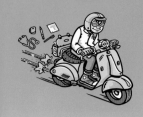

Preface

You too can pass finals!

Look at the PRHOs and SHOs that you've seen around you on your attachments—do you really think they were so different from you at medical school? They weren't. Crash Course: History and Examination is designed to get you through medical school with a few pearls of wisdom to help once you've qualified. It is a revision aid that will help you hone your skills in taking a history, examining a patient and thinking what to do next.

The process of discovering why a person has come to see their doctor is well established: you have a talk with them, asking specific questions on the way; do some tests (laboratory or radiological) and then stand back, think about all you have discovered and offer them your thoughts and possible ways to help. This book gives advice and assistance on how to approach and perfect this vital aspect of medicine.

At the end of the book are some handy hints on how to improve your exam technique. We've also included some sample questions including MCQs, OSCEs and EMQs to help guide your revision and test your knowledge.

Max Allan

In spite of the vast array of technology now available to assist doctors in their work with patients, and our ever-expanding understanding of the minutiae of disease processes, the role of the history and physical examination remains central in both diagnosis and management. Sir William Osler, arguably the most eminent physician of his time, exhorted his pupils in the early 20th century to 'listen to the patient, he is telling you his story' and, more recently, in the 1970s, George Engel said '...the interview is potentially the most powerful, sensitive instrument at the command of the physician.' The move in recent years towards a more patient-centred clinical method has, if anything, increased the importance of the history and examination. The benefits of good communication go well beyond making an accurate diagnosis – concordance with treatment is more likely, patient outcomes are improved, doctors feel more satisfied with their work and complaints and litigation are reduced. Similarly, the physical examination does more than help to confirm clinical hunches. It also enables the doctor to make a more discriminating use of diagnostic technology, something that demonstrates a professional approach to the patient and will be appreciated by both patients and the public purse.

This second edition of Crash Course: History and Examination, offers a comprehensive user-friendly guide to history taking and physical examination. A flexible and discriminating approach is encouraged; one that is sensitive to both the doctor's and the patient's needs. I am sure that this book will be useful to you not only in passing your exams (your main concern right now), but also beyond the dreaded OSCEs and long cases into 'real life'. Max Allan is to be congratulated for his efforts in revamping the text of the first edition.

John Spencer
Faculty Advisor

Over the last six years since the first editions were published, there have been many changes in medicine, and in the way it is taught. These second editions have been largely rewritten to take these changes into account, and keep Crash Course up to date for the twenty-first century. New material has been added to include recent research and all pharmacological and disease management information has been updated in line with current best practice. We've listened to feedback from hundreds of medical students who have been using Crash Course and have improved the structure and layout of the books accordingly: pathology and disease management material has been moved closer to the diagnostic skills chapters; there are more MCQs and now we have Extended Matching Questions as well, with explanations of each answer. We have also included references for 'further reading' where appropriate to highlight important papers and studies that you should be aware of, and the clarity of text and figures is better than ever.

The principles on which we developed the series remain the same, however. Clinical medicine is a huge subject, and teaching on the wards can sometimes be sporadic because of the competing demands of patient care. The last thing a student needs when finals are approaching is to waste time assembling information from different sources, or wading through pages of irrelevant detail. As before, Crash Course brings you all the information you need in compact, manageable volumes that integrate an approach to common patient presentations with clinical skills, pathology and management of the relevant diseases. We still tread the fine line between producing clear, concise text and providing enough detail for those aiming at distinction. The series is still written by junior doctors with recent exam experience, in partnership with senior faculty members from across the UK.

I wish you the best of luck in your future careers!

Dr Dan Horton-Szar
Series Editor

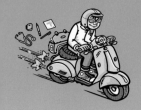

Acknowledgements

Fig. 1.1 adapted with kind permission from M A Stewart and D Roter. Communicating with Patients. Sage Publications, 1989

Figs. 5.1, 5.2, 5.12, 14.6, 14.7, 14.12, 14.13, 14.15, 14.19, 21.16   redrawn with permission from O Epstein, G D Perkin, D P deBono and J Cookson. Clinical Examination, 2nd edition. Mosby, 1997

Fig. 6.8 reproduced with permission from P M W Bath and K R Lees. ABC of arterial and venous disease. British Medical Journal 320, BMJ Publishing Group, 2000

Figs. 6.9, 17.5, 17.7, 17.13, 17.14, 17.16, 17.20, 17.24, 22.1,   reproduced with kind permission from D Lasserson, C Gabriel and B Sharrack. Crash Course: Nervous System and Special Senses. Mosby, 1998

Fig. 7.3 adapted with kind permission from, Advanced Life Support Group. Advanced Paediatric Life Support: The Practical Approach, 3rd edition. BMJ Books, 2000

Fig. 21.4 reproduced with permission from S V Biswas and R Iqbal. Crash Course: Musculoskeletal System. Mosby, 1998

Fig. 24.8 reproduced with kind permission from, P Kumar and M Clarke. Clinical Medicine, 5th edition. W B Saunders 2002

Fig. 24.9 reproduced with permission from J Weir and P H Abrahams. Imaging Atlas of Human Anatomy, 2nd edition. Mosby 2003

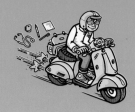

Dedication

To my wife and parents for their enduring love and support.

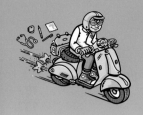

Contents

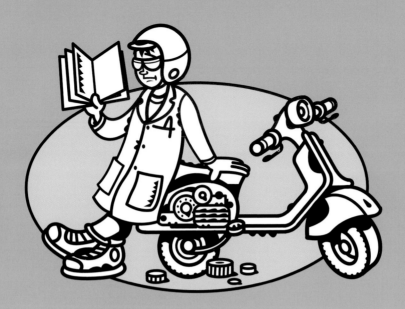

HISTORY TAKING

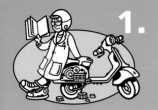

1. Introduction to History Taking

Overview

The first section of this book focuses on the history. After an introduction the basic structure of a medical history is given, detailing the bare bones. It is important to adopt a systematic approach so that all relevant information is obtained. The chapters which follow are used to illustrate the need to be flexible within that basic format, adapting your questions to different circumstances so that differential diagnoses can be explored. The examples of medical histories are not intended to provide a rigid checklist of questions. There are two kinds of history: those that you use in real life and those that you use in examinations. Beware of any institutional preferences when exam time comes. Histories in real life are context specific: what is appropriate for an 80-year-old woman who cannot cope at home is different from a young man who has just been stabbed. The examples provided are only a framework, and should be adapted to suit your own preferences, the individual patient and, of course, the exam format, e.g. the OSCE or long case.

Basic principles

The principal aims of medical clerking are to establish:
- What is wrong with the patient today?
- How do these problems impact on the person's life?

The standard approach is to obtain the history before conducting a physical examination and requesting appropriate investigations. Despite being presented here as separate chapters, these components of the clerking interlock with each other in a dynamic fashion from the moment that the doctor meets the patient.

The medical history has a traditional format, but it should not be considered as a rigid interrogation and checklist of questions. Effective history taking depends crucially on good communication skills. Although a structured approach is needed, it is important to adopt a flexible attitude, adapting your questions and differential diagnosis as information is received. The process of formulating a differential diagnosis starts as soon as the patient describes his or her presenting complaint. The symptom should be explored in detail so that possible diagnoses can be excluded, others can be introduced, and a balance of probabilities can be weighed up. Once the patient has described his or her main symptoms, specific questions should be asked to refine the differential diagnosis. Thus the process of history taking is an active skill, and not one of passive listening. If you have been unable to ascertain a differential diagnosis by the end of the history you will struggle to find signs on your examination to confirm your suspicions and will be unable to request appropriate investigations.

Obtaining and assessing information

Gleaning the important information is a fine art and takes years to master. Every medical student has experienced the frustration of taking a garbled, incoherent history from a rambling patient, only to see a consultant ask one or two seemingly simple questions that make the underlying diagnosis become embarrassingly dovious.

The traditional approach is to start by asking 'open' questions:
- 'Why don't you tell me about your pain?'
- 'Why have you come to hospital today?'

This gives patients the opportunity to tell you how they perceive their problems before the agenda is taken out of their hands, and your own prejudices take over. It is well recognized that doctors and patients often focus on different problems and/or have conflicting agendas. By careful steering and gentle coaxing, even the most garrulous patients can usually give full, clear and reasonably concise descriptions of their current symptoms. It is also necessary to ask 'closed' questions for further clarification, for example:

- 'Does your pain get worse after eating?'
- 'Did you black out completely or just feel lightheaded?'

It is a matter of judgement when to start interrupting and asking closed questions, but as a general rule, think twice before interrupting a patient in full flow. If specific questions are introduced too early, vital information may never come to light.

It is also important to obtain information on the impact the patient's illness has, not only physically, but also in a wider psychological and social context. The same pain or disability will restrict the activities of different people greatly (e.g. work, social interactions, hobbies). This information is vital for a full assessment and also reassures patients that the doctor is taking a genuine interest in them and not just their chest pain, arthritis, etc. Information to explore includes:

- *Ideas*. What does the patient think is wrong?
- *Concerns*. What does the patient worry might be wrong?
- *Expectations*. What does the patient think is going to happen in the consultation and regarding his or her future health? What might happen following the consultation? (e.g. investigations, operations).

To say that effective history taking is underpinned by good communication may seem to be stating the obvious. Yet there is considerable evidence to show that doctors' communication skills – *how* they elicit a patient's story – are wanting, particularly in respect of finding out what the patient thinks is wrong and what concerns them.

A useful way of looking at the medical interview is the Calgary–Cambridge framework, which is increasingly used in both undergraduate and postgraduate education, including in the design of OSCE stations. It divides the interview into distinct phases and identifies the key tasks and 'microskills' associated with each. In the context of history taking, as explored in this book, the 'explanation and planning' stage will not be addressed.

Calgary–Cambridge framework
1. Initiating the session
   - Establishing initial rapport
   - Identifying the presenting problem(s)
2. Gathering information
   - Exploration of problem(s)
   - Understanding the patient's perspective
   - Providing structure to the consultation
3. Building the relationship
   - Developing rapport
   - Involving the patient
4. Explanation and planning
   - Providing the correct type and amount of information
   - Aiding accurate recall and understanding
   - Achieving a shared understanding through incorporating the patient's perspective
   - Planning through shared decision making
5. Closing the session

Key skills areas for gathering information include:
- Attentive listening
  Eye contact, posture, nodding, facilitatory statements (e.g. 'Uh-huh' or 'Go on...')
- Appropriate use of questions. These can be classified as:
  Closed questions – are obviously necessary to ascertain facts, but generally invite a specific (often one-word) answer, and limit response to a narrow field
  Open questions – less focused but still direct patients to a specific area, but allow them more discretion
  Clarifying or probing questions – their purpose is self-evident. (e.g. 'What do you mean by that?' 'Can you tell me about the last time you had the pain.' 'What makes you say that?')
  The key issue is to use an appropriate balance of question types – all have a place
- Summarizing
  Summarizing periodically, and at the end of the interview, allows you to: check whether you've

heard the patient's story; review the story and deduce what else needs to be explored; help the patient carry on with their account; demonstrate that you have been listening; and close the interview in an appropriate way

Key skills areas for understanding the patient's perspective include:

- Asking about ideas, concerns and expectations
- Responding to cues, both verbal and non-verbal Interpersonal exchanges are loaded with messages, both non-verbal and verbal. These may give a clue to what's *really* going on, and responding to them directly ('You mentioned your mother ended up in wheelchair with her arthritis; do you think that's what is going to happen to you?') or using reflection ('I sense that you are really very upset about this') will usually provide important extra information. Sometimes simply repeating back the 'cue' to the patient will suffice ('...something could be done'...?' '...very worried'...?')

A patient-centred approach

The traditional medical history does not primarily aim to understand the meaning of the illness for the patient, focusing, as it does, on diagnosing disease in terms of an underlying pathology. The way that doctors have been taught to take a history in the past implied that if they simply asked the right number of (usually closed) questions about the functioning of an organ or system, they would gather all the information needed to make a diagnosis. Only lip service was paid to the impact the problem had on the patient's life beyond the symptoms themselves. This approach ignores the fact that the way in which a disease affects one person – their 'illness experience' – is very different from another person, emotionally, psychologically and functionally. Remember that accurately eliciting and addressing the patient's concerns and expectations is not only important for diagnosis, but will also have a major influence on concordance with treatment, patient satisfaction, detection of hidden problems, and some physical outcomes (e.g. glycaemic control in diabetics; pain relief after surgery).

The patient-centred approach aims to incorporate the patient's perspective and involves a parallel search of two frameworks – the 'illness framework', and the 'disease framework' (Fig. 1.1).

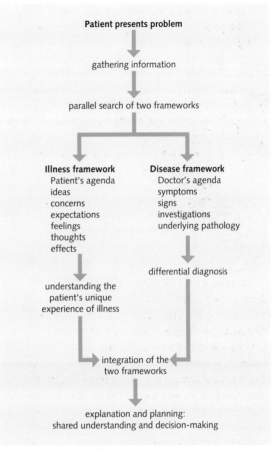

Fig. 1.1 The disease–illness model.

Relationship with the patient

The atmosphere and setting is important when taking a history. Patients should feel free to express their fears and concerns without fear or embarrassment. An air of absolute confidentiality should be created. At the same time, take note of any non-verbal signs (e.g. hostility, embarrassment). Often the most crucial information needs to be coaxed out of the patient. Never appear to be in a rush. Patients expect and deserve full attention and sympathy for their problems. It is not unusual for patients to express their real concerns just as they are leaving the consulting room.

 However tempting, do not ignore throwaway comments from the patient. They often carry the key to the whole problem. Never be in a rush. Time invested in taking a good history pays dividends in the long term.

It is often useful (even if potentially time-consuming), to ask patients at the end of a consultation if there is anything else they wish to discuss. If patients feel at ease with you, they will talk more freely. They should feel confident not only in your diagnostic abilities, but also in your sympathy, understanding and motivation. After all, you are acting as their advocate. This process should start as soon as you greet patients.

Remember that first impressions really do matter. Appear friendly, but professional. Patients must have confidence in your ability to act on their behalf.

Remember that the history is the most important part of the examination. If there is a language barrier, help the patient to relax, do not rush, explain everything clearly, and if necessary obtain an interpreter. If the patient is confused or unconscious, history taking is still vital. A relative, carer, nursing home worker, or other witness is usually available to provide information. This process is time consuming, but worthwhile.

There is no reason for yourself or any other member of staff to be harmed by a patient. Remember, there is no medical condition that cannot be managed in a police cell! There is, however, rarely any justification for resorting to a 'veterinary' approach. There will be times when you will hear stories that are difficult to cope with on an emotional level. Be professional with the patient but do not be afraid to discuss this with others. All of us need to share difficult experiences with one another. Anyone who tells you otherwise is trying to kid themselves.

Difficult consultations

In certain circumstances the history can be considerably more difficult to obtain, for example if:
- There is a language barrier.
- The patient is confused, hostile, or unconscious.

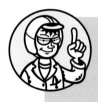

The history is the most important part of the patient's assessment and provides the information required to make a diagnosis in up to 80% of cash.

2. The History

Introductory statement

Before taking a detailed history it is essential to obtain some background information from the patient. This should include the patient's:

- Name (it might be Napoleon and hence a psychiatric problem).
- Age.
- Sex.
- What the person is like at their best.
- Occupation.
- Presenting complaint.

Ideally try to use the words that the patient has used (e.g. people never complain of dyspnoea, but will say that they feel 'short of breath'). This statement should be short and pithy, for example 'John Smith is a 56-year-old electrician complaining of chest pain'.

This information is vital as it helps you (and any listeners) form a thumbnail sketch of the person in front of you, so that appropriate questions can be anticipated if the patient does not volunteer the information. The process of forming a differential diagnosis should have already begun but at this stage it will, by necessity, be broad.

History of presenting complaint

This is the main component of the history. A detailed, thorough investigation into the current illness is performed. This is usually composed of two sequential (but often overlapping) stages:

- The patient's account of the symptoms.
- Specific, detailed questions by the doctor.

The relative proportion of each component depends upon the underlying problem, the communication skills of the patient, and listening skills of the doctor. Listening should be an active process. Ideally, the patient should be given every opportunity to talk freely at the start of the consultation with minimal interruption. A common mistake made by most students (and doctors) is to interrupt the patient and to intervene with closed questions too early.

Patients must feel that they are getting a fair hearing and have had an adequate opportunity to express themselves. They should be made to feel that the doctor is listening carefully and has a genuine concern for their problems. Subtle nuances are often missed if the doctor seizes the agenda too early.

A combination of art, experience, and patience determines when and how to interrupt a patient in full flow, but it is prudent to err on the side of caution and allow the patient to drift a little (especially when you are first taking histories), while making a mental note of the most important features of the narrative and issues that require clarification.

The full circumstances surrounding a single event or symptom need to be explored in a systematic manner so that a complete picture can be obtained.

A patient complains of pain

Explore in detail the circumstances surrounding the episode so that a complete picture can be obtained.

What was the patient doing immediately before the episode?

Ascertain exactly what the patient was doing at the time of the onset of the pain (e.g. running, arguing with wife, sitting in chair).

Speed of onset

Determine the rate of development of pain (e.g. seconds, minutes, hours, days). It may be helpful to draw a graph of symptoms versus time (Figs 2.1 and 2.2).

Time of onset

Try to obtain exact times and dates if appropriate.

Subsequent time course

Map out the fluctuations in symptoms with time.

Duration

How long did the pain last? Patients often overestimate the duration of symptoms.

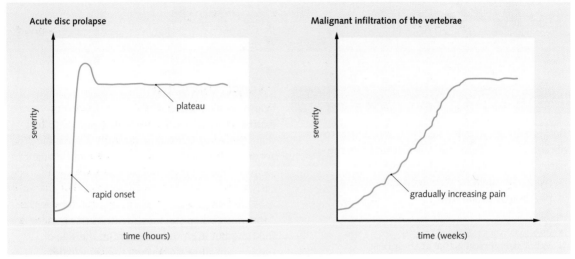

Fig. 2.1 Graphs illustrating the typical time course of two different types of back pain, which are of the same severity at presentation but of different aetiology.

Nature of pain

It is particularly useful to record direct quotations from the patient such as:

- 'Like a stabbing knife'.
- 'Like being compressed by a vice'.

They are often very descriptive, but some patients are less colourful in their language and may need help to describe a symptom. You could then provide examples such as 'Would you describe the pain as burning, stabbing, crushing, throbbing, or something else?' It can sometimes be useful to quantify the severity of the pain. The visual analogue pain score is a well established method (see Fig. 2.3).

Radiation

Radiation of pain is important and often gives clues to the aetiology. For example, the pain of a prolapsed intervertebral disc usually radiates down the back of one leg, whereas muscular strain is usually well localized.

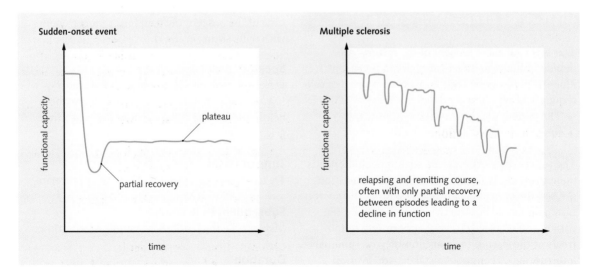

Fig. 2.2 Graph of the time course of functional capacity against time for a patient who has had a stroke or has multiple sclerosis. It is important to consider not only the speed of onset of a particular symptom, but its subsequent time course.

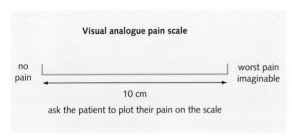

Fig. 2.3 Visual analogue pain score.

Associated symptoms

Pain rarely occurs in isolation. Associated symptoms are often characteristic of certain pathological processes. For example, if a patient describes pleuritic chest pain, ask about the presence of cough, dyspnoea, fever, haemoptysis, etc.

Aggravating features

Different types of pain have different aggravating factors. For example, mechanical back pain is often exacerbated by exercise, but inflammatory pain may be worse after a period of prolonged rest.

Relieving factors

Factors producing relief of symptoms may give clues to the aetiology or severity of the pain (e.g. the pain of intermittent claudication resolves rapidly on rest compared with the pain of critical limb ischaemia).

Recovery

Note the time and speed of recovery.

Residual symptoms

Once the pain has resolved, there are often ongoing symptoms; for example, after the pain of myocardial infarction the patient often reports ongoing fatigue, dyspnoea or palpitations.

Effect of any interventions

Ask about the effect of interventions, for example:
  'Did your chest pain get any better after taking a
     glyceryl trinitrate (GTN) tablet?'
  'Did the pain resolve when you stopped
     running?'

In the event of repeated symptoms additional information is also needed, for example frequency and pattern (e.g. getting progressively better or worse, more or less easily provoked).

Previous episodes

Ask the patient if he or she has had a similar episode of pain before.

Interpreting information

Do not accept the patient's (or the doctor's) interpretation of symptoms at face value. At this stage, you are most interested in what the patient was *actually* experiencing. If the patient has been given a label for the symptoms, it may be helpful to know by whom, and on what evidence. For example, if the patient says 'My doctor tells me I have angina!', find out whether the patient has had investigations such as an exercise test, angiography or electrocardiography, and if so what the results were.

Often different patients mean different things by the same phrase. Be wary! For example, dizziness may relate to vertigo, presyncope, muzziness, etc. This clearly has different implications for the underlying diagnosis. In addition, try to make your questions as clear and unambiguous as possible.

When recording the history try to keep it as brief and 'punchy' as possible. An example of a history obtained for chest pain could be 'He describes a sudden onset retrosternal chest tightness "like an elastic band" radiating to the jaw and left arm every time he climbs the staircase from the underground station (approximately 100 steps). He has a sensation that he needs to stop and rest immediately, and also feels mildly nauseated, short of breath and occasionally sweaty. He never has palpitations, lightheadedness nor syncopal episodes. The pain is relieved within 2 minutes of resting or seconds after placing a GTN tablet under his tongue, and he can then continue his daily activities. He has noticed that on a cold or windy day, the pain comes on earlier, but otherwise has been stable over the past two months.'

This illustrates the need to play an active role in the discussion, being always aware of:
- The differential diagnosis.
- How the symptoms interfere with functional activities.

Wherever possible, try to quantify the symptoms objectively. In addition, the presence of relevant 'negative' symptoms creates a more complete picture.

A long list of 'negatives' is very dull and judgement is needed when deciding which ones to include in the narrative. This is where experience helps when presenting the history. Try to imagine yourself as the listener, and consider carefully what information you would want to know.

Rounding off the history

Asking patients what they think the cause of their symptoms might be always provides an important insight. They are often worried about the consequences of what appears to be a trivial symptom to an objective observer. It is impossible to offer appropriate reassurance or counselling without this knowledge. Furthermore, if the patient's own judgement differs significantly from the doctor's, the doctor must reassess how he or she arrived at the differential diagnosis.

Often a history is very complicated or the patient appears to have given a contradictory account. It is helpful to read back your recollection of the history to the patient so that he or she can verify its accuracy – you will have opportunity to place your own interpretation at a later stage! You should both be in agreement about the facts before you introduce your own bias. It provides a message to the patient that you have been listening to his or her concerns. This is a useful way of focusing patients, especially if they are rambling. Finally, it is a good way of ending the history.

Summary

When taking the history of the presenting complaint:
- The primary objective is to obtain a comprehensive, but succinct account of the presenting symptom(s).
- Allow patients sufficient opportunity to describe their symptoms at the start.
- Resist the temptation to interrupt too early and too frequently.
- If patients drift, gently coax and steer them back on course to the main focus.
- Ask specific questions to clarify, obtain more detail, or to investigate potential diagnoses only after the patient has described his or her symptoms.
- Sometimes negative answers are more important than positive answers.

- Ask patients what they think may be causing the symptoms.
- If the history is complicated recount your interpretation of events back to the patient to ensure that your versions are concordant.
- Attempt to be as systematic and objective as possible. Look for collateral evidence to support any statement, especially if it is related to someone's interpretation of symptoms.
- Ask easily understood, unambiguous questions.
- If the patient presents with more than one presenting complaint this process may need repeating for each complaint.

Past medical history

This is important for placing the current illness in the context of past events, as they are often related. A review of the past medical history should include the points addressed below.

Previous hospital admissions

Outline essential information such as:
- Diagnoses/problems.
- Dates and places.
- Treatment and investigations.

Occasionally verification of previous events may be necessary, particularly if the patient has had a complicated hospital admission. This may prevent repetition of unnecessary (and sometimes harmful) investigations. The patient's recollection may be hazy, especially of events occurring within hospital (e.g. investigations for acute renal failure).

Operations

List procedures chronologically in a similar way.

Known medical or psychiatric conditions

Remember to have a healthy scepticism about diagnostic labels used by the patient. If necessary explore how a diagnosis has been established.

Problems related to underlying present illness

Ask about particular risk factors or associated diseases related to the primary complaint. For example, if a patient presents with chest pain, ask specifically about:

- Previous episodes of angina and myocardial infarction.
- Strokes and transient ischaemic attacks (TIAs).
- Diabetes mellitus.
- Hypertension, etc.
- Hypercholesterolaemia.

This is the component of the past medical history that takes the most skill. An awareness of the likely differential diagnosis is needed, illustrating that the history should be adapted to different circumstances. Listening should be active and relevant negative information often provides as much information as positive facts.

Drug history

A complete list of current medication with doses is essential. Taking a drug history is difficult and it may be necessary to phone the GP and find out what medications the patient should be taking. Remember that what we consider a drug and what the patient may consider a drug are two separate things. Commonly, patients don't consider their inhalers as drugs or many feel that the term drug refers only to illegal substances. One way to get round this is to ask the patient, 'what pills, potions and puffers do you use?'

Why is drug history important?
A detailed drug history is important because:
- It may give an indication of disease processes that the patient was either unaware of or has failed to mention (e.g. thyroxine suggestive of hypothyroidism).
- The drugs may be the cause of the present symptoms due to adverse effects or drug interactions (e.g. headache induced by nitrates used to treat angina). Try to establish a temporal relationship between the initiation or change of medication and the onset of new symptoms.
- Conversely, withdrawal of therapy may be responsible for the current symptoms (e.g. withdrawal of diuretics may lead to swollen ankles and orthopnoea).
- It provides an opportunity to explore the patient's understanding of the disease, often highlighting a need for further education (e.g. the controlled use and technique of inhaling steroids and bronchodilators by the asthmatic patient).

The potential therapeutic options for the presenting illness can be explored.

Check concordance and explore the reasons for non-concordance such as:
- Intolerable side effects.
- Perceived lack of efficacy.
- Ignorance.
- Poor communication from prescribing physician.
- Four times daily medication instead of once daily.

This exploration of concordance must be done very sensitively in an effort not to appear to be judgemental. Patients do not like admitting that they have not taken medication prescribed on their behalf. In a recent systematic review, the main factor contributing to non-concordance was whether or not the patient's beliefs about the medicine had been elucidated and discussed. Use statements such as 'Do you ever have difficulty taking your tablets?' or 'Do you ever forget to take your tablets?' Even when approached sensitively, few patients admit poor concordance. This is important because there is no point in inexorably increasing the dose of medication if it is not being taken. Frequent culprits include those taking antihypertensive agents.

Ask specifically about the use of over-the-counter (OTC) medication, herbal remedies, and (in women) oral contraceptives. These are often not considered to be 'medication'.

In the unconscious patient, check for the use of steroids, anticoagulants, anti-epileptics, insulin, etc. The patient may carry a card detailing this information or wear a 'medicalert' bracelet.

Ask to see the patient's medicines. This provides extra insight into the patient's understanding as well as concordance.

History of drug allergy

This follows naturally from the drug history. As with other sections of the history, a systematic approach is rewarded.

Many people think that they have an allergy to medication, but a healthy scepticism is needed when assessing this. Always enquire how the 'allergy' was manifested; for example 'stomach upset' after the use of antibiotics is common, but very rarely an allergic phenomenon. Skin rashes are much more likely to represent a true allergy.

It is important to clarify the circumstances of a suspected allergic reaction. Attempt to establish a 'temporal relationship' between the drug administration and the allergic manifestation. For example, it is not uncommon for a rash to be part of a viral illness or for a rash to be an epiphenomenon – patients with glandular fever who are prescribed amoxycillin will develop a macular erythematous rash. This is not an allergic phenomenon.

Enquire whether the patient has ever been 'rechallenged' with the same drug, and if so whether any reaction occurred. However, in most cases of uncertainty, it is usually safest to assume that the patient does have an allergy, and to avoid the suspected drug.

Finally, enquire about the presence of atopic conditions (e.g. eczema, hay fever, asthma, urticaria, etc.).

Social history

The social history is crucial for every patient as it provides information on how the disease and patient interact at a functional level. It is particularly important that it is detailed in elderly, frail, or socially isolated patients. Try to obtain a picture of daily activities, and consider the impact of the disease at each stage.

An elderly person presents with a hemiplegia
What is the structure of the home?
Consider the physical characteristics of the home as this will affect mobility and ability to function independently:
- Is it a flat or a house?
- If it is a flat, what floor is it on and is there a lift?
- How many bedrooms are there?
- What access is there to the house, bedroom, kitchen, toilet, etc? (e.g. stairs, ramps).

Who are the potential carers?
Enquire about the structure of the household and whether other members of the household are out of the house during the day and physically fit. Find out whether any family members live nearby. Are there any other potential local carers?

Can the patient perform the usual activities of daily living?
Assess the practicalities of routine activities such as:
- Getting in and out of bed.
- Dressing.

- Toileting (mobility and continence).
- Cooking and eating.
- Bathing.
- Shopping.

What level of social support is already provided for the patient?
The patient may already be known to the social services. Enquire specifically about community nursing, 'meals on wheels', home help, social worker, benefits, etc.

 In a hospital setting, discharge planning should begin from the first assessment so that potential problems can be anticipated before they arise.

Other patients may require the help of occupational therapists (e.g. patients with rheumatoid arthritis may need assessment for aids for eating, ramps for access to the home, stair rails, stair lifts, bath seats, etc.).

The young patient
Younger patients present different problems and an illness may interfere with their lifestyle or be a direct result of it. It is important to find out the following information.

Occupation
Consider whether the occupation may have predisposed to the current illness, for example:
- Backache in manual workers.
- Repetitive strain injury in keyboard operators.
- Non-specific chest pain in people presenting with stress and people who are stressed by their jobs.

Consider whether the present illness may interfere with the ability to continue with the patient's occupation, for example:
- Epilepsy or myocardial infarction in a heavy goods vehicle driver.
- Ischaemic heart disease or rheumatoid arthritis in a manual worker.

Do not forget that lack of employment may contribute to the presenting illness. There is a well-documented association with the onset of morbidity (both physical and psychological) and unemployment.

Hobbies

These may be the cause of the illness (e.g. pigeon-fancier's lung) or be precluded by the current illness (e.g. squash, if the patient has newly diagnosed angina).

Travel

World travel is increasingly common and it is therefore important to be aware of recent travel; for example you should consider:

- Malaria in a patient who has returned from an endemic area and presents with fever.
- Hepatitis A in a person with jaundice who has been to an endemic area.
- Schistosomiasis in a patient presenting with haematuria.

Other sources of stress

Common causes include financial difficulties, job insecurity, or strained relationships at home. The list, however, is endless and recognition depends upon great sensitivity by the doctor.

Recreational drugs

It is always appropriate to enquire specifically about the use of recreational drugs, the following should raise your suspicions:

- If immunodeficiency is suspected.
- Needle marks are spotted.
- The patient presents with a decreased level of consciousness.

Risk factors for human immunodeficiency virus (HIV) and hepatitis B and C

These diseases are becoming more common and an increasing index of suspicion is needed, especially for those patients with risk factors, for example:

- Intravenous drug users.
- Individuals partaking in unprotected sexual intercourse.
- Prostitutes and their partners.
- Haemophiliacs.
- Recipients of blood transfusion in Africa since 1977.
- Partners of the above groups.

Smoking

It is obligatory to ask every patient about cigarette smoking. A useful concept is 'pack years' (i.e. the number of packs of cigarettes smoked daily multiplied by the years of smoking). If the person tells you they are an ex-smoker always ask them when they stopped. Do not forget other forms of smoking.

There are very few diseases in adult patients for which a smoking history is not relevant.

Alcohol

Alcohol plays a contributory role in many illnesses. An attempt should be made to estimate consumption for every patient. This is usually quoted in units/week. One unit equals:

- $1/2$ pint of beer.
- 1 glass of wine.
- 1 single measure of spirit.

In certain circumstances, a more detailed history is appropriate. It is sometimes helpful to work through a typical drinking day for the 'heavier' drinker. Remember that patients often think that a doctor is likely to disapprove of heavy drinking, so denial is common. At this stage in the consultation it is not your job to be judgemental!

Nutrition

An attempt should be made to assess nutritional status. A detailed history is needed for certain patients (e.g. those presenting with weight loss or iron-, folate-, or vitamin B_{12}-deficient anaemia).

Family history

Information about the health and age of other family members is often instructive, particularly for young patients or those with a suspected inherited disease. It is helpful to draw a family tree (Fig. 2.4).

Some diseases have a predictable mode of inheritance (Fig. 2.5):

- Autosomal dominant (e.g. Huntington's chorea, adult polycystic kidneys).
- Autosomal recessive (e.g. cystic fibrosis).
- X-linked recessive (e.g. colour blindness).

Other disorders do not have a Mendelian mode of inheritance, but there is often a discernible genetic component, and family history is still significant. Such disorders include:

- Hypertension.
- Ischaemic heart disease.

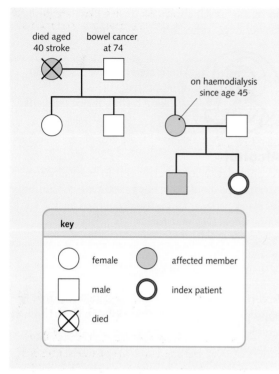

died aged 40 stroke   bowel cancer at 74

on haemodialysis since age 45

key

○	female	●	affected member
□	male	◎	index patient
⊗	died		

Fig. 2.4 A typical family tree written in hospital notes demonstrating family members affected by autosomal dominant polycystic kidneys.

- Schizophrenia.
- Breast cancer.

Even if the suspected disease has no recognized inheritable factor, it is useful to record a family tree with causes of death or major diseases. Doing this with the patient may open the door to some of the patient's concerns and may provide a useful insight into relationships within the family.

Review of symptoms

A brief review of symptoms in a systems enquiry is essential in a detailed history. It may suggest other disorders that have not been considered or highlight potentially serious complications that a patient may have considered to be trivial. In addition, it may be used as a screening process to highlight aspects of the history that require more detailed attention.

With practice, it is possible to cover this aspect of the history in a few minutes and this is time well invested.

It is helpful to consider this section in systems. When the presenting complaint appears to relate to one system, this system should be promoted to the detailed history of the presenting complaint, and a more detailed enquiry performed. The absence of particular symptoms attain a greater significance, for example when a patient describes chest pain, the presence or absence of dyspnoea or palpitations is clearly more relevant than when the presenting complaint is headache.

Since you have just spent some time exploring the history of the presenting complaint – usually the problem causing most discomfort distress for the patient – it may seem odd to them when you embark on a detailed enquiry about other parts of the body. 'Signpost' your intention; a sentence like, 'OK Mrs Thompson, I'm now going to ask you some questions about other symptoms', will suffice.

The systems enquiry is often the most difficult component of the history to interpret. The significance of each symptom and its relevance to the primary complaint needs to be analysed. This may lead to a review of the differential diagnosis and new questions to either confirm or refute new suspicions.

With a little practice, it is possible to draw up your own list of questions that can be asked and answered

Fig. 2.5 Examples of some inherited disorders.

Examples of some inherited disorders	
Pattern of inheritance	**Examples**
autosomal dominant	adult-onset polycystic kidney disease; neurofibromatosis; familial adenomatous polyposis
autosomal recessive	cystic fibrosis; sickle-cell anaemia; infantile polycystic kidney disease
X-linked recessive	colour blindness; haemophilia A
X-linked dominant	vitamin D-resistant rickets

Some screening questions for the cardiovascular system in the review of symptoms

Symptom	Questions
chest pain	explore in detail; in particular note the characteristics of the pain (e.g. cardiac, musculoskeletal, pleuritic, pericarditic, oesophageal, etc.)
short of breath	quantify exercise tolerance; ascertain whether predominant pathology is cardiovascular or respiratory
short of breath when lying flat	quantify number of pillows needed ('what would happen if you were forced to sleep with no pillows?'); enquire specifically about paroxysmal nocturnal dyspnoea ('do you ever wake up in the night gasping for breath and need to sit on the side of your bed?')
ankle swelling	duration; degree; presence of facial or genital oedema, ascites
fatigue	"when did you last feel completely well?"; "if I asked you to walk to the train station, what would make you stop?" (e.g. dyspnoea, chest pain, claudication, fatigue, etc.)

Fig. 2.6 Some screening questions for the cardiovascular system in the review of symptoms.

rapidly. It is helpful to consider each system of the body in turn. Some important symptoms and associated screening questions are listed in Figs 2.6–2.10.

Other general symptoms to consider include:
early morning stiffness,
mobility,
fevers
sweats
weight loss and
tiredness.

Summary

At the end of presenting the history, it is useful to provide a short summary of two or three sentences encompassing the most salient features. This will help you and the listener focus on the most relevant parts of the ensuing examination.

Some screening questions for the respiratory system in the review of symptoms

Symptom	Questions
dyspnoea	see Fig. 2.6
cough	duration; sputum production; constitutional symptoms (e.g. coryza, fever, malaise, weight loss); time of day (e.g. left heart failure or asthma may present with night-time cough)
sputum production	amount per day (e.g. teaspoonful, eggcupful, etc.); characteristics (colour, tenacity, etc.), foul taste (e.g. anaerobic infection); associated haemoptysis, chest pain
wheeze	provoking factors (e.g. exercise, cold weather, house dust, etc.)

Fig. 2.7 Some screening questions for the respiratory system in the review of symptoms.

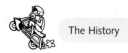

Some screening questions for the gastrointestinal system in the review of symptoms

Symptom	Questions
weight loss	'is your weight loss intentional?'; quantify; appetite; constitutional symptoms (e.g. fever, malaise, fatigue, etc.); diarrhoea, vomiting
nausea, vomiting	duration, frequency; time of day (e.g. early morning symptoms may indicate raised intracranial pressure!); obvious precipitating factors (e.g. drugs, alcohol, pregnancy, food poisoning); presence of haemoptysis
dysphagia	'where does the food appear to get stuck?'
abdominal pain	needs to be explored in detail; establish site, acute versus chronic; characteristics; relationship to food; indigestion; relieving factors, etc.
stool frequency	remember that different people have very different perceptions about the terms 'constipation' and 'diarrhoea'; establish the patient's usual bowel habit and what changes have occurred for both frequency and stool consistency; rectal bleeding; duration of symptoms; it is the change in frequency that is crucial

Fig. 2.8 Some screening questions for the gastrointestinal system in the review of symptoms.

Some screening questions for the genitourinary system in the review of symptoms

Symptom	Questions
urinary frequency	if abnormal, quantify the number of times that urine is passed during the day and night (e.g. day/night = 6-8/2)
poor stream dysuria	enquire about other features of prostatism (nocturia, hesitancy, terminal dribbling, etc.)
haematuria	timing during the urinary stream; constitutional symptoms; urinary frequency; appearance of urine (e.g. cloudy, blood, offensive smell); degree of blood clots, 'like claret', bloodstained, etc.)
menstruation	cycle length, duration of menstruation, pain, menorrhagia, etc.
sexual activity	many patients are not willing to discuss their sexual history and often it is not relevant; relevant questions may cover number of sexual partners, 'do you practise safe sex?', homosexual encounters, libido, impotence, etc.

Fig. 2.9 Some screening questions for the genitourinary system in the review of symptoms.

Some screening questions for the nervous system

Symptom	Questions
headache	explore features in depth including precipitating factors frequency, nature and location of pain, associated symptoms, timing during day, etc.
blackouts	if the patient describes a blackout, it is essential to devote time to exploring the event as this warrants investigation in its own right, regardless of other symptoms
fits	is the patient known to have epilepsy?; frequency and control, type of fits, duration of epilepsy, etc.
muscle weakness	duration, pattern of weakness, precipitating events
paraesthesia	distribution (e.g. dermatome, peripheral nerve, etc.)
change in vision	speed of onset, clarify visual acuity (e.g. 'can you read newspapers, watch television?' etc.); diplopia
dizziness	clarify exactly what the patient means by dizziness (e.g. vertigo, lightheadedness, muzzy feeling, etc.)

Fig. 2.10 Some screening questions for the nervous system in the review of symptoms.

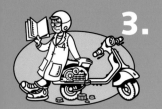

3. Presenting Problems: Cardiovascular System

Chest pain (cardiac)

Detailed history

Obtain a detailed account of the pain in a systematic manner, as described in Chapter 2, asking specifically about the features discussed below.

Site

Ask patients to indicate on themselves where exactly they experience the pain. Cardiac chest pain is typically retrosternal, but may only be present in the neck, throat, or arms (especially left arm) (Fig. 3.1).

Radiation

The pain may not radiate, but classically goes to the throat and left arm (see Fig. 3.1).

Nature of pain

It is helpful to write down the exact words used by the patient. Cardiac chest pain is usually described as 'tight', 'crushing', 'gripping', 'like a band across my chest', 'a dull ache'. Patients often have difficulty finding words to describe abstract sensations such as pain, but it is important to try and ascertain its nature. You could give alternatives, for example 'Would you describe the pain as burning, stabbing, tightness, tearing sensation?'. Remember to try and avoid leading the patient too much!

Often, patients have had angina for a long time and may describe a pain as 'like my angina, only worse', when experiencing a myocardial infarction.

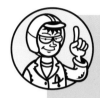

Your thumbnail sketch of the patient should include their risk factors for cardiovascular disease and at best, what the patient's exercise tolerance is.

Make an attempt to distinguish the pain from other types of chest pain (Fig. 3.2). The main types of pain are:
- Cardiac.
- Pleuritic – sharp, stabbing, aggravated by coughing, deep breathing, or occasionally posture.
- Gastrointestinal – often related to food ingestion, may be vague in character or described as burning, may be associated with an acid taste in the mouth.
- Musculoskeletal – usually easily recognized; the pain is often exaggerated by movement; there is often a good mechanical explanation, for example trauma or strain.
- Atypical diagnosis is partly by exclusion, partly by its atypical characteristics, e.g. sharp, lateral and may be precipitated by stress or anxiety.

Precipitating factors

Angina is typically provoked by exertion. If the pain is reproducible, try to find out the level of exertion necessary to induce it (e.g. walking up one flight of stairs, 200 metres on the flat). Note if this level of exertion has changed recently. Ask specifically about

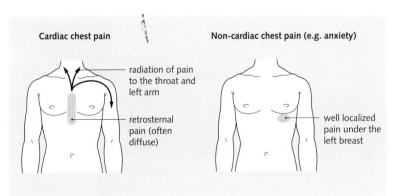

Fig. 3.1 Typical location of cardiac chest pain and non-specific chest pain in an anxious patient.

Cardiac chest pain

Non-cardiac chest pain (e.g. anxiety)

radiation of pain to the throat and left arm

retrosternal pain (often diffuse)

well localized pain under the left breast

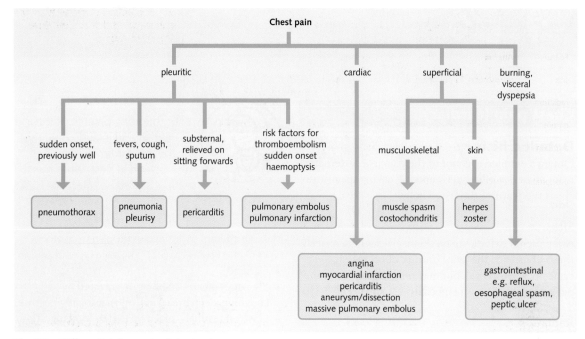

Fig. 3.2 Differential diagnosis of chest pain.

other precipitating causes (e.g. stress, excitement, sexual intercourse, meals).

If this is the first episode of pain or its nature has changed, it is important to know what the patient was doing 'immediately' before the onset of pain (e.g. stable angina is provoked by a predictable stress, but unstable angina and myocardial infarction often occur at rest).

Time course and relieving factors

Angina usually lasts for only a few minutes and is typically relieved by rest. Patients often describe an urge to slow down or stop if they are walking at the onset of pain. Ask the patient exactly how long the pain takes to subside on rest – angina will usually resolve within seconds or at most a few minutes. If the patient takes glyceryl trinitrate (GTN) tablets, enquire how quickly they seem to work. (Beware – some patients may have a false label of angina, and just because they are taking GTN tablets, it does not mean that the pain they are describing to you must be angina – keeping an open mind is is useful.) A myocardial infarction usually causes pain lasting for longer than 20 minutes. It would be rash to ascribe such pain to stable angina without other good evidence.

Associated features

Enquire specifically about any associated nausea, vomiting, sweating, shortness of breath, blackout or collapse during the pain. If the patient describes palpitations, it is crucial to know whether they preceded the onset of pain as occasionally a tachyarrhythmia may cause angina. Establish what the patient means by the term palpitation (ask them to tap out the rhythm). Make an attempt to distinguish between angina and myocardial infarction (Fig. 3.3).

Past medical history

Enquire specifically about the major risk factors for ischaemic heart disease:

- Previous episodes of angina or myocardial infarction. Record dates, events, and how the diagnosis was established (e.g. exercise test, hospital admission, angiography).
- What is the patient like at their best?
- Cigarette smoking. 'Pack years' is a useful concept (see Chapter 2). Current smokers have a significantly increased risk compared with ex-smokers.
- Hypertension.
- Diabetes mellitus.
- Hypercholesterolaemia.
- Positive family history of ischaemic heart disease.
- Other vascular disease (e.g. stroke, peripheral vascular disease).

Characteristics of angina and myocardial infarction		
Feature	Angina	Myocardial infarction
site	retrosternal, throat, left arm	retrosternal, throat, left arm
radiation	typically to the throat or left arm	typically to the throat or left arm
nature	'tight', 'gripping', 'a dull ache'	similar, but usually recognized as more severe
duration	short, usually a few minutes	usually greater than 30 minutes and only terminated by opiate analgesia
precipitation	exertion, stress, cold, emotion	usually none, but may have similar precipitants
relief	rest, GTN (rapid)	often none (opiates)
associated features	usually none	sweating, lightheadedness, palpitations, nausea, vomiting, sense of foreboding

Fig. 3.3 Characteristics of angina and myocardial infarction. GTN, glyceryl trinitrate.

The major risk factors interact and the probability of disease is greatly increased if more than one is present.

Consider factors other than coronary artery disease that can cause angina (e.g. anaemia, arrhythmia, previous valvular pathology, rheumatic fever).

Drug history

A full list of the medications the patient is currently taking is essential; however, it is important to also note the following:

- Have there been any recent changes?
- The effect of antianginal drugs on symptoms as well as side effects. In particular, does the pain resolve rapidly with sublingual GTN?
- Has concordance been good?
- Is the patient taking aspirin? Check that there are no contraindications (e.g. active ulceration, asthma provoked by aspirin).
- Consider the role of other drugs that might aggravate angina (e.g. theophylline, tricyclic antidepressants, wrong dose of thyroxine).

Social history

Enquire whether there have been any recent changes in lifestyle (e.g. financial difficulties, stress at home or work). These outside influences may be the precipitant for angina or a reason for developing a non-cardiac chest pain. Ask how the chest pain has interfered with normal lifestyle.

Review of symptoms

A brief review of symptoms is important for various reasons, for example:

- To exclude the gastrointestinal tract as the source of the symptoms (e.g. reflux oesophagitis).
- Associated neurological symptoms may be provoked by decreased perfusion.
- To assess potential risks when considering invasive investigations or treatment (e.g. angiography or thrombolysis).
- To assess whether the patient has the mobility to tolerate an exercise electrocardiogram (ECG).
- To assess whether activity is limited by cardiac status or other factors such as poor mobility, obesity or chronic lung disease.

Palpitations

Presenting complaint

Palpitation is an awareness of the heart beating. Different people mean different things when they say they have experienced palpitations.

Detailed history

It is essential to explore the event in great detail so that the underlying rhythm disturbance and functional consequences can be appreciated.

Nature of the palpitation

It is often possible to make a reasonable estimate of the underlying rhythm from the patient's description (Fig. 3.4), for example in response to questions such

Fig. 3.4 Characteristics of common arrhythmias causing palpitations.

Characteristics of common arrhythmias causing palpitations	
Rhythm	**Typical features**
ectopic beats	'I felt as though my heart missed a beat'; 'a heavy thud'; usually due to awareness of post-extrasystolic beat
atrial fibrillation	'fast, irregular beating'; may be associated with dyspnoea or chest pain, especially if fast rate
supraventricular tachycardia	rapid palpitation, often abrupt onset; may be associated with polyuria; may have rapid termination; patient may have learnt to perform vagal manoeuvres to terminate episode
ventricular tachycardia	often associated with shock, collapse, dyspnoea or progression to cardiac arrest; can be hard to distinguish from supraventricular arrhythmias as features overlap, and may even be asymptomatic; conversely, supraventricular tachycardia can cause shock, especially if rapid

as 'Can you describe what you experienced?', 'Can you tap out the heart beat on the table?' The rate of the heart during the palpitation often provides a clue to the primary electrical disturbance (Fig. 3.5).

Duration and frequency of episodes
The functional impact on the patient may be revealed, as well as the likelihood of being able to 'capture' the event on a 24-hour tape or event recorder.

Associated symptoms
Patients may have symptoms of cardiac decompensation, for example:

- Lightheadedness, fainting (syncope is due to poor cerebral perfusion and hypotension).
- Chest pain (angina).
- Sweating.

The presence of these symptoms should alert the physician and prompt more detailed investigation.

Events immediately preceding palpitation
It may be physiological to experience some palpitations after exertion or emotional stress, and this may be evident from the response to 'What were you doing immediately before the palpitations started?' If there was chest pain, find out whether

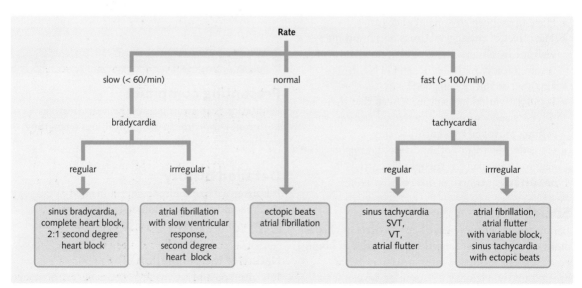

Fig. 3.5 Differential diagnosis of palpitations from the history. SVT, supraventricular tachycardia; VT, ventricular tachycardia.

the pain preceded the palpitation or coincided with its onset.

Past medical history

Review the possible underlying diseases that cause palpitations, including:

- Risk factors for ischaemic heart disease.
- Thyroid disease (especially atrial fibrillation).
- Rheumatic fever.

Drug history

This is very important. Particular attention should be paid to drugs with proarrhythmic effects such as tricyclic antidepressants, digoxin, β-blockers (and other antiarrhythmic agents), and theophylline. Review the response of the palpitations to therapy.

Social history

Particular attention should be paid to alcohol consumption, and caffeine-containing drinks. Use of recreational drugs (e.g. cannabis, ecstasy, amphetamines) may precipitate arrhythmias.

Summary of aims

The aims of the history for palpitations are as follows:

- To determine whether the rhythm is slow or fast, regular or irregular.
- To note any associated symptoms when the patient has the arrhythmia.
- To narrow down the differential diagnosis of the arrhythmia. This is usually possible, but ultimately a diagnosis can only be made by an ECG recording at the time of symptoms.
- To assess whether the episodes are long enough and frequent enough and the patient is capable of using an event recorder or whether a 24-hour ECG is more appropriate if further investigation is needed.

Heart failure

Presenting complaint

Acute

Acute heart failure presents with severe shortness of breath, severe distress, production of copious pink, frothy sputum and collapse.

Chronic

This presents with shortness of breath, limitation of exercise tolerance, ankle swelling and fatigue.

Detailed history

The features of heart failure are usually distinctive enough to be recognized from the history alone, but airway obstructions can sometimes be confused with heart failure and may coexist with it. Lung disease often coexists with heart disease. The detailed history will clarify the presence of heart failure and establish its severity and possible aetiology.

Chronicity of symptoms

Has the patient had a recent sudden decline suggestive of an ischaemic event? Ask the patient 'What are you like normally?', 'How many hospital admissions for this have you had in the past year?', and/or 'Have you had to go to your GP with worsening symptoms?'.

Severity of symptoms

Attempt to quantify the patient's impairment so that a reproducible assessment can be made. Focus on tolerance to exercise and the limiting factor for exercise.

Exercise tolerance

It is often difficult to be precise, but patients should, with assistance, be able to give quantitative answers to questions such as 'How many flights of stairs can you climb?', 'How far can you walk on the flat and uphill?', or 'Do you need help for any activities at home?'. Try to quantify what factor limits exercise capacity (e.g. fatigue, coexisting lung disease, claudication). The severity of the heart failure may be graded according to the New York Heart Association classification (Fig. 3.6).

Limiting factors

Try to establish the limiting factor for exercise (e.g. dyspnoea, fatigue, chest pain).

Evidence of left heart failure

Enquire about features of pulmonary oedema, for example:

- Paroxysmal nocturnal dyspnoea. This is a feature of acute pulmonary oedema. Ask 'Do you ever wake up in the night fighting for breath?'. Patients often describe having to sit upright on the edge of the bed and/or throwing open the windows.
- Orthopnoea. People may sleep with a few pillows for simple comfort or out of habit so it is important to find out if there has been any change. Ask 'How many pillows do you need to sleep with and has this changed from usual?'.

NHYA grading of severity of heart failure	
Grade	Severity of symptoms
I	unlimited exercise tolerance
II	symptomatic on extra exertion (e.g. stairs)
III	symptomatic on mild exertion (e.g. walking)
IV	symptomatic on minimal exertion or rest (e.g. washing)

Fig. 3.6 The New York Heart Association (NYHA) grading of severity of heart failure provides a simple, but reproducible assessment with interobserver agreement.

Evidence of right heart failure
Enquire about symptoms related to fluid overload, which may result in:
- Ascites.
- Peripheral oedema (in severe cases male patients may have scrotal oedema).
- Right upper quadrant discomfort (due to hepatic congestion).
- Nausea and poor appetite (due to bowel oedema).

Past medical history
The most relevant features include:
- Risk factors for ischaemic heart disease (see Chest pain (cardiac).
- Previous cardiac investigations (e.g. echocardiography, angiography, exercise test).
- Other causes of left heart failure (e.g. rheumatic fever, valvular disease, cardiomyopathy), high output states (e.g. thyroid disease, Paget's disease, arteriovenous shunt, anaemia).
- Other causes of right heart disease (e.g. chronic lung disease, pulmonary embolus).

Drug history
A full list of medication is needed, but focus on:
- Current therapy for heart failure, for example angiotensin-converting enzyme (ACE) inhibitors (cough may be a side effect or due to mild pulmonary oedema), diuretics (assess concordance and find out whether there has been a recent change in dose).
- Negatively inotropic drugs (e.g. β-blockers, verapamil, class I antiarrhythmic agents).
- Ask if the patient is on digoxin and if they are consider checking a level.

Social history
This section is very important. Assess daily activities, social support, mobility, etc. Review the patient's diet and appetite. Consider salt intake in oedematous states. Does the patient have sufficient mobility to cope with an increased diuresis and avoid incontinence?

Deep vein thrombosis

Presenting complaint
Deep vein thrombosis (DVT) is a common condition. It is often asymptomatic, however, the most common features of presentation include:
- Calf pain.
- Leg swelling.
- Increased temperature of the leg.

Red tender leg
The history should be directed at finding risk factors for developing a DVT (an asterisk denotes the more important ones), which include:
- Pregnancy or puerperium*.
- Prolonged immobility (e.g. long-haul air travel)*.
- Contraceptive pill*.
- Recent surgery*.
- Malignancy.
- Lower limb fractures.
- Heart failure.
- Dehydration.

Pulmonary embolism

Pulmonary embolus (PE) may be very difficult to diagnose, its presentation can vary from asymptomatic micro-emboli to sudden death caused by saddle embolism. The most common presentations are:
- Pleuritic chest pain.
- Shortness of breath.
- Haemoptysis.
- Collapse.

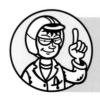
Thromboembolism is treatable and potentially fatal. It is under-recognized. A high index of suspicion is crucial.

Detailed history

If a PE is suspected, always ask specifically about risk factors suggestive of a DVT. In the presence of calf pain investigate its features systematically (see Chapter 2). In particular, note any preceding symptoms, the speed of onset, any associated symptoms, and whether the pain is unilateral or bilateral. Figure 3.7 highlights some of the more discriminatory features in the history.

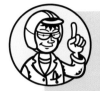

Almost 50% of DVTs do not produce local symptoms, so PE may be the presenting feature. Presentation may be non-specific, and the differential diagnosis is wide.

In the presence of pleuritic chest pain of undetermined aetiology do perform arterial blood gases and obtain a chest radiograph and an ECG.

Fig. 3.7 Differential diagnosis of leg swelling or inflammation other than venous thrombosis.

Differential diagnosis of leg swelling or inflammation other than venous thrombosis	
Condition	Features
infection (cellulitis)	subacute onset; fever; lymphangitis may be present; ask about portal of entry for infecting organism
ruptured Baker's cyst	preceding arthritis or swelling of knee; acute onset
torn calf muscle	acute onset, often during exercise
congestive cardiac failure	dyspnoea, fatigue, orthopnoea; risk factors for ischaemic heart disease; usually bilateral leg swelling
lymphatic obstruction	chronic; may be unilateral or bilateral
nephrotic syndrome	subacute or chronic leg swelling; bilateral; usually no features of inflammation

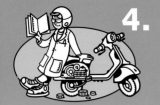

4. Presenting Problems: Respiratory System

Asthma

Presenting complaint

Can you actually obtain a history from the patient? If the patient cannot talk in sentences you have identified a medical emergency and you must seek senior help. However, the most common presentations include episodic wheeze, shortness of breath or a (nocturnal) cough.

 An acute astma attack is often frightening for both the patient and the attending physician. The patient is often too dyspnoeic to provide much history. The priority is to make a rapid assessment and institute effective therapy. A more detailed history can be obtained once the patient is stable.

Detailed history

If the patient presents with an acute attack, investigate this attack in detail. Obtain a systematic, chronological account of the recent deterioration focusing on:

- Severity – try to quantify in simple terms (e.g. unable to perform vigorous exercise, difficulty climbing stairs, unable to speak a complete sentence, being kept awake at night).
- Symptoms (e.g. wheeze, cough, dyspnoea).
- Time course (hours or days).
- Onset and precipitating events (e.g. exercise, emotional stress, viral illness, house dust, pets).
- Intervention during present attack, and response (e.g. nebulized bronchodilators, steroids).
- Reason for seeking medical attention at this stage.

Often asthma control has deteriorated chronically and insidiously. Ask either:

- 'Is there anything that you could do six months ago that you couldn't manage before this attack?'

or:

- 'Have you reduced your exercise over the past few months?'
- Has the patient been seeing their GP about their asthma?

Past medical history
Baseline asthma control

It is helpful to gain an awareness of the background control – in addition to allowing an assessment of disease severity, it may reveal information about the patient's understanding of the disease.
Ask about:

- Usual exercise tolerance. Try to quantify as described above. (Young patients should have unlimited exercise capacity. Older patients often have coexisting morbidity.)
- Frequency of attacks.
- Best recorded peak expiratory flow rate (PEFR). Ideally all asthma patients should have their own peak flow meter and know their baseline PEFR.
- Usual precipitating factors (e.g. pollen, stress, exercise, dust, pollution).
- Usual medication (see below).
- Usual response to therapy during exacerbations. For example ask 'Is this the worst attack you've ever had?', 'Would you normally expect your asthma attacks to get better after using a nebulizer?'.
- Previous hospital admissions. For example ask 'Have you ever been admitted to hospital with asthma?', 'Have you ever needed to be put on a ventilator?'.
- Attendance at their GP's asthma clinic, or for asthma review if relevant.
- Symptoms suggestive of poor baseline control. This is very important and under-recognized. (e.g. 'morning dips', poor sleep, nocturnal cough, time off work or school). An example of a peak flow chart from a child with poor control is illustrated in Fig. 4.1.

Other atopic conditions

Ask about other atopic conditions such as eczema, hay fever, urticaria.

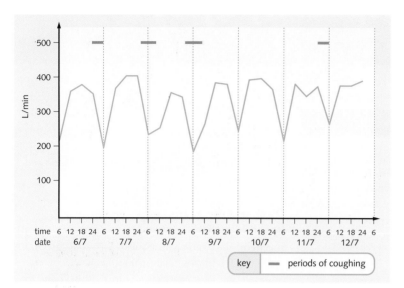

Fig. 4.1 An example of a peak flow recording from an adolescent with poor asthma control. Note the presence of cough at night and 'morning dips'.

Coexisting respiratory disease

Coexisting respiratory disease is particularly important in patients who present later in life, as it may be hard to distinguish asthma from chronic obstructive pulmonary disease (COPD) from the history.

Drug history

Obtain a full list of medication. Ask specifically:
- Do they have a nebulizer at home?
- Do they use bronchodilators?
- Do they take theophylline or aminophylline (phosphodiesterase inhibitors)? Have the drug levels ever been measured?
- Do they take steroids: inhaled, nebulized or oral?

Ask patients to demonstrate their inhaler technique. It is possible to quantify inhaler techniques as in Fig 4.2. Find out whether function tests have been performed to assess airway reversibility, and responses to different agents, especially for older patients for whom it may be difficult to define the relative components of asthma and COPD to the overall morbidity. Consider medication that may aggravate the symptoms (e.g. β-blockers, aspirin).

Social history

Review how the asthma is interfering with lifestyle for both older and young patients (e.g. school activities, absenteeism from work, limitation in sports, difficulty walking to the shops).

Always specifically enquire about smoking. During an exacerbation, it is timely to offer sensitive advice about smoking! Ask whether anyone in the patient's household is a smoker.

 No one with asthma should smoke!

Review of systems enquiry

Focus on other diseases that may limit exercise tolerance, especially cardiovascular, respiratory pathology and arthritis.

 Remember that asthma is a potentially fatal disease. The morbidity and mortality are high, and can be overcome by better supervision, objective assessment, better patient understanding and participation in his or her management, and appropriate use of steroids.

Inhaler Technique Scoring	
Prepares device (e.g. shakes inhaler)	1
Exhales fully	1
Activates and inhales	1
Holds breath for several seconds	1

Fig. 4.2 Inhaler technique scoring. (total out of 4)

Chronic obstructive pulmonary disease

Detailed history

Obtain a detailed history of chest symptoms. In an acute exacerbation patients usually present following a cold with a deterioration of dyspnoea in association with a productive cough and discoloured sputum. Outline a detailed history of the present attack following the usual systematic approach to explore:

- Time course.
- Treatment given and effects.
- Functional impact on lifestyle.
- Any hospital admissions in the last year for COPD.
- Has the patient been seeing their GP with the problem.

Obtain a thorough history of baseline function trying to be as objective as possible, for example ask:

- 'How far can you walk?'
- 'Can you climb one flight of stairs easily?'
- 'Do you get short of breath dressing?'
- 'Did you manage to walk to the outpatients' department without stopping?'

It is typical for a patient with COPD to have a pattern of chronically deteriorating exercise tolerance punctuated with acute declines during an infective exacerbation (Fig. 4.3). These may be seasonal, with an increased frequency in the winter months.

Sputum production and cough are characteristic. Try to quantify the usual amount per day and its characteristics (e.g. a teaspoonful, an eggcupful).

 Chronic bronchitis is defined on the basis of the history of cough productive of sputum on most days for 3 consecutive months for at least 2 years. Emphysema is a pathological diagnosis of dilatation and destruction of the lungs distal to the terminal bronchioles. In practice, these conditions coexist.

Consider the possibility of cor pulmonale in a patient with severe disease who describes ankle swelling.

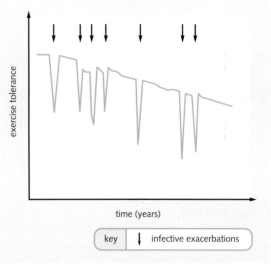

Fig. 4.3 Exercise tolerance in a patient with COPD.

Ascertain aggravating factors (e.g. cold weather, pollution, exertion).

 Many patients with COPD have a reversible component to their disease. This is under-recognized, but can be uncovered by a formal trial of steroids.

Find out whether a satisfactory attempt has been made to establish the diagnosis, for example:

- Have lung function tests been performed to assess airway reversibility?
- Have arterial blood gases been performed when the patient is well?

 Blood gases for assessment of COPD should be taken 3 months after any acute illness.

Past medical history

These patients may have multiple medical problems, which should be recorded, but specifically ask about:

- Previous admissions to hospital with acute exacerbations of COPD. Record the frequency, especially within the last year.
- Other smoking-related diseases (e.g. ischaemic heart disease, peripheral vascular disease, strokes, hypertension).
- Other causes of lung disease (e.g. occupational exposure to dusts, bronchiectasis due to, for example, previous tuberculosis, childhood whooping cough).
- Asthma. There may be a reversible component to the disease.

Drug history

Review medication prescribed for COPD, for example:
- Bronchodilators (inhalers and nebulizers).
- Home oxygen. Who initiated therapy and on what evidence? How many hours a day is it being used? Oxygen therapy should be used for 16 hours per day and its purpose is to prevent cor pulmonale. It is not for improving oxygen saturations *per se.*
- Theophylline. Have levels been measured recently?
- Steroids. Does the patient have a steroid card?
- Review inhaler technique.

Social history

This is particularly important for these patients as they often have significant limitation of exercise tolerance and rely heavily upon support from family, friends and state; e.g. are they receiving any benefits? Consider all aspects of daily living.

A detailed occupational history may be important if there is any doubt about the patient's ability to continue working or the aetiology of the lung disease, for example:
- Exposure to inorganic dusts (coal-miner's lung, silicosis, asbestosis).
- Occupational asthma (isocyanates, colophony fumes).
- Extrinsic allergic bronchiolar alveolitis (farmworkers, 'bird fanciers').

Obtain a detailed smoking history as this is undoubtedly a smoking-related disease in the vast majority of patients. Remember that the patient must not smoke if they are using home oxygen!

Review of systems enquiry

Many patients with COPD have multiple pathologies related to their smoking, so a thorough trawl of their symptoms may raise suspicions of previously unrecognized conditions (e.g. ischaemic heart disease, malignancy, renal disease, peripheral vascular disease).

Meticulous and realistic assessment of baseline function is essential – without this, it is impossible to make difficult decisions about appropriate treatment and to set realistic goals of therapy.

Chest infection

Detailed history

Perform a detailed enquiry about presenting symptoms adopting a methodical approach. Ask specifically about symptoms referable to the respiratory tract as follows:
- Cough – duration, whether productive or dry.
- Sputum production – quantity, colour, recent changes if the patient has a productive cough.
- Dyspnoea – obtain a quantitative account of exercise tolerance at baseline and during the current illness.
- Wheeze.
- Pleuritic chest pain – a common feature of pneumonia, but be aware of the possibility of a pulmonary embolus.
- Fever.

Ask about associated symptoms that have immediately preceded or coincided with the illness (especially gastrointestinal). These may give additional clues to the infecting organism causing pneumonia. Figure 4.4 illustrates how a detailed history may help to identify the microbiological cause of a pneumonic illness.

If symptoms are prolonged, recurrent, or associated with weight loss, consider the possibility of an underlying malignancy, especially in a smoker.

Clues to the underlying cause of pneumonia	
Organism	**Features from history**
Streptococcus pneumoniae*	most frequent identifiable infecting organism in community-acquired pneumonia; associated with herpes labialis, commonly prominent fever and pleuritic pain; often abrupt onset in previously fit individual
Mycoplasma pneumoniae*	occurs in epidemics with a 3–4-year periodicity; usually occurs in previously fit people; often young adults; may be preceded by a prodromal illness with headache and malaise; may be prominent extrapulmonary features (e.g. nausea, vomiting, myalgia, rash)
Haemophilus influenzae*	most common bacterial pneumonia following influenza; associated with underlying lung disease (especially COPD)
Legionella pneumophila	associated with institutional outbreaks (e.g. hospitals, hotels); may be associated with mental confusion or gastrointestinal symptoms; typically causes a dry cough
Coxiella burnetii	contact with farm animals
Chlamydia psittaci	contact with infected birds ('Do you have a sick parrot?')
Staphylococcus aureus	associated with preceding influenza, intravenous drug abusers, patient is often very ill
Gram-negative organisms	hospitalized patients; may be community-acquired in elderly or diabetics; *Branhamella catarrhalis* is associated with exacerbations of COPD
Pneumocystis carinii, cytomegalovirus, *Nocardia asteroides*, *Mycobacterium avium intracellulare*	acquired immunodeficiency syndrome (AIDS); transplant recipients; chemotherapy
Mycobacterium tuberculosis	weight loss, chronic cough, foreign travel, infected family member

Fig. 4.4 Clues to the underlying cause of pneumonia. Asterisks denote the more common organisms.

Drug history

Ask specifically about antibiotics used to treat this and any recent episode, and the duration of use as the response to therapy may give a clue to the infecting agent as well as the likelihood of obtaining a positive blood culture, for example:

- Resistance of *Mycoplasma* to penicillin.
- Resistance of tuberculosis or *Pneumocystis* to repeated courses of antibiotics.

Find out if the patient is taking immunosuppressive medication (e.g. those taking steroids, transplant recipients) (Fig. 4.4).

Social history

Relevant clues may be provided by a travel history and details of hobbies (e.g. involving pets), occupation, and risk factors (e.g. for HIV infection). Smokers are more likely to decompensate earlier in the course of the illness. Clearly it is important to assess the functional impact of the disease on patients and their families so that appropriate therapeutic and management decisions can be made.

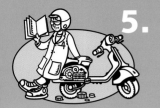

5. Presenting Problems: Abdominal

Detailed history

A very careful history needs to be elicited as it will form the foundation for a working hypothesis and differential diagnosis, and rational subsequent investigation.

On the basis of the history, abdominal pain can be divided into three types:

- Visceral.
- Somatic.
- Referred.

Visceral (deep) pain

This is dull, poorly localized pain referred to the midline. The site of pain is derived from its embryological origin (foregut, midgut, hindgut) (Fig. 5.1).

Somatic (peritoneal) pain

This is sharp, severe, and more precisely localized pain. It occurs when the disease process involves the surrounding peritoneum and mesentery.

Referred pain

This is the perception of sensory stimuli at a distance from its source (e.g. acute cholecystitis causing diaphragmatic irritation with the patient feeling pain over the right shoulder tip). The characteristics of the pain should be reviewed in a systematic manner as for other forms of pain (e.g. see 'Chest pain'

There are several key areas which should always be investigated and the outline of how to take a pain history is outlined in Chapter 2.

Site of the pain

Define the initial location of the pain and whether it has subsequently moved (e.g. acute appendicitis). This is of great importance as certain disease processes tend to cause pain localized to a defined region of the abdomen (Fig. 5.2).

Time and mode of onset

Sudden onset pain suggests a vascular event (e.g. rupture of an abdominal aortic aneurysm), or perforation of a viscus: 'One moment I was feeling fine, the next I was doubled up with pain!'

Frequency and duration

Colicky pain occurs when there is a pathological process in a smooth muscular tube (e.g. small and large bowel, ureter, fallopian tube). Ask whether the patient has had previous similar episodes.

Character

The pain may change character, indicating progression of the pathology (e.g. transition of colicky pain to constant pain suggests transition of visceral to peritoneal involvement in acute appendicitis).

Severity

Is the pain getting worse, better, or staying at the same intensity? 'If 0 equals no pain, and 10 is

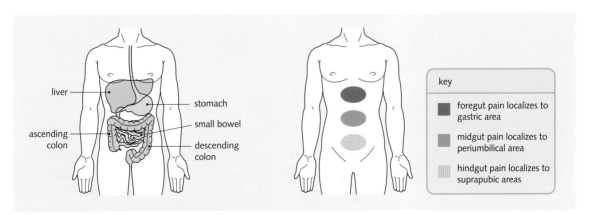

Fig. 5.1 The site of abdominal pain is related to the embryological development of the foregut, midgut, and hindgut.

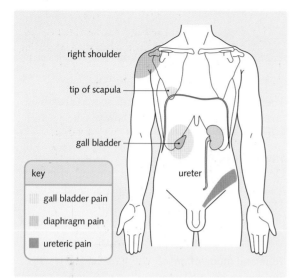

Fig. 5.2 Typical sites of radiation pain for pain originating in the gall bladder, diaphragm, and ureter.

the worst pain you have ever experienced, what value would you give this pain?'

Radiation
Loin pain, for example, radiates to the groin in renal or ureteric colic.

Aggravating factors
It is often apparent from first seeing patients what type of pain they have (e.g. patients with peritonitis lie still, patients with ureteric colic are often very restless). Certain foods may aggravate pain (e.g. fatty foods aggravate abdominal pain due to gallstones).

Relieving factors
The pain of pancreatitis is, for example, characteristically relieved by sitting forward, duodenal ulcer pain may be relieved by eating, and antacids or sleeping upright may relieve the pain of reflux oesophagitis.

Cause
Ask the patient what he or she thinks is the cause of the pain.

Other symptoms
Review other symptoms referable to the abdominal system:
- When were the patient's bowels last opened and when was flatus last passed? This is particularly relevant if partial or complete obstruction is suspected.

- Change in bowel habit. This is likely to reflect a large bowel pathology (e.g. carcinoma, inflammatory bowel disease.
- Vomiting. Establish the nature of the vomitus (i.e. blood, bile, 'coffee grounds', faeculent) and when it occurs in relation to eating.
- 'Do you still feel hungry?' This is useful for discriminating non-serious pathology as the majority of patients with serious intra-abdominal disease have anorexia.
- Abdominal distension.
- Appetite and weight loss. Chronic weight loss is suggestive of an underlying malignancy. It is useful to ask if the patient's clothes still fit them.
- Dysphagia. Ask the patient to point to where the food appears to stick. Establish whether the dysphagia is for food, or food and drink. Enquire whether there is associated pain on swallowing.
- Are there any foods that are particularly associated with pain e.g. fatty foods?
- Regurgitation, flatulence, heartburn, dyspepsia. Ask about these symptoms if there is a suspected peptic ulcer, gastro-oesophageal reflux or gallstone disease.
- Urinary symptoms. Frequency and dysuria may suggest a urinary tract infection. Nocturia, urgency, and hesitancy are consistent with prostatic enlargement.
- History of trauma. Have a low index of suspicion for a splenic or hepatic tear.

 Remember the five Fs as the causes of abdominal distension:
Fat.
Fluid.
Faeces.
Fetus.
Flatus.

Chapter 15 deals with how to take a gynaecological history from a women if such a cause is suspected.

 Consider the possibility of pregnancy in *all* women of childbearing age.

It is particularly important to include a cardiovascular and respiratory history as several medical conditions can cause acute abdominal pain (Fig. 5.3).

Past medical history

Obtain a detailed history, paying particular attention to:

- Previous operations – adhesions, recurrent pathology, etc.
- Recent myocardial infarction or cardiac arrhythmias – mesenteric embolus, especially in association with atrial fibrillation.
- Psychiatric history – patients will not volunteer this and a high index of suspicion together with old notes is needed for a diagnosis.
- Hypothyroidism
- Constipation.

Drug history

Obtain a full list of medication. Pay attention to non-steroidal anti-inflammatory drugs (NSAIDs) and steroids. Also consider drugs that may provoke constipation (e.g. opiates, tricyclic antidepressants, antimuscarinic agents, antiparkinsonism therapy).

Family history

There may be a positive family history of inflammatory bowel disease or bowel carcinoma.

Social history

Alcohol history is extremely important (e.g. for peptic ulcer, pancreatitis). For diarrhoeal illnesses consider foreign travel (e.g. amoebiasis, typhoid, giardiasis) or food poisoning (ask 'Are any of your friends or family also affected?'). The patient often has a strong inkling that symptoms have been caused by food and may be able to pinpoint exactly the suspect meal.

> If the patient may need an operation, do not forget to ask when he or she last had food or drink.
> In all cases it is mandatory to give analgesia at the earliest opportunity. It does not make interpretation of physical signs difficult, and patients give better histories if they are less distracted.

Acute diarrhoeal illness

Detailed history

Diarrhoea is a symptom and not a disease. Therefore it is important to establish the underlying cause. Ask about the nature of the stools, frequency, and events surrounding the episode. Important features to ask about include:

- Recent ingestion of undercooked meat, shellfish, unpasteurized milk, stream water (i.e. food poisoning).
- Associated abdominal pain and vomiting. Is the patient likely to need intravenous fluids?

Medical conditions that can mimic a 'surgical abdomen'	
Medical condition presenting as abdominal pain	Features
myocardial infarction (MI)*	especially inferior MI; may have paradoxical bradycardia; risk factors for ischaemic heart disease
angina*	usually epigastric
chest infection*	especially lower lobe pneumonia; previous respiratory symptoms; pleurisy
diabetic ketoacidosis*	especially young patient; decreased level of consciousness; preceding polyuria, polydipsia, weight loss; positive family history
acute pyelonephritis*	dysuria, haematuria, frequency; loin pain versus central abdominal pain; history of renal stones
hypercalcaemia	often elderly; 'bones, stones, moans and groans'
sickle cell crisis	ethnic origin, usually known history

Fig. 5.3 Medical conditions that can mimic a 'surgical abdomen'. The history may distinguish medical conditions masquerading as surgical problems. Asterisks indicate the more common conditions.

- Is the pain relieved by defaecation?
- Is there blood, pus, or mucus in the stool?
- Are the stools pale and frothy? (i.e. steatorrhoea).
- Duration of symptoms (e.g. hours, weeks, days – different illnesses may present acutely or subacutely).
- Weight loss or anorexia.
- Recent return from a foreign country (e.g. amoebiasis, giardiasis).
- Allergy to gluten products.
- Symptoms of thyrotoxicosis (e.g. heat intolerance, agitation, palpitations); thyrotoxicosis occasionally presents with diarrhoea.

Past medical history

Obtain a detailed history, paying particular attention to:
- Previous operations (e.g. short bowel syndrome, gastrectomy and vagotomy dumping).
- Inflammatory bowel disease.

Drug history

The drug history is particularly important as drugs commonly contribute to a diarrhoeal state. Common culprits include antibiotics, laxative abuse (may be surreptitious), and magnesium-containing antacids.

Family history

Enquire about inflammatory bowel disease, carcinoma of the bowel and coeliac disease.

Causes of diarrhoea
infective
Clostridium difficile (if recent use of broad-spectrum antibiotics),
viral,
Salmonella,
Shigella,
Campylobacter,
enterotoxic *Escherichia coli*,
inflammatory bowel disease
colorectal carcinoma
coeliac disease
drugs
anxiety states
miscellaneous
thyrotoxicosis

Fig. 5.4 Causes of diarrhoea.

Social history

An infective aetiology is suggested if friends or relatives have a similar illness. If the patient is dehydrated, frail, or responsible for child care consider whether admission is indicated.

The more common causes of diarrhoea are listed in Fig. 5.4.

Jaundice

Presenting complaint

Jaundice presents with yellow discoloration, which is initially often not noticed by the patient.

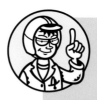

Painless jaundice in a patient over 55 should be considered to be a cancer of the head of pancreas until proven otherwise. In those under 55 it is most likely to be hepatitis A.

Detailed history

The history of a jaundiced patient is very challenging as the pathophysiology is so varied. It is helpful to review the pathophysiology of jaundice (Figs 5.5 and 5.6). Focus on the major features.

Onset

Who noticed the jaundice (e.g. patient, family, abnormal blood test)? Establish the time course (e.g. acute onset in fulminant hepatitis A, insidious progression in biliary stricture).

Associated symptoms

It is often possible to narrow down the differential diagnosis of jaundice by a detailed history. Many causes of jaundice have typical features. The usual classification is prehepatic, hepatocellular or posthepatic. Often the features of hepatocellular and obstructive jaundice overlap.

Prehepatic jaundice (haemolytic)

Jaundice is usually a minor component. The illness is often dominated by symptoms of anaemia, for example fatigue, dyspnoea, angina, and palpitations (in older patients). It may be associated with gallstones (pigment stones). On specific questioning patients report normal coloured stool and urine.

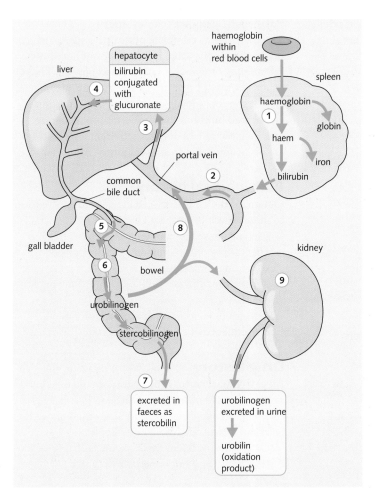

Fig. 5.5 The production, circulation, and clearance of bilirubin (see also Fig. 5.6).

Production and clearance of bilirubin		
Stage	Description	Example of pathology
1	haemoglobin within the red cells broken down within the spleen producing non-water-soluble unconjugated bilirubin	excessive breakdown (e.g. haemolytic anaemia)
2	unconjugated bilirubin transported in the blood to the liver	
3	uptake of bilirubin by the hepatocytes and transfer to the smooth endoplasmic reticulum	drug toxicity; Gilbert's syndrome; Rotor's syndrome
4	conjugation with glucuronate	Crigler–Najjar syndrome
5	excretion of conjugated bilirubin in the bile into the small bowel	biliary obstruction (defect may occur at level of hepatocyte, bile canaliculi, or bile duct)
6	breakdown within bowel to stercobilinogen (urobilinogen)	
7	oxidation of stercobilinogen to stercobilin (causes brown colouration of faeces) and excretion	white stool in cholestatic jaundice
8	absorption of urobilinogen; most goes through enterohepatic recirculation	
9	small amount of urobilinogen (water soluble) reaches systemic circulation and excreted via the kidney	large amounts of urinary urobilinogen detectable if severe haemolysis or liver damage saturates the liver's capacity for enterohepatic recirculation

Fig. 5.6   Production and clearance of bilirubin.

35

Patients may be transfusion-dependent. Consider the possible causes (i.e. abnormal red cells or immune-mediated haemolysis).

Examples of abnormal red cells occur in:
- Congenital spherocytosis (northern Europe).
- Glucose-6-phosphate dehydrogenase (G6PD) deficiency (West Africa, Mediterranean, Middle East, Southeast Asia).
- Sickle cell anaemia (sub-Saharan Africa).
- Thalassaemia (Mediterranean, Middle East, India, southeast Asia).

Causes of immune-mediated haemolysis include:
- Drugs (e.g. methyldopa, penicillin).
- Incompatible blood transfusion (acute onset).
- Warm auto-antibodies (e.g. systemic lupus erythematosus, lymphoproliferative disorders).
- Cold agglutinins (e.g. infectious mononucleosis, *Mycoplasma*).

Hepatocellular jaundice (inability to excrete bilirubin into the bile)

This is often dominated by symptoms of liver dysfunction (e.g. malaise, anorexia, right upper quadrant discomfort, abdominal distension, loss of libido, confusion). The list of diseases that may be responsible is vast, but the more important causes are illustrated in Fig. 5.7.

Posthepatic jaundice (cholestatic)

The patient may complain of pruritus due to the deposition of bile salts. It is usually, but not always, relentlessly progressive rather than episodic. There is often a history of pale stools and dark urine due to a lack of stercobilinogen in the stool and retention of conjugated bilirubin. It is important to recognize extrahepatic causes of obstructive jaundice as these are often amenable to surgical intervention (Fig. 5.8).

Past medical history

Obtain a detailed history, paying particular attention to more recent events, for example:
- Alcohol abuse – recent bingeing
- Ulcerative colitis – may suggest the presence of sclerosing cholangitis.
- Recent viral illness – Gilbert's syndrome, hepatitis A or B.
- Gallstones – either a cause of jaundice or a consequence of chronic haemolysis.

Drug history

An extremely careful drug history should be taken as drugs may have precipitated the jaundice. In addition, certain drugs need to be avoided or used with care in liver disease. For example:
- Drugs causing haemolysis – acting as haptens (e.g. penicillin, sulphonamides), direct

Causes of hepatocellular jaundice	
Cause	Examples
viral*	hepatitis A* (common, especially in endemic areas may occur in epidemics; may present acutely); hepatitis B* (common in endemic areas, e.g. Southeast Asia; ask specifically about risk factors for bloodborne infections); hepatitis C* (becoming more common; ask about blood transfusions, shared needles in drug addicts; usually chronic insidious illness)
alcoholic*	common; often presents as acute hepatitic illness
drugs*	common in hospitalized patients (e.g. rifampicin, isoniazid, prolonged course of antibiotics, paracetamol overdose, etc.)
cirrhosis*	of any aetiology (e.g. alcohol, biliary, haemochromatosis, etc.)
malignant infiltration*	primary or secondary (especially bronchus, bowel, breast)
congenital	for example Gilbert's syndrome* (common and mild); Crigler–Najjar syndrome
acute fatty liver of pregnancy	rare
inherited disorders	for example α-1-antitrypsin deficiency, Wilson's disease, etc.

Fig. 5.7 Causes of hepatocellular jaundice. Asterisks indicate the more common causes.

Causes of post hepatic jaundice	
Cause	**Features from the history**
gallstones*	common; often intermittent history of biliary colic or rigors 'fat, female, forty, fertile'
carcinoma of head of pancreas*	weight loss; pain; relentless progression
pancreatitis*	acute onset; patient often very ill
benign stricture of common bile duct	may mimic carcinoma of the pancreas
sclerosing cholangitis	associated ulcerative colitis
cholangiocarcinoma	

Fig. 5.8 Causes of posthepatic jaundice. Asterisks indicate the more common causes.

autoimmune effect (e.g. methyldopa), precipitating haemolysis in G6PD deficiency (e.g. primaquine, nitrofurantoin).

- Drugs causing hepatocellular damage – for example, paracetamol overdose, alcohol, isoniazid.
- Drugs causing intrahepatic cholestasis – for example, oestrogens, phenothiazines.
- Drugs causing gallstones – for example oral contraceptives, clofibrate.

Social history

Reviewing the patient's lifestyle may provide many clues to the aetiology. A detailed alcohol history is essential for acute alcoholic hepatitis and cirrhosis. A travel history is particularly pertinent (e.g. to an area where hepatitis A is endemic). Risk factors for bloodborne infections (e.g. intravenous drug abuse, unprotected persistent sexual intercourse, multiple blood transfusions) should be considered (e.g. for hepatitis B or C, or HIV infection). Cigarette smoking may point to malignant disease. Social contacts with hepatitis A may be apparent if there has been an epidemic.

Finally, review the patient's occupation and hobbies (e.g. leptospirosis in sewage workers or farmers, exposure to toxins by workers with organic solvents, hepatitis B in health care workers on dialysis units).

Family history

A family history is particularly relevant for younger patients (e.g. for Gilbert's syndrome, haemoglobinopathies, Wilson's disease).

Review of systems enquiry

The differential diagnosis is broad, so a complete systems enquiry is needed.

The differential diagnosis of jaundice is broad. A detailed history is needed to focus further investigations.

Anaemia

Presenting complaint

May be insidious, with lethargy, pallor, tired all the time or an incidental finding on blood test.

Detailed history

Review symptoms related to anaemia. Ask specifically about:
- Lethargy.
- Exercise tolerance.
- Palpitations.
- Angina and intermittent claudication (older patients).
- Dyspnoea.

Try to establish the duration of symptoms; the causes of acute and chronic anaemia are different. For example ask 'When did you last feel completely well?' Obtain the results of previous laboratory investigations – they may help in differentiating acute and chronic causes (Fig. 5.9).

Usually the result of the blood film will be available. It is helpful to categorize anaemia according to the mean corpuscular volume (MCV) (Fig. 5.10) as:
- Hypochromic microcytic.
- Normochromic normocytic.
- Macrocytic.

37

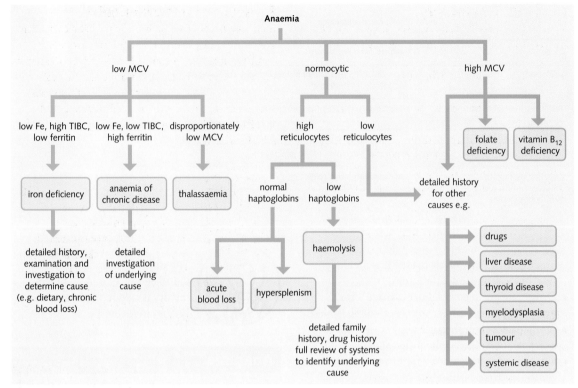

Fig. 5.9 Algorithm for the differential diagnosis of anaemia based on the mean corpuscular volume (MCV). Fe, iron; TIBC, total iron binding capacity.

Causes of anaemia	
Causes	**Features**
hypochromic	
iron deficiency*	overwhelmingly the most common cause of anaemia, usually a chronic insidious pattern (e.g. dietary, chronic blood loss)
thalassaemia trait and disease	disproportionately low MCV; Mediterranean; family history
anaemia of chronic disease*	may have normal MCV
congenital sideroblastic anaemia	rare
normochromic normocytic	
haemolytic anaemia*	often variable red cell indices
aplastic anaemia	may have variable MCV due to reticulocytosis (e.g. G6PD deficiency, drug-induced, etc.)
anaemia of chronic disease	usually multifactorial causes (e.g. malignancy, chronic renal failure, connective tissue disease, etc.)
macrocytic	
vitamin B_{12} deficiency*	common, megaloblastic (e.g. pernicious anaemia, veganism)
folate deficiency*	common, megaloblastic (e.g. nutritional, malabsorption, pregnancy)
alcohol*	the most common cause of an elevated MCV
hypothyroidism	
liver disease	
reticulocytosis	
myelodysplasia	rare
acquired sideroblastic anaemia	rare

Fig. 5.10 Causes of anaemia. Asterisks indicate the more common causes. G6PD, glucose-6-phosphate dehydrogenase.

Past medical history

Take an extensive history. Ask specifically about the following conditions, including symptoms relating to:

- Peptic ulceration or indigestion – blood loss causing iron deficiency.
- Malignancy – chronic disease, marrow infiltration, blood loss.
- Renal disease – chronic disease, blood loss, haemolysis, erythropoietin deficiency.
- Connective tissue diseases.
- Thyroid disease – previous treatment with radioiodine.
- Diseases associated with pernicious anaemia – for example, vitiligo, diabetes mellitus, thyroiditis.
- Jaundice – alcohol abuse, chronic liver disease, haemolysis.

Drug history

A particularly detailed drug history is important as often drugs can cause or exacerbate anaemia. Drugs can cause anaemia in many ways, for example:

- Blood loss – aspirin or NSAIDs.
- Haemolysis – immune-mediated (e.g. quinidine, methyldopa), glucose-6-phosphate dehydrogenase (G6PD deficiency (e.g. antimalarials, dapsone, favism).
- Aplasia – cytotoxic chemotherapy, idiopathic (e.g. sulphonamides).
- Megaloblastic anaemia – phenytoin, dihydrofolate reductase inhibitors (trimethoprim, methotrexate).
- Sideroblastic anaemia – isoniazid.

Family history

Consider the possibility of an inherited haemolytic anaemia (especially in the appropriate ethnic group), for example:

- Sickle cell anaemia – especially in sub-Saharan Africans and malarial areas.
- Thalassaemia – especially in those from the Mediterranean, Middle East, India, southeast Asia.
- Hereditary spherocytosis – northern Europeans.
- G6PD deficiency – in people from west Africa, Mediterranean, Middle East, southeast Asia.

Social history

Focus on the diet, especially if there is iron, folate or vitamin B_{12} deficiency. In addition, alcohol can cause anaemia in many ways.

Review of systems enquiry

As the cause of anaemia is often multifactorial, the systems enquiry is often fruitful. In particular, consider causes of chronic blood loss (e.g. dyspepsia, melaena, menorrhagia) and symptoms suggestive of systemic disease (e.g. weight loss, fevers, sweats).

If a particular cause of anaemia is suspected, specific questions relating to that system should be asked in detail.

Anaemia is often multifactorial, so a detailed history is essential to elucidate different components. A diagnosis of iron deficiency is inadequate. The underlying cause for the deficiency must be found.
Always ask about the use of aspirin or NSAIDs.

Acute gastrointestinal bleeding

Presenting complaint

Typical presentations include vomiting blood (haematemesis), dyspepsia, abdominal pain, and 'tarry black stools', which are very often smelly (melaena).

Detailed history

This is a medical emergency and should be assessed via the ABC approach.

The most common causes of acute upper gastrointestinal (GI) bleeding include the following, those with an asterisk being the most common:

- Gastric ulcer*.
- Duodenal ulcer*.
- Gastric erosions and gastritis*.
- Mallory–Weiss syndrome.
- Oesophageal varices.
- Haemorrhagic peptic oesophagitis.
- Gastric carcinoma (rarely presents with an acute GI bleed).
- Hereditary haemorrhagic telangiectasia (rare).

39

Acute lower gastrointestinal bleeding may be due to:

- Bleeding piles.
- Diverticulosis.

The presence of melaena indicates that the source of blood loss is probably proximal to and including the caecum. It is not enough to accept a history of melaena. A digital per rectum (PR) examination must be performed to positively confirm or refute this.

You only have time to ask specifically about symptoms suggestive of haemodynamic instability if you are receiving the history second hand, e.g. as a triage telephone conversation in a GP surgery, including:

- Faintness and loss of consciousness.
- Sweating.
- Palpitations.
- Confusion.

Obtain a detailed history, focusing on symptoms referable to the gastrointestinal tract. Ask specifically about abdominal pain, dyspepsia and heartburn, vomiting and nausea, weight loss, and early satiety.

Ask about the duration of symptoms. It is worth enquiring whether the patient has experienced any symptoms suggestive of anaemia (e.g. lethargy, angina, palpitations, unexplained fatigue).

There may be a periodicity and relationship to food or identifiable precipitating events, for example an alcoholic binge, vomiting (e.g. Mallory–Weiss syndrome, pyloric stenosis).

Past medical history

Ask about pre-existing GI tract pathologies and investigations (e.g. endoscopy, barium meals). Liver disease or jaundice may suggest gastritis or oesophageal varices in the presence of portal hypertension.

Drug history

Ask specifically about:

- Aspirin and NSAIDs (common causes of gastritis).
- Steroids (may exacerbate pre-existing ulcer).

- Use of antacids, histamine H_2 blockers, proton pump inhibitors.

Family history

Patients with peptic ulceration often have a positive family history.

Social history

Cigarettes are associated with peptic ulceration. Alcohol is strongly associated with liver disease and gastritis. Binge drinkers may have been vomiting and have produced Mallory–Weiss tears.

The underlying cause of the bleed is often indicated from the history, but subsequent confirmation by endoscopy is almost invariably indicated.

Change in bowel habit

Presenting complaint

Patients may present with either a change in their normal stool frequency or a change in the nature of the stool.

Detailed history

The main conditions producing a change in bowel habit are illustrated in Fig. 5.11. Find out what the normal pattern of bowel movements are for the patient. A normal pattern varies from one stool every three days to three stools a day. Enquire specifically about the frequency of stools and do not accept terms such as 'diarrhoea' or 'constipation' without clarification.

Ask about the duration of symptoms. A very short history of a few hours is likely to indicate an infective aetiology, whereas altered bowel habit for many years is more likely to indicate irritable bowel disorder in a young patient. Ask specifically about weight loss, anorexia, fatigue, etc., and their onset.

Associated abdominal pain may suggest an anatomical site of pathology (e.g. left iliac fossa pain is common with disease of the sigmoid colon).

Enquire about the presence of blood in the stool. The colour and relationship to the stool may reveal its origin, as follows:

- Bright red blood on the surface of the stool occurs with rectosigmoid lesions (e.g. polyp, carcinoma) or haemorrhoids.

Fig. 5.11 Causes of change in bowel habit. Asterisks indicate the more common causes.

Causes of change in bowel habit	
Condition	**Features**
colorectal carcinoma	weight loss; chronic history; blood in the stool
inflammatory bowel disease	Crohn's disease; ulcerative colitis; ask about systemic manifestations (e.g. arthropathy, oral ulcers, weight loss, etc.)
diverticular disease	very common; older patients; hard to diagnose from the history and examination alone
colonic polyps	may have mucoid discharge
infective colitis	usually acute, explosive history
irritable bowel syndrome	colicky abdominal pain; bloating; mucus; related to stress; absence of any sinister features in the history; very common

- Red blood mixed with the stool is a feature of colorectal lesions (e.g. polyp, carcinoma, inflammatory bowel disease, diverticular disease).
- Altered blood or clots almost always implies significant pathology (e.g. colorectal lesion such as polyp, carcinoma, inflammatory bowel disease, diverticular disease).

Enquire about the presence of mucus or slime in the stool (Fig. 5.12). If it is associated with blood, the most likely causes are inflammatory bowel disease or colorectal carcinoma. If mucus or slime occurs in isolation, irritable bowel syndrome may also be a cause.

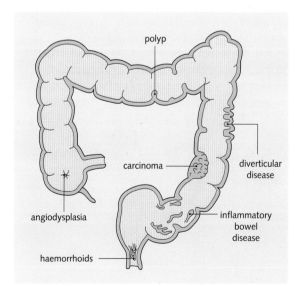

Fig. 5.12 Potential sources of rectal bleeding.

Finally ask about other characteristics of the stool. For example:
- Reduced calibre stools occurs in low strictures.
- Fatty, floating, difficult to flush, offensive stools suggest steatorrhoea.
- Pellet-like or 'stringy' stools occur in diverticular disease or irritable bowel syndrome.

Past medical history

A detailed history is essential, but previous surgical or medical problems may elucidate the cause of the change in bowel habit, for example:
- Previous colonic polyps, abdominal surgery.
- Thyroid disease.
- Malabsorption syndromes (e.g. pancreatitis).
- Diabetes mellitus (autonomic neuropathy).

Drug history

Many drugs can cause a change in bowel habit, for example:
- Constipation – opiates, anticholinergic agents, tricyclic antidepressants.
- Diarrhoea – thyroxine, laxative abuse, magnesium salts, broad-spectrum antibiotics (specifically consider pseudomembranous colitis).

Family history

Some diseases causing a change in bowel habit have a genetic component, for example:
- Familial adenomatous polyposis.
- Inflammatory bowel disease.
- Carcinoma of the bowel.

41

Social history

Ask about foreign travel for amoebiasis, giardiasis and typhoid. If there is unexplained diarrhoea, consider the patient's risk factors for HIV infection.

Dysphagia

Detailed history

Dysphagia refers either to difficulty in swallowing or pain on swallowing. Although the cause usually requires specific investigations (e.g. barium swallow, endoscopy, and biopsy), the history is important in directing these investigations. The main causes of dysphagia are indicated in Fig. 5.13.

What does the patient mean by dysphagia?

It is important to clarify exactly what patients mean when they say that they have difficulty in swallowing. It is not acceptable to write 'Patient complains of dysphagia' in the medical notes.

True dysphagia almost always indicates the presence of an organic lesion. It is important to distinguish dysphagia from 'globus hystericus' (the sensation of a lump or fullness in the throat associated with chronic anxiety states).

How bad is the dysphagia?

 Weight loss is a useful indicator of a serious underlying organic disorder and should always be asked about specifically.

Try to assess the functional impact. Dysphagia often progresses from solid food to soft food and liquid.

Ask the patient to describe exactly which foods cause difficulty. Ascertain whether there is complete obstruction (e.g. regurgitation immediately after attempting to swallow food, vomiting).

Duration and time course of symptoms

Ask patients how long they have had difficulty swallowing.

- Malignancy often presents over weeks or months and is typically progressive.
- An oesophageal ring may present over a similar time course, but produces a more intermittent pattern.
- Other causes may be present for years without any obvious systemic disturbance (e.g. globus hystericus).

Clues to underlying pathology

Specifically enquire about previous dyspepsia, proven peptic ulcer disease, or reflux. Ask about symptoms of heartburn such as acid taste in the mouth, retrosternal burning, relationship to posture. These symptoms suggest the presence of a benign oesophageal stricture.

Look for risk factors for oesophageal cancer such as:

- Cigarette smoking.
- Barrett's oesophagus.
- Old age.
- Heavy alcohol use.
- Significant weight loss.

Dysphagia to solid foods alone suggests a mechanical obstruction, dysphagia to liquids to a greater extent than solids suggests a neuromuscular cause.

Ask the patient where the food appears to get stuck. Symptoms such as difficulty initiating swallowing, coughing, choking, or nasal regurgitation suggest an oropharyngeal pathology. A sensation of

Fig. 5.13 Causes of dysphagia in the oesophagus.

Causes of dysphagia in the oesophagus	
Type of lesion	**Example**
obstruction within the lumen	carcinoma of the oesophagus; peptic stricture; foreign body; lower oesophageal ring
extrinsic compression of the oesophagus	mediastinal lymphadenopathy
motility disorder of the oesophagus	achalasia of the oesophagus; oesophageal spasm, scleroderma; Chagas' disease; diabetic autonomic neuropathy

food sticking after swallowing suggests an oesophageal lesion (Fig. 5.14).

Acute renal failure

Presenting complaint

Patients may present in various ways and these include the following:

- With symptoms directly referable to the renal tract (relatively rare presentation) (e.g. with haematuria, loin pain).
- With the consequences of renal failure (e.g. oedema, uraemic symptoms, hypertension).
- As an incidental finding from laboratory investigation (e.g. biochemical profile from investigation of other disease).

Detailed history

Ask specifically about uraemic symptoms as these may indicate the need for haemodialysis. Ask about:

- Nausea, vomiting.
- Anorexia.
- Malaise, lethargy.
- Pruritus.
- Hiccupping.

Note that many of these symptoms are non-specific. Specifically enquire about symptoms referable to the urinary tract as these may indicate the aetiology of the renal dysfunction, for example:

- Prostatism – may suggest outflow obstruction.
- Haematuria – enquire specifically about the colour if haematuria is present (often described as 'like cola' in glomerulonephritis; bright red usually implies lower urinary tract bleeding).
- Dysuria, frequency (may suggest infective aetiology).
- Oliguria or anuria (may suggest prerenal disease or severe renal failure).

Complications of renal failure

These may be present, for example:

- Peripheral oedema.
- Hypertension.
- Dyspnoea due to pulmonary oedema.

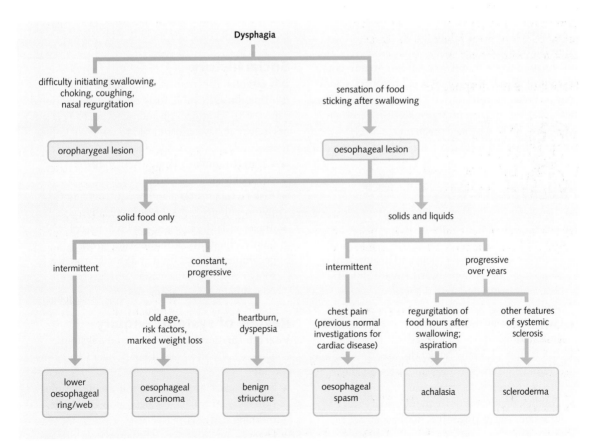

Fig. 5.14 Features from the history to aid the differential diagnosis of dysphagia.

Duration of disease

It is often difficult to elicit the duration of the disease as often the symptoms begin insidiously and are usually very non-specific. Clues may be obtained by asking specifically about, for example, change in weight or fatigue. Ask 'When did you last feel completely well?' 'Have you been more tired than usual lately?'. This may date the onset of renal failure, but usually renal pathology remains clinically silent until decompensation occurs or it is discovered incidentally. However, a meticulous history may help date the original renal insult in different circumstances.

Hospitalized patients

Most cases of acute renal failure occur in hospital. Create a flow chart of the blood results (especially biochemical profile) dating back to the decline in renal function. It is usually possible to identify within one or two days when the creatinine started to rise. At this point, focus on events that might have provided a critical insult to the kidneys (e.g. period of hypotension or dehydration, toxic levels of aminoglycosides, coexisting infection).

New referral from the community

Almost invariably, there is less immediate information to chart, but it is still essential to obtain historical records of previous renal function. Clues may be obtained from various sources (e.g. previous blood test results, results of urinalysis for women who have previously been pregnant). The GP is a source of useful information. A quick telephone call can reveal all.

Past medical history

As the causes of renal failure are numerous, detailed past medical history is essential. In particular consider:

- Diabetes mellitus – duration, and presence of neuropathy or retinopathy, which are almost invariably associated with diabetic nephropathy.
- Hypertension – did it predate or postdate renal dysfunction?
- Risk factors for renovascular disease, for example, claudication, aortic aneurysm, ischaemic heart disease, hypercholesterolaemia.
- Childhood enuresis or frequent urinary tract infections suggesting reflux nephropathy.
- Renal stones or colic.

- Autoimmune diseases, for example, systemic lupus erythematosus (SLE), rheumatoid arthritis, scleroderma.
- Jaundice, for example, hepatitis B, hepatitis C-associated glomerulopathy, leptospirosis, hepatorenal syndrome.
- Recent infections, for example, post-infectious glomerulonephritis (rare), presentation of IgA nephropathy with haematuria following a sore throat.

Drug history

Again a detailed drug history is essential. Very often, drugs have precipitated the renal failure. Remember to ask about over-the-counter medication and herbal remedies.

Drugs may precipitate renal failure by various mechanisms (Fig. 5.15). Other drugs must be used with caution in renal failure. For example:

- Renally excreted drugs (aminoglycosides).
- If there is an accumulation of metabolites due to failure of clearance (opiates).

Family history

Consider inherited conditions (e.g. polycystic kidneys, Alport's syndrome).

Social history

It is essential to obtain as much background information as possible to assess normal functional capacity. In addition, consider whether the patient's lifestyle may have contributed to the renal failure, for example:

- Cigarette smoking (renovascular disease).
- Alcohol (hepatorenal disease).
- Risk factors for HIV and hepatitis B, and C (glomerulonephritis, hepatorenal disease).
- Travel and ethnic origin – many forms of glomerulonephritis demonstrate great geographical variation (e.g. IgA nephropathy is more common in Caucasians, SLE is more common in Afro-Caribbeans).

Review of systems enquiry

Vital information may be omitted if a systems enquiry is not performed. In particular, consider:

- Symptoms suggestive of autoimmune aetiology – skin rash, arthralgia, myalgia, alopecia, early morning stiffness.
- Fevers – any infective or inflammatory disease.

Mechanisms of drug-induced renal dysfunction	
Pathology	**Drugs**
decreased renal perfusion	diuretics* (hypovolaemia); NSAIDs* (also cause interstitial nephritis, hyperkalaemia, and rarely papillary necrosis)
decreased glomerular filtration pressure	ACE inhibitors*
nephrotic syndrome	gold; penicillamine
acute tubular necrosis	aminoglycosides* (especially if toxic drug levels); antibiotics (e.g. cephalosporins); contrast agents (especially in diabetics); chemotherapy (e.g. cisplatin)
interstitial nephritis	NSAIDs*; antibiotics* (e.g. penicillin, sulphonamides)
renal stones	cytotoxic agents (especially in lymphoma)
electrolyte disturbances	diuretics* (especially hypokalaemia); renal tubular acidosis (acetazolamide); inappropriate ADH secretion (carbamazepine, chlorpropamide); hyperkalaemia (NSAIDs, ACE inhibitors, diuretics acting on distal tubule)
retroperitoneal fibrosis	methysergide

Fig. 5.15 Mechanisms of drug-induced renal dysfunction. Asterisks indicate the more commonly implicated drugs. (ACE, angiotensin-converting enzyme; ADH, antidiuretic hormone; NSAID, non-steroidal anti-inflamatory drug.)

Chronic renal failure

Presenting complaint

It is assumed that the patient will already be on dialysis or is being reviewed in the predialysis clinic and that the cause of renal disease has already been investigated (see previous section).

Detailed history
Dialysis

Assess symptoms indicative of inadequate dialysis or need to commence dialysis such as:
- Anorexia.
- Nausea, vomiting.
- Fatigue, malaise.
- Pruritus.
- Confusion, drowsiness.

Although many of these symptoms are non-specific, if no other cause is found, assume that they represent uraemia.

Dialysis-related problems

Dialysis is associated with a number of specific problems or issues, which need to be considered, whether the form of dialysis is peritoneal dialysis or haemodialysis. Review the mechanics and complications of dialysis (Fig. 5.16).

Fluid balance

There are many common problems of chronic renal failure and these should always be addressed. Review fluid balance as this is central to the management. It is essential to ask about the following:
- Does the patient have a target 'dry' weight? Fluctuations from this weight in the short term usually indicate fluid shifts.
- Urine output and daily fluid restriction, which is usually 500 ml more than daily urine output.
- Interdialytic weight gains. Large gains may indicate poor compliance and understanding of self-management.

Anaemia

Review symptoms (e.g. dyspnoea, lethargy, decreased exercise tolerance). Many patients will be taking recombinant erythropoietin. Always specifically enquire about and record:
- The dose.
- Side effects (e.g. hypertension, hyperkalaemia).
- Reasons for lack of response to erythropoietin (e.g. iron deficiency, intercurrent infection, hyperparathyroidism).

Renal osteodystrophy

Renal osteodystrophy is a common problem of chronic renal failure and should be explored. From the notes and patient account review:

45

Features of peritoneal dialysis and haemodialysis to elicit from the history		
Parameter	Peritoneal dialysis	Haemodialysis
mode of dialysis	continuous ambulatory peritoneal dialysis (CAPD); automated peritoneal dialysis (APD)	hospital haemodialysis; home haemodialysis
dialysis dose	number and type of bags (e.g. 'light/heavy'); volume of fluid (typically 2L)	hours on dialysis; frequency (typically 4 hours three times weekly)
access	PD exit site	arteriovenous (AV) fistula; temporary catheter (e.g. 'vascath'); AV shunt
complications of dialysis	peritonitis; exit site and tunnel infections	dialysis disequilibrium; hypotensive episodes; difficulty needing fistula; exit site infections: vascular stenosis

Fig. 5.16   Features of peritoneal dialysis (PD) and haemodialysis (HD).

- Calcium and phosphate balance.
- Diet.
- Calcium carbonate dose.
- Biochemical evidence for hyperparathyroidism.

Transplant status

Review plans for discharging the patient from this form of dialysis. In particular, consider (at every visit) the appropriateness for transplantation, taking into account the patient's wishes and knowledge. Review intercurrent medical issues that may preclude transplantation: for example, age, infection, malignancy, severe vascular disease, untreated ischaemic heart disease, active peptic ulceration.

Blood pressure control

Review the documentary evidence of blood pressure measurements, for example from dialysis charts or recordings made at home (before erythropoietin dosing) or by the GP.

Past medical history

This is usually well known. Do not forget the original cause of the renal failure!

Drug history

A meticulous drug history is essential. Very often, the patient will have a long list of medication. Enquire specifically about:

- Antihypertensive agents.
- Erythropoietin (see above).
- Phosphate binders and vitamin D.
- Iron supplements.
- Over-the-counter medication.

Consider drugs to be used with caution in renal failure (see 'Acute renal failure').

Social history

A detailed assessment should be made, especially in the predialysis patient, when considering whether dialysis would be appropriate, and if so, which form.

If considering haemodialysis:
- Will transport be needed to the hospital?
- Does the patient have motivation and space at home, and a partner for home haemodialysis?

If considering chronic ambulatory peritoneal dialysis (CAPD):
- Does the patient have space at home to store boxes containing peritoneal dialysis fluid?
- Does the patient have the manual dexterity needed to change bags?
- Does the patient have the motivation and intelligence to manage the care so that there is not an undue risk for developing peritonitis or exit site infections?
- Is the patient obese?

Review the patient's nutrition and diet. This is often specialized, and referral to a renal dietician is indicated.

Review of systems enquiry

This is particularly important as often these patients are multisymptomatic and renal failure is associated with so many other diseases (e.g. ischaemic heart disease, arthritis, gastrointestinal bleeding).

Chronic renal failure results in mutisystem dysfunction. Assessment needs to be detailed. It is pointless to rush. Always allow enough time. In predialysis patients check that adequate plans have been made for the initiation of dialysis so that the transition can be as smooth as possible. Consider patient education, mode of intended dialysis, access for dialysis, and estimated time to dialysis initiation.

Haematuria

Detailed history

Haematuria is a common symptom and may be due to a wide variety of pathologies (Fig. 5.17). Take a full history of the presenting symptom.

Ascertain that true haematuria is present

Some patients with uterine bleeding mistakenly believe that they have haematuria.

Duration

Note whether the haematuria is an acute presentation or has been present for many years or months.

Nature

A small amount of blood produces visible discoloration of the urine. Try to establish how much blood is present in the urine. It may be helpful to ask:

- 'Are there any blood clots in your urine?'
- 'Is your urine bright red or stained like blackcurrant juice?'
- 'Does your urine appear cloudy or like cola?' (glomerulonephritis).

The timing of blood during the urinary stream may provide a clue to the origin of bleeding. For example:

- Bleeding at the start of the urinary stream suggests a urethral lesion.
- Bleeding through the whole stream suggests a source in the bladder or higher in the urinary tract.
- Bleeding at the end of the urinary stream suggests a source in the lower bladder.

Associated urinary symptoms

Other symptoms referable to the urinary tract often provide useful clues to the cause of haematuria. Specifically ask about:

- Dysuria and frequency with small quantities of urine – urinary tract infection.
- The above symptoms in association with fever and loin pain suggest pyelonephritis.
- Colicky loin pain is indicative of renal stones.
- Symptoms of renal disease such as ankle swelling or uraemic symptoms.
- Terminal dribbling, hesitancy, and poor stream are common in prostatic obstruction.

Past medical history

A detailed past medical history is important. In particular, ask about:

- Previous renal disease.
- Abdominal trauma (e.g. renal capsular tear).
- Renal stones or previous episodes of colic.
- Previous cystoscopies.
- Prostatectomy (in men).
- Sickle cell anaemia (papillary necrosis).

Drug history

Some drugs may aggravate or cause haematuria. For example:

- Cyclophosphamide (haemorrhagic cystitis, carcinoma of the bladder).
- Warfarin (bleeding diathesis).
- Analgesic abuse (papillary necrosis).

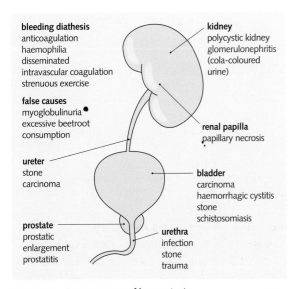

bleeding diathesis
anticoagulation
haemophilia
disseminated
intravascular coagulation
strenuous exercise

false causes
myoglobulinuria
excessive beetroot
consumption

ureter
stone
carcinoma

prostate
prostatic
enlargement
prostatitis

kidney
polycystic kidney
glomerulonephritis
(cola-coloured
urine)

renal papilla
papillary necrosis

bladder
carcinoma
haemorrhagic cystitis
stone
schistosomiasis

urethra
infection
stone
trauma

Fig. 5.17 Some causes of haematuria.

Family history

Many renal diseases have a familial tendency. For example:

- Polycystic kidney disease (adult variety is autosomal dominant).
- Alport's syndrome (X-linked recessive). Ask about deafness.
- IgA nephropathy. Ask about the relationship of macroscopic haematuria to infections.
- Sickle cell anaemia.

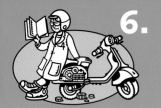

6. Presenting Problems: Nervous System

The unconscious patient

Detailed history
The history is especially important in the evaluation of the unconscious patient, even though it may not come from the patient. Obtain the history from relatives or friends, the ambulance crew, or police, if appropriate. Try to establish the following.

Time of onset of unconsciousness
Who found the patient unconscious, and when? When was the patient last seen conscious? Where was the patient found?

Duration of illness preceding unconsciousness
Had the patient been well before being found unconscious? Was the illness sudden, e.g. minutes, gradual (hours) or chronic (days to weeks)?

Nature of the preceding illness
It is helpful to consider the differential diagnosis, so that questions can be more focused (Fig. 6.1).

Past medical history
Obtain a full history. There may have been previous episodes. Enquire specifically about:
- Diabetes mellitus (hypoglycaemia, hyperglycaemic coma).
- Risk factors for cerebrovascular disease (stroke).
- Epilepsy and other neurological disorders.
- Head trauma – no matter how mild and how much in the past; a subdural haematoma may be preceded by a history of a trivial head injury, especially in the elderly.
- Preceding headaches – for example, meningitis, intracranial mass lesion, subarachnoid haemorrhage.
- Renal failure.
- Liver failure.
- Vomiting.

Drug history
Consider all drugs that may depress the conscious level if taken in therapeutic or toxic amounts. Remember to ask about analgesic agents and psychotropic medication.

Social history
This is particularly important, especially in younger patients. Ask specifically about:
- Alcohol (very important).
- Drugs of abuse (very important).
- Possible reasons for deliberate self-harm.

Do not underestimate the importance of the history, even if the patient cannot provide one directly. The differential diagnosis is broad, but can usually be narrowed down with the aid of a well-taken history from a 3rd party. Detailed history taking often needs to be deferred until appropriate resuscitation or stabilization has been carried out.

Blackouts

Detailed history
A common problem for admitting medical teams is the investigation of a patient who has had a blackout. The history is central to the diagnosis. It is imperative to find out what the patient means by the term 'black out.' Follow the usual systematic approach to investigate circumstances of the blackout. It is helpful to consider the differential diagnosis of blackouts (Fig. 6.2).

Investigate the episode chronologically. Find out what the patient was doing immediately before blacking out, whether the patient had any warning symptoms, and how the patient felt immediately after regaining consciousness (Fig. 6.3).

Did anyone witness the episode?
This is probably the most useful piece of information. If so, ask specifically about:

Clues from the history on the underlying cause of unconsciousness

Description	Indications
vascular* subarachnoid haemorrhage* intracerebral bleed* massive infarction* brainstem stroke*	preceding headache; sudden onset; often young adult; may have had 'herald bleed' risk factors for cerebrovascular disease (hypertension, diabetes mellitus (DM), ischaemic heart disease, age, family history, etc.)
metabolic* DM* drugs and toxins* hypoxia, hyponatraemia hypothyroidsm* uraemia, hepatic encephalopathy	hyperosmolar coma (type II DM); diabetic ketoacidosis (type I—may be presenting feature of disease); hypoglycaemia alcohol*; sedative drugs (opiates, benzodiazepines, barbiturates, etc.) often present non-specifically
sepsis generalized, meningoencephalitis brain abscess	usually preceding illness; ask about rash, photophobia, fevers, headache, vomiting, etc.
subdural*/extradural haematoma	may be history of trauma (often absent)
postictal	may find bottle of anti-epileptic tablets
intracranial mass lesion	ask about features of raised intracranial pressure (e.g. increasing morning headache, vomiting, developing focal neurological problems)
factitious/hysteria	often unusual presentation; past psychiatric history

Fig. 6.1 Clues from the history on the underlying cause of unconsciousness. Asterisks indicate the more common causes. DM, diabetes mellitus.

Differential diagnosis of blackouts

epilepsy*

decreased cerebral perfusion
vasovagal episode*; cardiac disturbances* (e.g. arrhythmia, aortic stenosis, ischaemia); postural hypotension*; TIA (especially in posterior circulation); micturition syncope (decreased venous return during breath holding); cough syncope (decreased venous return); carotid sinus hypersensitivity

metabolic disturbances
hypoglycaemia; hypocalcaemia

psychological
panic attacks*; hyperventilation*; factitious

drugs
alcohol*; recreational drugs of abuse; prescribed medication (e.g. decreased threshold for epileptic fit, sedative, β-blockers provoking profound bradycardia, etc.)

Fig. 6.2 Differential diagnosis of blackouts. TIA, transient ischaemic attack.

- How long the blackout lasted (seconds, minutes, or hours).
- What was the patient doing during the episode? (e.g. lying still, shaking, appearing confused, purposeful movements).
- The presence of any incontinence or shaking to suggest an epileptic fit.
- Did anyone feel the pulse either during or immediately after the blackout? A normal pulse during the blackout would exclude an arrhythmia.

Clues from the history on the underlying pathology responsible for an episode of loss of consciousness	
Clues from the history	**Possible underlying cause of blackout**

'What were you doing immediately before blacking out?'
    standing up quickly
    turning head sharply
    trauma
    completely at rest
    standing still in hot environment
	postural hypotension
	cervical spondylosis (occlusion of vertebral artery)
	subdural haematoma; extradural haematoma; contusion injury
	arrhythmia; cerebrovascular disease, etc.
	vasovagal

'Did you have any warning that you were going to blackout?'
    aura
    palpitations, chest pain
    lightheadedness
    sweating, hunger
	epileptic fit
	cardiogenic; panic attack
	vasovagal, etc.
	hypoglycaemia

Fig. 6.3 Clues from the history on the underlying pathology responsible for an episode of loss of consciousness.

Remember to evaluate the competence of the person who felt the pulse.

Try to establish whether the episode was a true syncopal attack (loss of consciousness and motor tone) or just a period of lightheadedness. Very often people say that they have blacked out when they do not completely lose consciousness: ask for example 'Did you lose any time?', 'Were you out cold?'.

Enquire about the immediate period following recovery of consciousness. Symptoms at this stage may give clues to the precipitating event, for example:
- Immediate recovery – vasovagal.
- Confusion and disorientation e.g. postictal.
- Weakness – Todd's paralysis, transient ischaemic attack (TIA).

Past medical history
Ask about previous blackouts and investigations performed. Consider clues from the past history that may increase the probability of certain underlying problems, for example:
- Risk factors for epilepsy – for example, head injury, cerebrovascular disease, meningitis.
- Cardiac diseases.
- Diabetes mellitus – enquire about medication, diabetic control and previous episodes of hypoglycaemia.

Drug history
A full drug history is essential. In particular, consider:
- Recent changes to prescribed drugs.
- Negative chronotropic and inotropic agents (e.g. β-blockers).

- Drugs likely to cause arrhythmias (e.g. tricyclic antidepressants, theophylline).
- Insulin (hypoglycaemia).
- Antihypertensive agents (postural hypotension).
- Glyceryl trinitrate (GTN) syncope.
- Illicit drug use.

Social history
Investigate whether the home environment is safe for someone who may blackout unexpectedly (e.g. are there any carers at home?). The patient's lifestyle may suggest underlying risks for a blackout (e.g. alcohol consumption, unusual stresses at home or work).

Review of systems enquiry
Blackouts may result from a wide range of pathologies, so a review of systems may reveal unexpected pathology. Focus on the cardiovascular, neurological, metabolic, and locomotor systems.

 The key to diagnosing the cause of a blackout is a well-taken history. The most useful information comes from an eyewitness account.

Headache

Detailed history
Consider the following common causes of single and recurrent headaches:
- Tension headache (by far the most common).
- Migraine (common).

- Hangover (apparent from the history).
- Subarachnoid haemorrhage (rare, but consider for any sudden-onset headache).
- Meningitis, encephalitis.
- Raised intracranial pressure (e.g. tumour, hydrocephalus).
- Temporal arteritis.

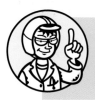 Twenty percent of headaches presenting in A&E are subarachnoid haemorrhages; the most common mistake is to diagnose them as migraine.

Obtain a detailed history about the frequency of headaches, for example recurrent headaches are typically tension headaches or migraine, while a headache every morning can be due to raised intracranial pressure associated with a tumour.

 For any new-onset headache, always ask specifically about photophobia, neck stiffness, rash, fever, and vomiting.

Obtain information about the onset, nature, and location of headache. It is often possible to identify the cause of a headache from these parameters (Figs 6.4 and 6.5).

Past medical history
Ask specifically about previous malignancy if raised intracranial pressure is suspected.

Drug history
Ask about medication taken to relieve symptoms and efficacy. It is often hard to assess the severity of headache as people can rarely give a quantitative description. It may be worth asking 'If 0 is no pain, and 10 is the worst headache you have ever had, what score would you give this pain?'. Ask girls and women about the use of oral contraceptives (may precipitate or worsen migraine particularly in the pill-free week).

Social history
For recurrent headaches, it is essential to ask about stresses, for example at home and work, that may be precipitating chronic non-specific headaches. The patient's alcohol history is also relevant. Eliciting the patient's ideas and concerns about their headache is especially important as many are worried about serious pathology, e.g. brain tumour or stroke.

Features of different types of headache	
Headache	Characteristics
tension headache	most common recurrent headache, typically described as 'throbbing', 'pressure', etc. often identifiable precipitating factor (e.g. stress, depression)
migraine	common cause of recurrent headache; usually presents in young adults; prodrome—often visual (e.g. scotomata, teichopsia), tingling, etc.; headache—often starts unilaterally; associated symptoms (e.g. nausea, vomiting, photophobia, etc.)
subarachnoid haemorrhage	may have had 'herald bleed' with milder 'subclinical' episodes; typically sudden onset 'like a hammer hitting the back of my head'; may have associated neurological deficit or decreased level of consciousness
hangover	preceding alcohol consumption; associated nausea
meningitis	photophobia; neck stiffness; fever; rash
raised intracranial pressure	usually subacute onset; relentless; present on waking; aggravated by coughing, sneezing, stooping, associated nausea
temporal arteritis	pain over superficial temporal arteries, especially on touching area (e.g. combing hair); may have associated malaise, proximal muscle weakness, and stiffness, and visual loss; usually older than 60 years

Fig. 6.4 Features of different types of headache.

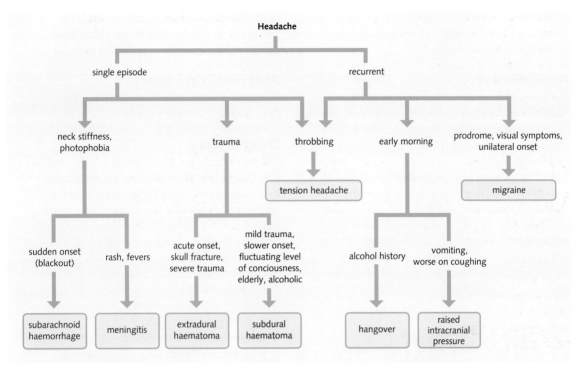

Fig. 6.5 Differential diagnosis of headache.

 Headache is a universal condition. The principal aim is to distinguish non-serious benign headaches from those that may represent serious underlying pathology needing further investigation so that appropriate reassurance can be given.

Always consider headaches representing serious disease. Alarm words may include:

Scalp tenderness, proximal limb stiffness – temporal arteritis.

Rash, fever, photophobia, neck stiffness – meningitis.

Sudden-onset occipital headache – subarachnoid haemorrhage.

Early morning headache, nausea – raised intracranial pressure.

Epileptic seizure

Presenting complaint

Epilepsy may present as an unwitnessed blackout (single or recurrent) or as an eyewitness account of a fit. More rarely it may present with behavioural changes.

Detailed history

Start with the patient's own recollection of the event, recording the following chronologically.

Prodrome

Ask 'Did you have any warning that you were going to blackout?'. Typical auras include sensations the patient may find difficult to describe, including strange thoughts, emotions, or hallucinations (e.g. smell, taste, vision). They often follow a predictable course for the individual patient.

Seizure

Ask 'Tell me what you remember about the attack?' 'Did you blackout and lose consciousness?'. The answers to these questions may help distinguish between generalized and partial seizures. If the patient was conscious during the episode, ask him or her to describe exactly what happened. If the patient has experienced a partial seizure, the symptoms are often characteristic of the site of epileptic focus, for example:

- Jacksonian motor seizures.
- Temporal lobe epilepsy (déjà vu, jamais vu, hallucinations of smell or taste, etc.).

It is usually possible to distinguish partial seizures, generalized seizures, and partial seizures with secondary generalization.

Postictal period

Ask 'How did you feel when you came around?' It is usual to experience a headache, 'muzziness', lethargy, confusion, and non-specific malaise, etc. A focal weakness may be present for up to 24 hours (Todd's paralysis).

Obtain an eyewitness account if possible. This is invaluable, and can provide diagnostic information.

If the episode was a single blackout, the most common difficulty is distinguishing between epilepsy and syncope. Look for an identifiable precipitant for syncope (e.g. emotional stress, prolonged standing, cough, micturition syncope), gradual onset and recovery, and pallor and flaccidity during the episode.

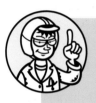

Generalized seizures imply widespread abnormal electrical activity in the brain while partial seizures imply a discrete area of abnormal electrical activity which may or may not spread.

Beware that a convulsion or urinary incontinence rarely occurs during syncopal episodes.

On the basis of the history, try to decide on the type of epilepsy (Fig. 6.6). If the patient has had multiple fits, ask about seizure control (i.e. frequency of fits, duration of fits). Ask about precipitating factors (e.g. flickering lights).

Past medical history

Consider possible underlying causes of fits (Fig. 6.7).

Drug history

Ask about drugs used to control epilepsy, and their side effects (e.g. phenytoin, sodium valproate, carbamazepine). Ask specifically about symptoms suggestive of overdose (e.g. drowsiness, ataxia, slurred speech). Review concordance, especially if there is evidence of poor seizure control, and consider the need to check drug levels (phenytoin has a narrow therapeutic index).

Consider medication that may:
- Interact with anticonvulsants (e.g. oral contraceptives, warfarin).
- Lower the seizure threshold (e.g. phenothiazines, tricyclic antidepressants, amphetamines).

Family history

In younger patients, there is often a positive family history.

Social history

There are multiple social issues surrounding epilepsy. Often, patients feel stigmatized and socially isolated. School performance is often poor. The reasons for this should be explored (e.g. poorly controlled seizures, drug intoxication, social isolation and

Fig. 6.6 The history often reveals the type of epilepsy. Asterisks indicate the more common causes.

Historical features of different types of epilepsy	
generalized seizures	
tonic–clonic seizure (grand mal fit)*	most commonly perceived form of epilepsy—'convulsions'
absence seizures (petit mal)*	especially in childhood; brief (few seconds) loss of consciousness; no fall; no convulsion
myoclonic seizures	especially in childhood; usually symmetrical
tonic seizures	especially in childhood; loss of consciousness; usually underlying organic brain disease
akinetic seizures	no prodrome ('drop attacks')
partial seizures	
simple partial seizures*	remains fully conscious during attack (e.g. Jacksonian fit)
complex partial seizures*	originates in the temporal lobe; often complex sensory hallucinations, déjà vu, jamais vu, lip smacking, chewing, behavioural disturbances; etc.
partial seizure with secondary generalization*	as above, but progresses to tonic-clonic seizure

Underlying pathology causing seizures

cerebravascular disease*
  most common cause in older age group; risk factors (e.g. hypertension, smoking, ischaemic heart disease, diabetes mellitus, etc.)

alcohol and drug withdrawal*

drugs*
  for example tricyclic antidepressants, phenothiazines, amphetamines, etc.

head injury and neurosurgery

tumours

encephalitis

degenerative brain disease

metabolic disorders
  for example hypoglycaemia, hyponatraemia, hypocalcaemia, uraemia, liver failure, etc.

fever
  NB febrile convulsions are not epilepsy

Fig. 6.7 Underlying pathology responsible for epileptic fits can often be identified. Asterisks indicate the more common causes.

bullying, underlying brain disease). Parents are often understandably overprotective. Consider sensible restrictions on activities for children while allowing a full social life (e.g. avoiding known precipitants such as strobe lighting at discos, bathing in a locked bathroom, or dangerous sports such as rock climbing).

Review occupational problems (e.g. use of dangerous machinery, employers who do not understand the disease).

Consider the restrictions on driving. This may affect the decision to start withdrawing medication in patients with well-controlled disease if driving is particularly important to them. Consult the *Medical Aspects of Fitness to Drive* handbook for further information.

In common with many other neurological events, try to obtain a good eyewitness account of a typical episode as very often the patient is asymptomatic and has no physical signs on presentation to a doctor.

Stroke

Strokes are common and take up large amounts of NHS resources. They are the third most common cause of death in the developed world. Eighty percent of all strokes are embolic events and 10% of people with infarcts will die within 30 days. (See Gubitz & Sandercock, *Br Med J* **320**, 692-6.)

Detailed history

Establish that the described event is a stroke. It is usually obvious from the history that a stroke has occurred. Try to work out where in the cerebral circulation the stroke has occurred as this has prognostic value (see Figs 6.8 and 6.9).

A stroke is an acute focal neurological deficit due to a vascular lesion, lasting longer than 24 hours. A TIA is a focal neurological deficit due to a vascular lesion that resolves within 24 hours.

Onset

Obtain a chronological account of the onset and progression of neurological disability. Ask 'What were you doing immediately before this happened?'. Typically it occurs at rest, but patients may wake up to find that they cannot move a limb. The onset is typically immediate, but may evolve over a few hours – 'One moment I was fine, and the next, I was unable to move my right arm'.

Symptoms and signs of stroke	
Anterior circulation strokes	**Posterior circulation strokes**

• Unilateral weakness
• Unilateral sensory loss or inattention
• Isolated dysarthria
• Dysphasia
• Vision:
  Homonymous hemianopia
  Monocular blindness
  Visual inattention
	• Isolated homonymous hemianopia
	• Diplopia and disconjugate eyes
	• Nausea and vomiting
	• Incoordination and unsteadiness
	• Unilateral or bilateral weakness and/or sensory loss
	Non-specific signs
	• Dysphagia
	• Incontinence
	• Loss of consciousness

Characteristics of subtypes of stroke				
	Lacunar	**Partial anterior circulation**	**Total anterior circulation**	**Posterior circulation**
Signs	Motor or sensory only	2 of following: motor or sensory; cortical; hemianopia	All of: motor or sensory; cortical; hemianopia	Hemianopia; brain stem; cerebellar
% dead at 1 year	10	20	60	20
% dependent at 1 year	25	30	35	20

Fig. 6.8 Symptoms and signs of stroke, and characteristics of subtype.

Define the neurological disability, for example ask 'What can't you do now that you could manage before this happened?'. This is important because:

- It provides a baseline to assess recovery or subsequent deterioration.
- The anatomical site of the lesion can be identified. The neurological disability typically corresponds to the vascular territory of the occluded or haemorrhaging artery (Figs 6.8 and 6.9).
- It allows an assessment of whether the event is likely to be a stroke or a TIA and any evidence of recovery between the onset and presentation.

Past medical history
Consider the possible aetiology of the stroke as this will affect subsequent management (Fig. 6.10). Ask specifically about previous TIAs and transient loss of sight, PVD.

Drug history
Ask specifically about warfarin, aspirin, and heparin if an intracranial bleed is suspected.

Reviewing the list of medication may highlight a risk factor that the patient or his or her relatives may have forgotten.

Social history
An extremely detailed social assessment is necessary to ascertain if and when the patient can be discharged home. Remember that discharge planning should begin at the point of admission to hospital.

The diagnosis of stroke is usually apparent on presentation, but an attempt should be made to define its aetiology and severity. There is as yet little proven medical therapy to limit the neurological deficit. The bulk of treatment will be supportive to aid rehabilitation. This relies upon an adequate initial assessment and the detailed social history is essential for coordinating the various members of the multidisciplinary team (e.g. physiotherapist, occupational therapist, social worker, dietician, speech therapist).

 When stroke is diagnosed, coordinate all members of the multidisciplinary team as soon as possible. Discharge planning should begin on admission to hospital.

'Off the legs'

Detailed history
Elderly people often present in a non-specific manner with difficulty functioning at home with their normal day to day activities. The ability to compensate for relatively minor physiological derangements is impaired in the elderly. The differential diagnosis is enormous, and represents one of the greatest challenges in history taking. Consider some of the more common underlying disorders listed below that may present non-specifically as confusion or inability to cope at home (the more common are denoted with an asterisk):

- Infection* (e.g. urinary tract infection*, chest infection).
- Drugs* – very common (e.g. diuretics causing electrolyte disturbances, sedatives, antihypertensives).

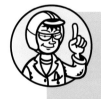

Fig. 6.9 The vascular territories of the main cerebral arteries.

A

anterior cerebral

middle cerebral — posterior cerebral

B

anterior cerebral

middle cerebral — posterior cerebral

key	
A	**B**
■ anterior cerebral distribution	▦ frontal pole
▦ middle cerebral distribution	▦ cuneus
▦ posterior cerebral distribution	

- Metabolic – for example hypothyroidism*, hyperthyroidism, diabetes mellitus (new presentation or established disease), electrolyte disturbances* (e.g. hyponatraemia, hypernatraemia, hypercalcaemia), dehydration.
- Neurological (e.g. dementia*, Parkinson's disease, subdural haematoma*).
- Cardiovascular – for example cerebrovascular disease*, myocardial infarction* (e.g. heart failure*, hypotension*), arrhythmias* (especially atrial fibrillation*).
- Haematological (e.g. anaemia due to peptic ulceration, bowel cancer, vitamin B_{12} or folate deficiency).
- Liver disease.
- Psychiatric (e.g. depression*).

Often the history from the patient is vague or uninformative. A collateral history from friends, family, or other carers is invaluable.

Almost the whole medical dictionary can be added to this list, including apparently mundane conditions (e.g. urinary retention, constipation).

Try to obtain a chronological, systematic history in the usual way, focusing on:

- Time course.
- Rate of decline (e.g. a sudden decline may be suggestive of a vascular event, acute may suggest

Common causes of stroke	
Pathology	Features in the history
ischaemic stroke*—thrombosis*, embolism*	by far the most common; ischaemic heart disease, diabetes mellitus, hypertension, smoking, valvular heart disease (especially mitral stenosis/prosthetic heart valve), atrial fibrillation, family history, older age; hyperviscosity (e.g. polycythaemia, Waldenstrom's macroglobulinaemia)
cerebral haemorrhage*	common; as above, but hypertension is often pronounced; headache is often a prominent feature as is a disturbed level of consciousness
extradural haematoma	severe head injury
subdural haematoma	history of head injury (often mild); alcoholic; old age
subarachnoid haemorrhage	'herald bleeds', sudden-onset headache; loss of consciousness common; meningism
vasculitis	giant cell arteritis, systemic lupus erythematosus (SLE), Wegener's granulomatosis, sarcoidosis, etc. (consider features of above diseases)
infections	syphilis, infective endocarditis (rare)

Fig. 6.10 Aetiology of strokes. Asterisks indicate the more common causes.

an infective or metabolic disorder, a chronic decline may be due to dementia).
- Pattern of dysfunction (e.g. stepwise deterioration, sudden decline, relapsing and remitting).
- Functional skills. Ask 'What does he (or she) have difficulty doing now that he (or she) could manage last week?'.

Past medical history

A detailed past medical history should be obtained. The dysfunctional state may result from deterioration of a pre-existing condition or a new event superimposed on a pathological process. In particular ask about:
- Ischaemic heart disease and cerebrovascular disease (including risk factors).
- Diabetes mellitus.
- Psychiatric disorders (dementia, depression).
- Malignancy.

Drug history

The drug history is particularly important. Often the carer may not be aware of the detailed past medical history and the patient may not be in a state to provide one, so a look at the patient's medication may offer clues about pre-existing conditions. Alternatively, the drugs often contribute to the presentation. Concentrate on:

- Newly prescribed medication – why? when? effect?
- Psychotropic medication (e.g. sleeping tablets, antidepressants).
- Antihypertensive medication (especially if newly prescribed).
- Drugs that may cause electrolyte derangement (e.g. diuretics).

Social history

Obviously, the social history is central to a full assessment. It is important to understand the normal pattern of daily activities and how they are normally negotiated (e.g. dressing, bathing, cooking, toileting, shopping, managing medication, social interaction).

The social support usually provided, and the possibility that this could be improved should be assessed (e.g. family, friends, home help, 'meals on wheels', community nurse, previous social worker involvement and benefits).

Consider other factors in the patient's lifestyle that may have contributed to decompensation, for example:
- Alcohol is a surprisingly common contributory factor in declining social functioning in elderly patients.
- Smoking history may highlight risk factors (e.g. for cardiovascular disease, chest disease, malignancy).
- Diet and nutrition are often inadequate in elderly patients.

Elderly patients often present in a non-specific manner with an inability to cope in their home environment. A thorough assessment should be made to elucidate the reason(s) behind this. Usually there are multiple pathologies. Try to diagnose each individual problem and consider which ones are active and which are responsible for the current presentation. Do not ignore apparently trivial illnesses! Review the home circumstances in detail and consider whether the home is safe in the short term or a more detailed assessment is needed (e.g. by occupational therapists and social workers).

Review of systems enquiry

There are few circumstances when it is more important to perform a thorough review of systems enquiry. Inability of elderly people to cope in their home environment is usually due to the interaction of multiple pathologies reaching a critical level and resulting in decompensation. If adequate time is allowed, it usually becomes apparent that the patient was polysymptomatic from different systems before this presentation. For example, you could have an elderly man with:

- Osteoarthritis affecting his hips and limiting mobility.
- Early Alzheimer's dementia.
- A peptic ulcer resulting in iron deficiency anaemia.
- Urinary retention due to prostatism.
- Recently prescribed tricyclic antidepressant.

It is sometimes difficult to distinguish symptoms relevant to the current presentation, but that is part of the skill and challenge of good history taking!

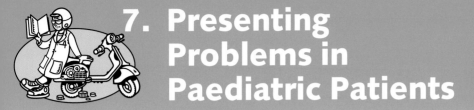

7. Presenting Problems in Paediatric Patients

Paediatrics includes a wide range of patients from the newly born to the adolescent verging on adulthood. Clearly, a uniform approach to clinical evaluation is not applicable.

It is useful to distinguish the following age groups:

- Fetus: in utero.
- Neonate: birth to 28 days.
- Infant: birth to 1 year.
- Toddler: 1–3 years.
- Preschool: 3–5 years.
- School child: 5–16 years.
- Adolescent: 12–18 years.

A clinical approach for two important categories of paediatric patient is set out here:

- The toddler and preschool child aged 1–5 years.
- The newborn infant.

Taking a history

For the majority of paediatric patients the history will be mainly from a parent, usually the mother. The general format is the same as that in adult medicine, but with some very important differences in emphasis. Set out below is a scheme for paediatric history taking. During the history taking:

- Remember parents, especially mothers, observe their children very closely.
- Never ignore or dismiss parental observations.
- Listen carefully: the diagnosis and the parent's concerns are usually apparent in the history.
- Avoid leading questions.

On taking a history be comprehensive: if you don't ask, they won't tell. Formulate a differential diagnosis by the end of the history. Examine the patient with your diagnosis in mind.

Introductions

On meeting the patient:

- Introduce yourself and get down to the same level as the patient (this makes you less intimidating.)

- Identify the patient (find out name, age and sex in advance), e.g. 'Is this Billy? How old is he?'
- Confirm the relationship of the accompanying adult, e.g. 'Are you his mother?' (it could be the au pair, older sister, social worker, etc.).

Presenting complaint

Give a prompt to allow the parent to have their say, e.g. 'What has been your main worry?'

Listen carefully and patiently and then follow up with specific questions to elicit the full details of presenting symptoms. Ask about any treatment such as medicines from the GP or chemist.

Previous history

This should include:

- Birth history: 'Where was the child born? Was the pregnancy and delivery normal? Was the baby early or late? What did the baby weigh? Were there any problems in the newborn period?'
- Immunizations: 'Has the child had all immunizations?' (see Fig. 7.1).
- Medical: 'Any hospital admissions or operations?'

Developmental history

Have there been any problems or concerns about the child development (either from their parents or doctors/health professionals)? See Fig. 7.2 for developmental milestones.

Family history

- Age and sex of siblings? 'Do you have other children?' What is the relationship between the parents looking after the child? 'Are you John's Mum or step Mum?'
- Family illness, e.g. TB, asthma, epilepsy? 'Do any illnesses run in the family?'

Social history

Build up a picture of the family circumstances. Identify socioeconomic deprivation. 'Are you or your partner working at present? Any problems with your housing? Does anyone help to look after him?' If appropriate, 'As a lone parent, what support do you have?' or 'How is he getting on at school?'.

Immunization schedule
at 2, 3 and 4 months DTP (diphtheria, tetanus and pertusis) HIB (*Haemophilus influenzae* B) Meningococcal group C Polio
at 12–15 months MMR (measles, mumps and rubella)
Before school or nursery DTP booster Polio booster MMR booster
at 10–14 years BCG
before leaving school Diphtheria and tetanus booster Polio booster

Fig. 7.1 Immunization schedule. These guidelines change so check the British National Formulary (BNF) close to exams for up-to-date information.

Systems review

This is a set of questions used to identify key symptoms; it is similar to the adult system, with the emphasis on the system implicated by the presenting complaint:

- Respiratory system: breathing difficulties or does she have any difficulty breathing whilst feeding?
- Cardiovascular system: syncope, breathlessness or cyanotic episodes?
- Gastrointestinal system: appetite, vomiting, bowel habit, or abdominal pain, frank weight loss or crossing centiles?
- Genito-urinary tract: excessive thirst, polyuria or dysuria?
- Central nervous system: headache, regression (loss of skills) or fits and funny turns?

Examination

The key word in a paediatric examination is opportunistic. While in adult examination you can have a system to work through in paediatrics you must be flexible enough to examine what you can in the circumstances. Young infants and school-age children are relatively easy to examine, but the most commonly encountered patient in general paediatric practice is an uncooperative toddler in the 1–3 year age group. In this group particularly, the following 'dos and don'ts' apply.

Do:

- Be friendly and cheerful: try to smile and keep up some idle chatter (unless of course the child is acutely and severely ill).

- Be gentle: rapport is lost if you cause pain or discomfort.
- Be opportunistic: if asleep auscultate the chest; if screaming inspect the tonsils.
- Explain or demonstrate what you are about to do: auscultate a doll or teddy.
- If appropriate or feasible try and distract the child whilst examining them, e.g. shining a pen torch whilst examining the lung fields.
- Leave unpleasant procedures until last: examination of ears, nose, and throat, rectal examination (rarely necessary), blood pressure measurement.

Don't:

- Tower over the child.
- Stare at the child: avoid looking too intently at toddlers.
- Separate the child from the mother: a toddler is best examined sitting on the mother's lap.
- Undress the child: ask the mother to take off outer layers while the history is taken, but don't strip the child naked – a certain way to make toddlers cry is to undress them and lie them on a cold couch.

The features unique to a paediatric examination of a 9-month to 5-year-old child are outlined below; the frame work of 'inspection, palpation, percussion and ascultation' still hold true. For a detailed description of examination please see the specific system chapter. The following should be read in conjunction with the specific system chapter.

Inspection

Careful initial observation should be made to assess:

- Severity of illness: is this child well, unwell or ill?
- Growth: is the child well grown and well nourished? Height, weight, and head circumference should be entered on the centile chart.
- Appearance: are there any dysmorphic features? Is the child clean and well kempt?
- Fever or rash: infection?
- Major signs relating to specific systems: level of consciousness, pallor or bruising, cyanosis, tachypnoea, or jaundice.

Hands/neck/pulse

The first touch on the hands should be gentle, so as to be non-threatening, as should be palpation of the

Developmental milestones				
Age	Gross motor	Fine motor and vision	Hearing and speech	Social behaviour
Newborn	Symmetrical movements in all four limbs, normal muscle tone	Fixes on mother's face	Cries	Settles on being picked up
6 weeks	Good head control, presence of the Moro reflex, transiently holds head in horizontal plane when held in ventral position	Follows mother's face	Loud noises will startle them, makes contented noises	Has started to smile
8 months	Sits unsupported, starting to crawl	Palmar grasp, moves objects from hand to hand, eyes follow a dropped toy	'Dadda' and 'Mamma', reacts to name, positive distraction test	Stranger anxiety, separation anxiety, plays 'peek-a-boo'
18 months	Walks, climbs onto chair	Pincer grip, builds 3-brick tower	Three-word sentence, comprehends simple commands	Begins toilet training, uses spoon
3 years	Runs and jumps, manages stairs, kicks a ball	Builds 8-brick tower, copies lines and circles	Short sentences	Dry by day, Plays with other children, dresses under supervision
5 years	Heel–toe talking, catches ball	Draws man with features	Comprehensive language skills	Can play games, tells time

Fig. 7.2 Developmental milestones.

neck for cervical lymphadenopathy. The radial or brachial pulse can be palpated for rate, rhythm, and volume.

Chest

This will include examination of the cardiovascular and respiratory systems. Important signs common to both will have been noted on initial inspection:

- Cyanosis.
- Tachypnoea (Fig. 7.3).
- Clubbing (rare).

Respiratory system

Look for:

- Intercostal or subcostal recession.
- Nasal flaring.
- Use of accessory muscles.

Paediatric vital signs			
Age	Respiratory rate	Heart rate	Systolic BP
<1	30–40	110–160	70–90
1–2	25–35	100–150	80–95
2–5	25–30	95–140	80–100
5–12	20–25	80–120	90–110
>12	15–20	60–100	100–120

Fig. 7.3 Paediatric vital signs.

- Chest shape and movement specifically, Harrison sulcus, and asymmetrical movements.

Percuss (but this is seldom helpful in very young infants).

Auscultate and note:
- Breath sounds.
- Added sounds, e.g. wheeze and crackles.

The cardiovascular system should be examined as described in Chapter 3. Detailed evaluation will include:
- Measuring blood pressure (this is quite unpleasant for a child and so should be left until the end if possible).
- Checking for hepatomegaly: this is an important sign of cardiac failure in infants.

Additional features in the examination of the abdomen
Inspect for:
- Distension this could be because of intestinal obstruction or ascites.
- Peristalsis, which is a useful sign in pyloric stenosis.
- Inguinal region and genitalia (hernia, hydrocele, testicular torsion).

Palpate the abdomen for tenderness or guarding.

Masses – organomegaly
Auscultate and listen to the bowel sounds, which are:
- Increased in obstruction and acute diarrhoea.
- Reduced in ileus.
- Absent in peritonitis.

Rectal examination may be indicated in suspected appendicitis or intussusception. Remember that this is an unpleasant procedure. Try to have a parent in the room with you for reassurance and use your little finger.

Nervous system
Important signs noted on inspection include:
- Level of consciousness.
- Which developmental milestones have been met (as in Fig. 7.2).

In infants, it is important to:
- Measure occipitofrontal head circumference.
- Palpate the anterior fontanelle: this is a window in the skull that allows assessment of intracranial pressure and levels of dehydration to be assessed. It closes at about 12 months.

If indicated, more detailed evaluation may include the same features as would be examined in a adult: tone, power, coordination, sensation and reflexes (see Chapter 17).

Ears and throat
Usually left to the last, as their examination is not enjoyed by toddlers, mothers or doctors. The key to success is parental help in holding the child. The child should be seated on the mother's lap and held firmly by her with one hand on the forehead and one around the trunk and both arms.

Examine the ears first and the throat last; the occasional child will cooperate by 'opening wide'. In some cases it is necessary to insert a wooden spatula between clenched teeth onto the tongue.

History in an infant
Before examining the infant, details of the mother's health, the pregnancy, and labour should be ascertained.

Maternal health
Conditions that may affect the baby
Ask about:
- Diabetes mellitus type I.
- Autoimmune disorders, e.g. hyperthyroidism.

Maternal drugs
Find out about drug use, e.g. which drugs has she taken during pregnancy (prescribed and illicit plus cigarettes and alcohol). The BNF is a great reference book and is kept up to date. Check the drugs she mentions in it to find out if there are likely to be adverse effects.

Maternal infections
Infections that may affect the fetus include:
- Rubella.
- Cytomegalovirus.
- *Toxoplasma gondii*.
- Chickenpox.
- *Listeria monocytogenes*.
- *Treponema pallidum* (syphilis).
- HIV.

Pregnancy
Ask about:
- Length of gestation.
- Complications, e.g. pre-eclamptic toxaemia, intrauterine growth retardation.
- Antenatal diagnoses.

Birth
Ask about:
- Mode of delivery.
- Intrapartum complications.

The mother should be encouraged to express any concerns or questions about her infant. Enquire about the mode of feeding, e.g. if breast fed then for how long and when did weaning take place.

Examination of the infant

Routine examination

As soon as a baby is born, the midwife (obstetrician or paediatrician if present) will check that the baby is pink, breathing normally, and has no major congenital malformations. Obviously, if the infant is of low birthweight (<2500 g) or ill (e.g. after-birth asphyxia), admission to a special care baby unit will be required.

About 95% of babies are born at term and appear healthy. However, they all need a full medical examination within the first 24 hours of life. The purpose of this is:

- To give the parents a chance to ask any questions about their baby.
- To identify any problems anticipated as a result of maternal disease or familial disorders, e.g. congenital infection, maternal diabetes mellitus.
- To detect congenital abnormalities, which may not be immediately obvious at birth, e.g. cataract, cleft palate, heart murmur, undescended testes, dislocatable hip.

A scheme for the routine examination of the normal term infant is outlined below.

Neonatal screening

On day 6 of life, at which time feeding has been established, all babies have a blood sample from a heel prick taken on to a card (the Guthrie test). This is analysed to detect two inborn errors of metabolism:

- Phenylketonuria: 1:6000 births.
- Hypothyroidism: 1:3000 births.

Look hard but unobtrusively before you touch. Careful observation is the key to success. Vital information is obtained just from looking.

Upper airways noises are readily transmitted to the upper chest in infants. They can be difficult to distinguish from coarse rhonchi.

Watch a child's face for grimaces as you palpate the abdomen.

Putting the child's hand under yours may enhance cooperation.

In the first 24 hours, many babies have a quiet systolic 'flow' murmur. Features suggesting a significant murmur:

- Loud murmur.
- Diastolic murmur.
- Associated cardiac signs.
- These should be investigated with CXR, ECG, and echocardiogram.

To test for congenital dislocation of the hip (Fig 7.4) use the:

- Barlow manoeuvre -stabilise the pelvis with one hand and with the other abduct the hip to 45°. If the hip is dislocated, forward pressure with your middle finger will cause the femoral head to slip back into the acetabulum.
- Ortolani Manoeuvre -with the child on their back, flex their hips to 90° and also bend the knees to 90°. Place your middle finger over the greater trochanter and your thumb on the inner aspect of the thigh over the lesser trochanter. The child has a dislocated hip if, slow abduction causes a palpable or audible jolt. A click is more commonly felt and isn't diagnostic of a dislocated hip.

After the child has been discharged from hospital they should have a 6–8 week check at their GP's. This will include:

- Weight and head circumference.
- Hips again.
- Testes and penis.
- Heart sounds.
- Primitive reflexes.
- Muscle tone.
- Smiling.
- And most importantly, any parental concerns?

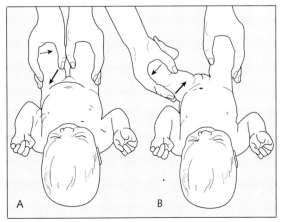

Fig. 7.4 Examination of the hip in newborn infants (A) the Barlow manoueuvre (B) the Ortolani manoueuvre.

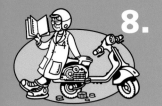

8. Presenting Problems in Psychiatric Patients

Introduction

Psychiatry can be a challenging area of medicine. It also makes up more of the work load than you may at first imagine. Around a quarter of the population may experience some form of psychiatric symptom in a year. At any given time roughly 7% of the population will have depression and the lifetime risk of schizophrenia is 1% (remember schizophrenia carries a 10% lifetime risk of suicide for those affected). Patients with physical disease may also (and often do) develop mental distress as part of their reaction to ill health.

Around one quarter to one third of patients presenting to GP have psychiatric symptoms.

With psychiatric problems, more so than any other area, history taking is key. It can be very difficult as patients may be too distressed or unwilling to communicate. Developing a rapport is essential but can be very challenging.

Remember your safety. It may be advisable to have a chaperone with you but this is not always possible or appropriate: always make sure that the patient does not come between you and the door.

The following is an outline of the format of a psychiatric history and the mental state examination.

A thumbnail sketch

This should include the patient's name, age and occupation.

Referral method

Who referred the patient? Was it self referral, via concerned family, the GP or even the police. Note the legal state of the patient, e.g. informal or under which part of the Mental Health Act they are being held, if appropriate.

Presenting complaint

Always ask open questions, 'What brought you to see a psychiatrist?' or 'Why do you think you're here?'. As with all histories it is important to use the words that the patient used, e.g. 'Life just isn't worth living'.

History of the presenting complaint

As discussed in Chapter 2 it is important to formulate an idea of how long this has been going on. Is it gradual in onset or is it acute? Have there been any clear precipitants, e.g. drug induced psychosis? Does anything make this better, does anything make it worse? How often does this happen? Is it weekly, daily or even monthly. It is important to get an idea of how severe an impact on the patient's life the problem is having. Ask if it is interfering with employment and relationships.

Past psychiatric history

Has this person had contact with psychiatric services previously? For example, have there been depressive episodes or deliberate self harm? What was the form of this? Have they previously been sectioned under the Mental Health Act and if so, how many times? Have they been admitted to hospital and have they ever had psychotherapy or counselling? Each episode should be investigated and detailed. Many psychiatric disorders are chronic and so there has often been multiple contacts with the patient. You might also ask about on-going contact with psychiatric services (e.g. Community Psychiatric Nurse (CPN), Community Mental Health Teams, partial hospitalization and or regular attendance at their GPs).

Family history

This is generally split into two sections.

Relationships with parents and siblings

Do they get on with their family and what contact do they have with them? Is home a safe and supportive place to be? What have been the learnt coping mechanisms that they have developed; for example you might ask, 'In the past when you felt down what actions have you taken?'. Do any family members have criminal convictions and if so what for? The answer might be 'Dad has spent the last 10 years in prison'.

Family psychiatric history

As many psychiatric illnesses have a genetic component it is important to know if any family members have psychiatric illnesses.

Personal history
Early development

Were there any problems during pregnancy, at birth and did they meet their developmental milestones (see Chapter 7). If the patient is young enough you may have access to their parents to ask these questions, otherwise you will have to ask the patient if they can recall their Mum discussing their early childhood.

Childhood behaviour

Did they play with other children or were they antisocial? You will need to explore the possibility that the person may have been abused at some point in their childhood. This is a difficult area to broach and not everyone will volunteer the information at the first time of asking. Direct questioning in such a sensitive and distressing area is often misappropriate and ineffective. A more oblique approach, for example using a statement instead of a question may help, e.g. 'sometimes distressing experiences in childhood can make people feel this way'.

School history

What kind of school did they go to, e.g. was it single sex, boarding, young offenders' institution, etc. Were they bullied or did they do the bullying. Did they manage to make and maintain friendships at school, did they play truant and what was their disciplinary record like (e.g. suspensions and expulsions). Were there any family upheavals during these years (e.g. divorce, deaths in the family, etc).

Occupational history

Ask how many jobs have they had, how long did they hold them down and why did they leave (e.g. the 16-year-old boy who went into mining and was then made redundant and has not found work in the past 10 years).

Sexual history

This includes sexual orientation, number of partners (including use of prostitutes) and whether or not the relationships have been successful.

Relationship/marriage

Often this is quite different from the above. Has this person been in a stable relationship that has recently ended and so they have lost their social support network?

Children

How many children do they have and with how many partners? What sort of contact do they have with the children and how do they feel about this?

Forensic history

Have they ever been in trouble with the police and if so how much contact was there? Have they been to prison and if so for how long and how many times? Do they have a case pending?

Current social circumstances

With whom are they living with at present? Where are they living? Are they owner occupier or is it rented accommodation and is it private or council owned? How many people live there? The answers to these questions can be quite revealing.

Premorbid personality

It is important to ask the patient how they perceived themselves before they became ill. Ask them about the following topics.

Social relationships

Do they feel they get on with people? Did they have a social support network? How were their friends and how did they perceive the relationships?

Hobbies/interests

For example, find out if they like sport or have a hobby like model railways? Are they members of any clubs?

Predominant mood

Would they describe themselves as predominantly anxious, pessimistic, depressed, happy or optimistic? It's amazing the number of people who will describe themselves as happy-go-lucky!

Character

Would they describe themselves generally as irritable, self-centred, obsessive or suspicious?

Habits

Do they drink alcohol and if so how much? Do they use recreational drugs? If so which drugs do they use, e.g. amphetamines, ecstasy, cannabis, heroin and tobacco. It is important to quantify drug use. A full and comprehensive drug history is essential.

Past medical history

This is no different from taking a history in any other setting but remember particularly to ask about previous head injuries and epilepsy. Medical problems can have psychological presentations or sequelae (e.g. hypothyroidism). Ask about their medication as this can also cause psychiatric problems.

A full psychiatric history can take upwards of an hour to take. Do not worry if the patient chooses to terminate the interview. Very often more than one interview is required to build a rapport, and thus obtain a full picture.

The mental state examination

This is the psychiatrist's equivalent of the physical examination. It begins when you first meet the patient and continues through the interview. It is your assessment of their mental state at the time you see them and not the history of their illness. It includes a few specific tests, e.g. testing memory (see Fig. 8.1). It is broken down into the following categories:

- Appearance.
- Hygiene.
- Clothes, signs of self neglect (this may indicate depression, dementia or schizophrenia) or strange or inappropriate behaviour, e.g. in mania.
- The state of their nutrition can be a sign of alcoholism or anorexia nervosa.

Mini-mental test
1. time of day (to nearest hour)
2. year
3. age
4. birthday
5. place
6. recognize two people
7. dates of Second World War
8. name of the monarch
9. count backwards from 20 to 1 with no mistakes
10. recall an address given 5 minutes earlier

Fig. 8.1 The mini-mental test. Score 1 point for each correct answer. Scores of less than 7 indicate well-established dementia.

- Facial expression, e.g. smiling, Parkinsonism dyskinesia and posture.
- Tremors – are they at rest, on movement and are they fine or coarse.
- How much eye contact they have during the interview.

Behaviour

You should mention the quality of the rapport generated with the patient. You should also mention how the patient behaved. Most will be pleasant and cooperative but they may also be:

- Aggressive.
- Restless or agitated.
- Slow/withdrawn.
- Overly familiar or frankly sexually disinhibited.
- Catatonic, e.g. when the patient is mute, stuperous or adopts bizarre postures.
- Unusual mannerisms, e.g. repetitive hand actions.

Speech

You should consider the patient's speech with respect to:

- Amount, e.g. how much talking is the patient doing?
- Intonation, e.g. is the patient monotonous in their speech or does the pitch rise and fall naturally?
- Rate (pressure of speech or slow speech).
- Dysphasia/dysarthria.
- Quality; does the patient use proper words or are they using made-up words (neologism), attaching different meanings to proper words (paraphasia), or are they repeating words spoken by another person (echolalia)?

Mood

A subjective and objective assessment of the patient's mood should be made. If the two fail to match the patient is said to be 'mood incongruent.' Patients may be:

- Blunted – the patient cannot externalize emotions fully.
- Flat – no emotional reactivity.
- Depressed – feels down.
- Irritable.
- Euphoric.
- Angry.
- Anxious or worried.

Thought

The patient's thoughts should be assessed for both form and content.

Form

Disorders of thought form reflect a disturbance in the process of formulating and expressing thoughts. Thoughts may be classified as:

- Loosening of associations – here there is a link between the patient's thoughts but it can be difficult to see it.
- Disordered – one thought follows the next with no obvious connection.
- Knight's move thinking – here the patient's associations are tortuous, at best.
- Word salad – this is when the patient is speaking a jumble of unrelated words.
- Flight of ideas – this is common in manic patients where they jump from one idea to the next with some discernible association.
- Thought insertion/withdrawal/block/broadcast. Here the patient may feel that someone or something is putting thoughts into their head or taking them out or stopping them having thoughts. In thought broadcast the patient feels everyone can read their thoughts.

Content

The content of a patient's thoughts must be assessed, although this will largely have occurred during the history taking. It is important to ask if the patient has any thoughts that are troubling them or that they do not think others would have. Thoughts content disorders include:

- Preoccupations. Does the patient have something that they cannot stop thinking about.
- Obsessions. An obsession is a recurrent thought or feeling which is unpleasant and cannot be got rid off.

- Delusions. This is a fixed and false belief abnormal to society.
- Over-valued idea. These are thoughts that the patient places an abnormal emphasis on.
- Depressive. Is the patient depressed? Do they have predominantly unhappy thoughts?
- Suicidal ideation. You must ask all patients if they are considering taking their own life. Most patients will answer honestly. Beware of patients who are vague in their answers.

 You must ask directly about suicidal ideation at some point. Failure to do so will be considered negligent.

Perceptual abnormalities

Remember that hallucinations are perceptions without stimulus while illusions are the misinterpretation of a stimulus. You should identify which sensory modality is affected (visual, auditory, somatic, etc.). For auditory hallucinations you should identify where the voice or voices come from (for example, inside the patient's head or outside), and how many of them there are and whether the first second or third person is used.

 Visual hallucinations point towards an organic problem whereas auditory hallucinations are commonly associated with schizophrenia.

Cognitive functions

The patient's cognitive state is assessed under the following divisions:

- Orientation in time, person and place.
- Memory (short and long term).
- Concentration.
- Attention.
- Intellect.

Insight

This is the final section of the mental state examination and deals with the patient's understanding of whether they are ill or not. It also includes the patient's willingness to accept treatment, and which treatments they are prepared to accept.

Once you have taken the history and mental state you need to pull it all together so it can be succinctly presented. Figure 8.2 shows how to do this. The case should be presented along the following lines.

A case summary

- The differential diagnosis you have reached.
- The aetiology.
- The management plan.

In this section we will consider some common psychiatric problems that, as a junior doctor, you will be exposed to and will be expected to deal with. They are deliberate self harm and suicide risk assessment, depression and acute confusion.

Deliberate self harm and suicide

Deliberate self harm is a self-initiated act in which the individual person injures themselves in a way that does not result in death. Suicide is a self-initiated act that leads directly to the person's death.

After the patient has been stabilized and any medical complications treated, an assessment of suicidal intent *must* be made.

Figure 8.3 shows the widely used Beck Suicide Intent Scale.

Key points to ascertain are:
1 A clear intention to die and remorse at having failed.
2 Detailed planning of the event.
3 Attempting to avoid detection.
4 Not seeking help after the event.

5 Using traumatic means.
6 Undertaking final acts, e.g. changing a will, paying off bills.

Risk factors for suicide
- Men>Women
- Older
- Single, divorced, widowed
- Psychiatric illness
- Chronic illness
- Traumatic means.

Depression

Depression as an isolated symptom is one of the commonest presenting complaints that GPs see. It often presents in both hospital and community settings with vague physical symptoms, e.g. tiredness. It is easily missed and accurate diagnosis depends upon the communication skills of the doctor. When taking a history from a depressed patient open and closed questions are needed. It is important to elucidate any of the symptoms listed in Fig. 8.4 and *must* include suicidal intent. It is a myth that asking a patient about suicidal ideation will precipitate the thought in their minds. It is negligent to fail to ascertain any such ideation. It is often possible to ask a direct question (e.g. 'Have you ever been so unhappy that you've thought about ending your life?'), but it may be more appropriate to ask in a more oblique fashion (e.g. 'Sometimes when people are so unhappy they feel that they can't go on?'). It is important to differentiate between real suicidal intent and the more common feeling that a

Sample case summary for a psychiatric patient				
	Biological	Psychological	Social	Example
Predisposing	(? ? ?)	(? ? ?)	(? ? ?)	Family history, personal childhood
Precipitating	(? ? ?)	(? ? ?)	(? ? ?)	Bereavement, disaster, divorce
Perpetuating	(? ? ?)	(? ? ?)	(? ? ?)	Organic damage, self-esteem
Example	Genetic, biochemical, drugs, endocrine	Stress, coping strategy, mental mechanisms	Poverty, social class, culture, institutions	

Fig. 8.2 Sample case summary for a psychiatric patient. Try to fill in the 'question boxes' (? ? ?) table for every patient you see. It makes pulling the history together easier and will enable management plans to be formulated.

Suicide Intent Scale		Circumstances related to suicidal attempt
1. Isolation	0	Somebody present
	1	Somebody nearby or in contact (as by phone)
	2	No one nearby or in contact
2. Timing	0	Timed so that intervention is probable
	1	Timed so that intervention is not likely
	2	Timed so that intervention is highly unlikely
3. Precautions against discovery and/or intervention	0	No precautions
	1	Passive precautions e.g. avoiding others but doing nothing to prevent their intervention. (Alone in room, door locked)
	2	Active precautions, such as locking doors
4. Acting to gain help during or after the attempt	0	Notified potential helper regarding attempt
	1	Contacted but did not specifically notify potential helper regarding the attempt
	2	Did not contact or notify potential helper
5. Final acts in anticipation of death	0	None
	1	Partial preparation or ideation
	2	Definite plans made (e.g. changes in a will, taking out insurance)
Self report		
1. Patient's statement	0	Thought that what he had done would not kill him
	1	Unsure whether what he had done would kill him
	2	Believed that what he had done would kill him
2. Stated intent	0	Did not want to die
	1	Uncertain or did not care if he lived or died
	2	Did want to die
3. Premeditation	0	Impulsive, no premeditation
	1	Considered act for less than one hour
	2	Considered act for less than one day
	3	Considered act for more than one day
4. Reaction to the act	0	Patient glad he has recovered
	1	Patient uncertain whether he is glad or sorry
	2	Patient sorry he has recovered
Risk		
1. Predictable outcome in terms of lethality of patient's act and circumstances known to him.	0	Survival certain
	1	Death unlikely
	2	Death likely or certain
2. Would death have occurred without medical treatment?	0	No
	1	Uncertain
	2	Yes

Fig. 8.3 The Beck Suicide Intent Scale. Scores of 0–3 indicate a low risk of repeat, 4–10 indicate a moderate risk and those of 11 and over indicate high risk. Scores of 18 and over indicate a very high risk of repeat in the short term.

patient wishes they were dead but has no intention of taking their life. This may require direct but sensitive probing.

Acute confusional state

Up to 20% of hospital inpatients will manifest some degree of acute confusion, and early on in your medical career as a newly qualified house officer you will be asked to come and sedate a patient (usually an elderly lady) because they are disturbing the night staff. Be warned that sedating

them is a last resort and should *only* be done if they are presenting a danger to themselves and/or to others. Ask your SHO for guidance before prescribing anything. Common clinical features of acute confusion are:

- Impaired consciousness, the level of this commonly fluctuates.
- Disorientation to time, person, place.
- Incoherent or rambling conversations.
- Patient may develop perceptual disturbance, e.g. illusions or hallucinations.
- There will be a diurnal variation in the symptoms and the sleep/wake cycle if often disturbed.

Symptoms of depression

Mood
Low mood for most of the time
Anhedonia
Anxiety (common)

Speech and thought
Suicidal ideas and/or intent
Slow speech
Poverty of thought
Pessimism, hopelessness
May develop delusions (mood congruent)

Biological function
Disturbed sleep (often with early morning wakening)
Anergia
Reduced appetite/weight loss
Reduced libido

Perception
May develop hallucinations if severe

Behaviour
Avoids social interaction
Self neglect
May show psychomotor retardation or agitation
Actions in preparation for suicide

Minimum time for diagnosis
2 weeks

Fig. 8.4   The symptoms of depression. (Courtesy of Dr Brian Lunn, Department of Psychiatry, University of Newcastle upon Tyne)

- Their behaviour is quite out of character, e.g. a normally quiet elderly lady becomes abusive and violent.

Try to identify and treat the underlying problem (e.g. a urinary tract infection or an upper respiratory tract infection). The best method of managing the patient is with good nursing care. Nurse the patient in a well lit, single room. Provide plenty of reassurance and repeated explanations.

High risk groups include the very young, very old, alcohol and drug abusers and those with dementia.

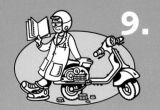

9. Presenting Problems: Locomotor System

Back pain

Detailed history

Back pain is extremely common. It is the largest single cause of lost working hours in the developed world amongst both manual and sedentary workers; in the former it is an important cause of long-term disability. The history is used to highlight potentially serious or treatable causes of the pain. Consider the differential diagnosis of back pain (Fig. 9.1).

Ask patients what they consider is causing the pain. This is always extremely informative. Take a detailed history in the usual systematic manner, focusing on the factors below.

Location of the pain

Most back pain is in the lumbar region. Thoracic pain is usually due to an organic cause (e.g. tuberculosis, osteoporotic crush fracture, myeloma).

Radiation of the pain

For example, radiation down the distribution of the sciatic nerve after lumbar disc prolapse.

Speed of onset

This may be acute (e.g. disc prolapse, crush fracture), insidious (e.g. malignancy, infection, inflammatory causes), or chronic for years (non-specific back pain).

Aggravating and relieving factors

Mechanical pain is often exacerbated by exercise. Inflammatory pain is often worse after a period of inactivity. Spinal stenosis may be worse on walking, but relieved by leaning forwards or resting.

Pattern of severity with time

For example, is the patient experiencing chronic unrelenting pain (e.g. inflammatory disease, psychogenic), intermittent or relapsing pain (e.g. disc disease)?

Associated symptoms

A full review of systems enquiry should be performed as the back pain may be part of a systemic disease such as ankylosing spondylosis (polyarthritis, dyspnoea, etc.), malignancy, renal failure (hypercalcaemia, etc.)

Past medical history

A detailed past medical history may elicit a potential underlying cause for the pain. Consider psychiatric disorders, especially depression, which may be a cause or result of the pain (e.g. somatization or lowered pain threshold).

Drug history

Ask patients what analgesics they have taken in an attempt to relieve the symptoms and their efficacy.

Social history

Explore how the pain limits functional activity. Ask specifically about time off work due to the pain. For suspected non-specific pain or psychogenic pain, explore current social pressures being experienced by the patient.

Review of systems enquiry

It is essential to consider systemic illnesses that may have precipitated the pain. In particular, consider weight loss, fevers, sweats, features suggestive of malignancy, polyarthritis, etc.

Back pain is very common. A good history is the key to efficient diagnosis and can prevent unnecessary and occasionally expensive or unpleasant investigations, which may reinforce illness behaviour.
Try to distinguish between systemic disease and mechanical pain. Symptoms such as thoracic pain, weight loss, fevers, systemic symptoms, or new-onset pain should trigger alarm bells.
Psychogenic back pain is not a diagnosis of exclusion. An attempt to make a positive diagnosis should be made as management can be tailored to this.

Differential diagnosis of back pain

Fig. 9.1 Differential diagnosis of back pain. Asterisks indicate more common causes.

Inflammatory
ankylosing spondylitis*; psoriatic arthropathy; enteropathic arthropathy

Bone disease
osteoporosis*; osteomalacia; renal bone disease; malignancy

Disc disease and osteoarthritis
spondylosis*; acute disc prolapse*; tuberculosis and septic discitis

Mechanical disease
posture* (pregnancy, obesity, scoliosis, etc.); spondylolisthesis; spinal stenosis

Soft tissue disease
'fibrositis'*; muscle strain*
Back pain is unlikely to have a serious cause when:
• the patient can get on & off the examination couch without discomfort
• there is no associated spasm of the spinal muscles and/or local tenderness
• the spine has a full range of movement

Non-specific back pain*
the most common cause; usually has a mechanical basis

Referred pain
chronic pancreatitis; posterior duodenal ulcer; abdominal aortic aneurysm, etc.

Rheumatoid arthritis

Detailed history
Rheumatoid arthritis is a multisystem disease and the history should be taken in a systematic manner.

Background disease
Ask about age of onset (typically 25–40 years) and usual pattern of arthritis etc. About 5–10% of patients will have a positive family history.

Current disease activity
Attempt to assess whether the patient has active synovitis and try to distinguish it from secondary osteoarthritis due to burnt out rheumatoid disease. Enquire about the time pattern of disease activity (e.g. relentless progression, disease flares separated by periods of remission) and the presence of red or swollen joints. If so, note the response to analgesics and non-steroidal anti-inflammatory drugs (NSAIDs) and the duration of early morning stiffness (> 30 minutes is significant). Map out the joints that the patient thinks are inflamed (Fig. 9.2).

Functional impact of the disease
Consider how current disease activity has altered functional ability. For example ask 'Is there anything that you have difficulty doing now that you could manage a few weeks ago?'. Consider mobility, grip, doing buttons, climbing stairs, etc. Ascertain whether activities are limited by pain, weakness, or other factors.

Extra-articular features of the disease
Rheumatoid arthritis should be considered as a systemic disease. For each system, consider how disease activity may be manifested:
• Lung – dyspnoea (e.g. due to rheumatoid nodules, pleural effusion, bronchiolitis obliterans).
• Skin – rash, vasculitic leg ulcers, rheumatoid nodules.
• Nervous system – paraesthesiae (especially carpal tunnel syndrome), symptoms of peripheral neuropathy.
• Eyes – dry eyes (Sjögren's syndrome) especially if associated with a dry mouth, red eye (scleritis).
• Renal – proteinuria or known dysfunction (e.g. due to amyloid, medication).
• Anaemia – many patients will have an anaemia of chronic disease; this may be exacerbated by anaemia due to blood loss if the patient is on NSAIDs.

Drug history
A particularly detailed drug history is absolutely essential. Concentrate on drugs currently being used

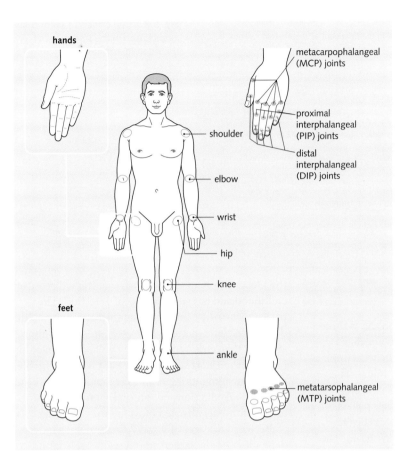

Fig. 9.2 Simple diagrams can be used to illustrate the distribution of active synovitis. Shaded circles represent inflamed joints.

hands

metacarpophalangeal (MCP) joints

proximal interphalangeal (PIP) joints

distal interphalangeal (DIP) joints

shoulder

elbow

wrist

hip

knee

feet

ankle

metatarsophalangeal (MTP) joints

to control the disease (e.g. steroids, analgesics, NSAIDs, disease modifying agents). Often, a multitude of drug combinations has been used previously. Try to chart previous experiences objectively so that an assessment can be made about changing agents, if necessary, to improve control of disease activity. For each disease modifying agent, chart:

- Acceptability of agent to the patient.
- Time period of use.
- Efficacy – use objective and subjective parameters if possible, for example what did the patient think of it, early morning stiffness, erythrocyte sedimentation rate (ESR), progression of joint erosions radiologically.
- Reason for discontinuation – for example side effects, lack of response.
- Doses used – especially cumulative dose.
- If on NSAIDs have they had any gastrointestinal side effects and had they tried selective cyclo-oxygenase-2 (COX2) antagonists?

All second-line agents have side effects (Fig. 9.3). Ask specifically about the use of steroids.

Social history

It is important to investigate the functional impact of the disease on daily life, exploring the home environment as well as occupation. Many aids to living are available, and specialist use of physiotherapists and occupational therapists may be invaluable. As with many long-term disabling conditions, it is easy to concentrate on symptom control, and practical issues; enquire how the patient is feeling and coping, and what they are worried about. This is equally important.

Remember that rheumatoid arthritis is a chronic (and often disabling) condition. Patient education and motivation are crucial for optimal rehabilitation. It is particularly important that an air of mutual trust is fostered between the patient and doctor.

Fig. 9.3 Side effects of second-line agents used in the treatment of rheumatoid arthritis.

Side effects of second-line agents used in the treatment of rheumatoid arthritis	
Drug	**Side effects**
gold	proteinuria (membranous nephropathy); thrombocytopenia and agranulocytosis; skin rash (approximately 25%); stomatitis
penicillamine	proteinuria (common); nephrotic syndrome; thrombocytopenia; agranulocytosis; anorexia; nausea (early in treatment); rash
methotrexate	bone marrow suppression; oral ulceration; gastrointestinal disturbances; hepatotoxicity (especially prolonged use); teratogenic
azathioprine	bone marrow suppression; increased risk of malignancy; infections; gastrointestinal disturbances
sulphasalazine	nausea; vomiting; skin rash; blood dyscrasia (rare)
hydroxychloroquine	retinopathy (especially long-term use)

Osteoarthritis

This is the commonest joint condition and is three times more common in women than men and normally presents at about 50. It usually occurs as a primary feature, but may occur after injury. The patient will normally complain about pain on exertion which is relieved by rest. Their pain is often worse at the end of the day. This process begins insidiously and develops over years. With time the relief with rest is less complete. The patient may also complain about stiffness after periods of rest. Unlike the inflammatory joint diseases, however, there are no systemic features of osteoarthritis.

Ask the patient what joints are particularly affected. (In order) it is the distal interphalangeal joints, first metacarpophalangeal, first metatarsophalangeal joints which are most commonly affected. The hip and knees are also commonly affected. Determine what the patient's current level of function is and what exactly stops them doing more. It is useful to find out if they have had any joint replacements and whether they feel them to have been successful. As the patient will often complain about pain, it is important to take a drug history to determine what analgesics they use and which they find most effective. Refer to Chapter 21 on investigations for detail about the X-ray changes associated with osteoarthritis.

Perthes' disease

This condition is a subject much loved of orthopaedic surgeons as it demonstrates the changing anatomy of

the blood supply to the hip with age. It is a disease of childhood and has an incidence of 1:10 000. The patient is usually a boy between the ages of 4–8 with delayed skeletal maturity. (Boys are four times more affected than girls.) Initially they will complain of hip pain and then start to limp. The joint will be irritable; thus all movements are diminished and painful at the extremes. Abduction and internal rotation are the most commonly affected movements.

Between the ages of 4 and 7 the femoral head is dependent on the lateral epiphyseal vessels for its blood supply. Their course makes then susceptible to occlusion by pressure from any effusion around the hip. After the age of 7 the blood vessels in the ligamentum terres are developed and supply the femoral head.

The pathology is a three-stage process. Initially, there are one or more episodes of ischaemia causing bone death. Revascularization and repair then occurs but there is then distortion and remodelling of the femoral head and neck. This can then lead to the incomplete covering of the femoral head by the acetabulum.

Slipped upper femoral epiphysis

A slipped upper femoral epiphysis is basically a fracture through the hypertrophic zone of the cartilaginous growth plate. The patient is usually a pubertal boy who will present with referred hip pain (e.g. knee pain, groin pain, anterior thigh pain and limping). They can present with acute pain following trauma, chronically or with acute-on-chronic pain. These patients are very often unusually tall and thin, or fat and sexually under-developed. On examination the leg will be externally rotated and shorter and all movements will be painful.

pressure sores, DVT and PEs. If the patient is to make a successful recovery operative management is mandatory to facilitate early mobilization.

Fractured neck of femur

This usually happens to older women who have osteoporosis. It often follows a simple fall; however, care should be taken to ensure that there is no medical cause for the fall. The patient cannot normally weight bear but some will be able to walk albeit with considerable pain. On examination, the affected limb will be shortened and externally rotated. This condition has a 1-year mortality of approximately 50%. The fractures are classified according to Garden's classification (Fig. 9.4; see also Chapter 21 on investigations). Patients are often frail and susceptible to hospital-acquired pneumonia,

Garden's classification of fractured neck of femur	
Type 1	Inferior cortex not completely broken but trabecule lines are angulated
Type 2	Inferior cortex clearly broken but trabecule lines are not angulated
Type 3	Obvious fracture line and rotation of head in acetabulum
Type 4	Fully displaced fracture

Fig. 9.4 Garden's classification of fractured neck of femur.

10. Presenting Problems: Endocrine System

Detailed history

Review presentation with diabetes mellitus

The most important features of diabetes mellitus are:

- Age of onset.
- Presenting symptoms (e.g. weight loss, polyuria, polydipsia, coma).

Form of diabetes mellitus

Note the class of disease, as complications and management strategies will vary, for example:

- Type I – lack of insulin.
- Type II – insulin resistance.
- Secondary (due to glucocorticosteroids, pancreatitis, Cushing's disease).

Diabetic control

This is the cornerstone of managing diabetes mellitus, so much of the time available at consultation should be devoted to this. Review the form of blood sugar control (e.g. diet alone, oral hypoglycaemic agents, insulin). Try and ascertain their concordance. Be sensitive in inquiring for example, 'Do you ever forget to take your tablets?' or 'Do you have dietary lapses?'.

Establish how the patient monitors glycaemic control. Check the form of monitoring (e.g. measuring blood glucose, urinalysis), frequency of measurements, and the levels attained. Most patients will have a book charting the blood glucose level. This should be reviewed to assess general control and fluctuations at different times of the day. It also provides an additional insight into the patient's concordance. In an analogous way to checking inhaler technique, it is often informative to observe a patient performing a blood glucose estimate. While patients may try to improve their diabetic records, they cannot fake the glycosylated haemoglobin (Hb_{A1C}), which is a measure of long-term glucose control. This is produced by the attachment of glucose to Hb. The measure of the glycosylated fraction gives the average glucose concentration over the lifetime of the Hb molecule (120 days, normally 4–8%).

In type I diabetes, patient education and motivation are crucial to the long-term prognosis. Good long-term control is pivotal for reducing the long-term complications of diabetes mellitus. Focus on risk factors for ischaemic heart disease and always ask specifically about visual problems and foot care.

Complications of diabetes

Review the frequency of acute complications of therapy or hyperglycaemia, for example:

- Hypoglycaemic attacks.
- Diabetic ketoacidosis (DKA).
- Hyperosmolar non-ketotic coma.

Have they required hospital admissions for any of these?

Ask specifically about symptoms suggestive of poor control, for example:

- Weight loss, malaise, fatigue.
- Polyuria, polydipsia (due to osmotic diuresis).
- Blurred vision (refractive changes in the eye).
- Balanitis, pruritus vulvae, thrush.

Macrovascular complications

Diabetes mellitus is strongly associated with macrovascular disease. It is imperative that any coincident risk factors such as hypertension, hyperlipideamia are identified and minimized. Check for symptoms related to the three main forms of macrovascular disease:

- Ischaemic heart disease (ask specifically about chest pains, myocardial infarction).
- Peripheral vascular disease (e.g. claudication).
- Cerebrovascular disease.

Microvascular complications

Long-term disease is associated with relentless progression of microvascular disease. Good control is clearly associated with a decreased likelihood of microvascular complications. Early recognition may allow specific therapy to be instituted. Ask about the three main forms of microvascular disease:

- Retinopathy – ask about visual symptoms, laser therapy.
- Neuropathy – paraesthesiae.
- Nephropathy – proteinuria and hypertension.

Other complications

Diabetes mellitus is associated with other complications, which may be multifactorial. Specific enquiry should be made about:

- Impotence – rarely spontaneously volunteered by the patient, but common so always ask.
- Staphylococcal skin infections – for example boils, carbuncles.
- Gastroparesis – nausea, vomiting, early satiety.
- Foot ulcers – neuropathy and vasculopathy this normally manifests as numbness, pain and paraesthesia. 'Do you feel like you're walking on cotton wool?' 'Do you know where you're putting your feet?'

Past medical history

Review the other risk factors for ischaemic heart and cerebrovascular disease. Consider other possible autoimmune diseases (especially thyroiditis, pernicious anaemia, vitiligo, Addison's disease), renal failure, and systemic infections.

Drug history

Review the agents used to control the diabetes and drugs that may be related to complications, e.g. antihypertensives, angiotensin-converting enzyme inhibitors, statin etc.

Oral hypoglycaemic agents

Consider whether it is appropriate for the patient to be on an oral hypoglycaemic agent. Beware of metformin in the presence of renal dysfunction (metformin is contraindicated as it may cause lactic acidosis). Consider whether it is more appropriate to use agents that are hepatically metabolized or renally excreted.

Insulin

Review the form of insulin used (e.g. long- or short-acting, porcine or human). Assess whether the dose needs to be modified. Ask about problems at injection sites (e.g. lipohypertrophy, scarring).

Review the use of other medication that may aggravate diabetic control (e.g. glucocorticosteroids, thiazide diuretics). It may be possible to improve diabetic control by appropriate adjustment of other medication.

Family history

This is usually positive for patients with type II diabetes mellitus.

Social history

Review home circumstances, for example:

- Is the patient's eyesight good enough to read BM sticks?
- Does the patient have sufficient manual dexterity (especially if he or she had neuropathy) to monitor his or her own therapy?

Education and motivation are central to the long-term outlook for the diabetic patient. An appropriate diet is essential for improving the control of all diabetic patients, especially those who are obese. Help from a dietician may be indicated. It is particularly important that the patient understands the unacceptable risks of smoking.

Diabetes is a condition in which a 'patient-centred' approach has been shown to positively influence outcome.

In diabetes mellitus, patient education and motivation are crucial to the long-term prognosis. Good long-term control is pivotal for reducing the long-term complications of diabetes mellitus. Focus on risk factors for ischaemic heart disease and always ask specifically about visual problems and foot care.

Thyroid disease

Presenting complaint

Hypothyroidism and hyperthyroidism may present in many ways, and form part of the differential diagnosis of a variety of disorders. Some of the more common presentations are shown in Fig. 10.1. A high index of suspicion may be needed to diagnose these conditions as presentation is often non-specific.

Detailed history
Hyperthyroidism

Ask about symptoms of hyperthyroidism. Enquire specifically about palpitations (see Fig 10.1).

Presenting features of thyroid disease	
Hypothyroidism	**Hyperthyroidism**
weight gain*	weight loss despite good appetite*
general slowness	
mental slowing, poor memory	poor concentration
anorexia	
cold intolerance*	heat intolerance*, excessive sweating
depression	agitation*, restlessness*
coma	
constipation	diarrhoea
altered appearance	eye changes
	palpitations

Fig. 10.1 Presenting features of thyroid disease. Asterisks indicate the more common or discriminatory features.

The common causes of atrial fibrillation are ischaemic heart disease, hyperthyroidism, and mitral valve disease.

Hypothyroidism and hyperthyroidism can produce a multitude of symptoms. A high index of suspicion is needed, particularly in the context of mental changes, palpitations, changes in weight, altered conscious level, or cardiac disease. The most discriminatory features from the history are cold and heat intolerance and weight changes despite contradictory dietary history. A relative may provide invaluable clues as the patient may not spontaneously report symptoms.

The following specific features may suggest underlying Graves' disease:
- Eye disease (diplopia, proptosis).
- Goitre (ask about difficulty swallowing or breathing).
- Pretibial myxoedema.

Hypothyroidism

Ask about symptoms of hypothyroidism (see Fig. 10.1) tiredness, general slowing down and deepening of the voice. In particular, enquire about weight gain, fertility problems, menstrual difficulties, and cold intolerance. The symptoms are often insidious and are not noticed by patients or their immediate family, but may be observed by occasional visitors or general practitioners.

Past medical history

Ask about:
- Other autoimmune disorders (e.g. diabetes mellitus, Addison's disease, vitiligo, myasthenia gravis).

- Previous partial thyroidectomy or treatment with radio-iodine if there is suspected hypothyroidism.

Also consider treatable causes of thyroid disease (Fig. 10.2) and the presence of ischaemic heart disease in hypothyroid patients as thyroxine therapy will then need to be more cautious.

Secondary causes of thyroid disease	
Hypothyroidism	**Hyperthyroidism**
dietary iodine deficiency	
antithyroid drugs used at inappropriate dose or on resolution of hyperthyroid state	over-dosage with thyroxine
post-thyroid surgery	
radio-iodine therapy	thyroid carcinoma (rare)
tumour infiltration (rare)	TSH-secreting tumours (rare)
hypopituitarism	
post-subacute thyroiditis	acute thyroiditis (e.g. infective, autoimmune)

Fig. 10.2 Secondary causes of thyroid disease. TSH, thyroid-stimulating hormone.

Try to assess thyroid status clinically in treated patients as biochemical tests lag behind therapeutic responses by several weeks.

Drug history

Review the use and dose of antithyroid medication and thyroxine. Consider drugs that may aggravate symptoms (e.g. β-blockers causing bradycardia in hypothyroidism). In addition, consider drugs that may interfere with interpretation of thyroid function tests (e.g. oestrogens increase thyroid-binding globulin concentration). Thyroid-stimulating hormone (TSH) levels are usually (if not always) needed in addition to total thyroxine concentration, when interpreting thyroid function tests.

Review of systems enquiry

A detailed screen of systemic symptoms is essential as many features are non-specific. It is often fruitful to concentrate on psychological changes, e.g. symptoms of depression.

The common causes of atrial fibrillation are ischaemic heart disease, hyperthyroidism, and mitral valve disease.

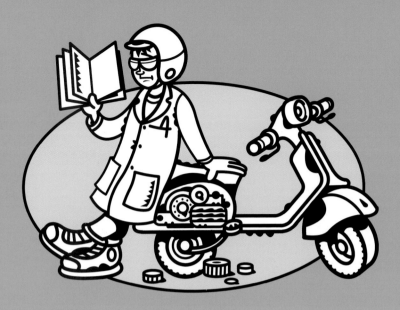

EXAMINATION

11. Introduction to Examination

Overview

This section of the book is divided into the individual systems of the body. The first part of each chapter describes the routine examination of that system. The second part illustrates the process described above in practice by providing examples of pathologies or presentations related to the system. These examples are intended to provide a skeleton for the student's examination, illustrating the important features. When it comes to exams, there is a set way in which your examiners will expect you to examine patients. Failure to use this approach will unsettle examiners and they may not appreciate the visionary methods you are using! This is especially true in the OSCE environment where marks are awarded for doing a specified task. It is important to get as much feedback as possible on your examination technique. Take every opportunity for someone more experienced to be present, watch what you are doing, and give you constructive feedback.

Setting

A good physical examination relies upon a cooperative patient and a well-lit room. It is important to engender an atmosphere of trust and professionalism during the history taking and to explain the steps of the examination appropriately, and if necessary what information you hope to elicit from the process. This will help to avoid any misunderstanding and will reassure the patient, taking away some of the mysticism that may surround the doctor–patient relationship.
It is good practice to start any examination with the hands. It is much more socially acceptable to have your hands examined than your abdomen. As the examination progresses up the patient's arm you have time for the patient to relax and trust in your professionalism. It is important to be sensitive to the patient. It is always appropriate for a chaperone to be present; however, it may be inappropriate for the patient's partner to be in the room during the examination.

The patient must be appropriately positioned, comfortable, and in a well-lit warm room. Ensure that there is adequate privacy. It is clearly unacceptable for a semi-clad patient to be examined on a couch without screens if the door to the examination room is potentially going to be opened without warning or for the patient to be examined on a ward without curtains pulled round.

Examination routine

Although the examination is described as a separate process from the history, a good assessment should start as soon as the patient walks into the examination room (Fig. 11.1). There are countless other observations that can be made, and a rapid inspection of the patient will put the subsequently elicited history into context. For example, does the patient look ill or well? Have they apparently lost weight? Are there any obvious facial features? (the staring eyes of thyrotoxicosis, yellow sclera of jaundice, etc.).

The examination, like the history, should be performed in a systematic manner, but again it is vital to be aware of the differential diagnosis as each sign is elicited. It is also important to think about what you expect to find from the history – it's easier to find something if you know what you're looking for. In many clinical examinations, including OSCEs and long cases, you may be asked to describe what you're doing and why, so it is a good idea to get into the habit. However, it is also

---

Points to consider when the patient walks into the room

Does the patient look ill or in pain?

Is the patient cachectic or overweight?

What is the patient's ethnic/cultural background?

Does the patient have a normal gait?

Is the patient short of breath on walking into the examination room?

Does the patient require help to get out of a chair?

Fig. 11.1 Points to consider when the patient walks into the room.

necessary to keep an inquiring mind, as it is not difficult to convince yourself you've found the sign(s) you expected, when in fact they're not actually present!

Once again the process is active. The examination routine usually follows a strict order. For most systems, the order of examination is as follows:

- Inspection.
- Palpation.
- Percussion.
- Auscultation.

Or in orthopaedics:

- Look.
- Feel.
- Move.

The most important component of the examination is inspection.

Examining a system

When examining any system, try to answer the following three questions.

What is the pathology?

This process requires interpretation of the physical signs so that a deviation from normality can be recognized and the individual signs integrated.

What is the aetiology of the pathological process?

It is not enough to identify that a patient has a pleural effusion. An attempt should be made to find the underlying cause (e.g. lymphadenopathy and hepatomegaly suggesting malignancy, a third heart sound and elevated jugular venous pressure suggesting heart failure and fluid overload).

What is the severity and functional impact on the patient?

For example, severe aortic stenosis is an indication for valve replacement. This may be assessed clinically by measuring the pulse pressure and noting the presence of a slow-rising pulse.

Physical signs

Many physical signs are subtle, or simply represent a variation in the normal. It is essential that the doctor has an appreciation of the wide range of normality so that any signs can be placed into context. There are no short cuts. To gain this ability requires practice.

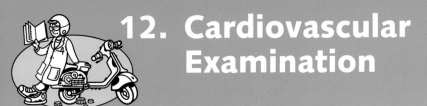

12. Cardiovascular Examination

Examination routine

As with all examinations the cardiovascular examination follows the format of inspection, palpation, percussion and auscultation. Many cardiovascular pathologies produce multiple signs, which when integrated allow assessment of the severity and aetiology of the lesion. It is particularly important to perform the examination in a systematic manner so that physical signs can be put into context with each other.

Patient exposure and position

Ensure adequate lighting. The patient should be comfortable and seated at 45 degrees to the horizontal, and stripped to the waist. Female patients should remove their bra. (It is difficult auscultating through clothing!) It is courteous to provide a blanket as the patient may wish to remain covered until examination of the praecordium.

General inspection

In all systems, the specific examination should be preceded by an inspection of the patient. Vital clues are often found.

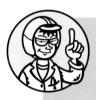 It is essential to know in advance what you are looking for, or it will not be found! Prepare a mental checklist. The whole process need only take a few seconds.

General features

Note any obvious features on general observation including:

- Age, sex, general health.
- Body habitus (obese or cachectic).
- Breathlessness (observe the effort required to climb onto the couch).
- Position in bed (is the patient comfortable, or do they seem to need to sit up or forward).

Listen for any clicks of prosthetic heart valves. Inspection can then be performed from the head downwards.

Eyes

A brief inspection will reveal abnormalities such as arcus senilis (significant in young adults, suggesting hypercholesterolaemia) or xanthelasma (suggestive of hyperlipidaemia). The patient may be obviously jaundiced.

Face

Look for evidence of cyanosis particularly around the lips or under the tongue, or plethora (e.g. due to superior vena cava obstruction, polycythaemia). The patient may have a typical facies for a pathological process, for example: Malar flush (mitral stenosis).

Always inspect the mouth (dental hygiene in infective endocarditis).

Neck

Note any visible pulsations.

Praecordium

Observe the shape of the chest for:

- Any obvious deformity (e.g. pectus excavatum in Marfan's syndrome).
- Visible collateral veins (e.g. in superior vena cava obstruction).
- Visible apex beat (e.g. left ventricular hypertrophy).
- Presence of any scars (Fig. 12.1).

Also look in the brachial and femoral regions for scars from cardiac catheterization.

Ankles

Briefly look for swelling suggestive of peripheral oedema. This can be confirmed by later examination.

 Adequate inspection is neglected at your peril! If omitted, simple diagnoses can be easily overlooked. It also helps to anticipate subsequently elicited physical signs and to put them in perspective.

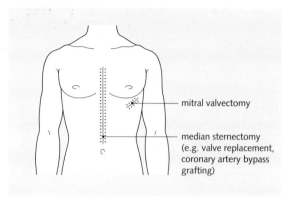

mitral valvectomy

median sternectomy
(e.g. valve replacement,
coronary artery bypass
grafting)

Fig. 12.1 Position of scars related to cardiovascular pathology on the praecordium.

toes. Hold the nail up to the plane of your eyes to facilitate detection. Although a non-specific sign, its presence should alert the physician to underlying disease (Fig. 12.3). You must be able to tell your examiners the causes of clubbing.

New-onset clubbing is highly significant. If detected, ask the patient whether he or she has noticed any recent change in the shape of their nails.

Specific examination

Specific examination can now be performed.

Hands

Careful examination of the hands often reveals clues of underlying cardiovascular disease. Feel the temperature and look for peripheral cyanosis. Note the shape of the hands (e.g. arachnodactyly in Marfan's syndrome).

Clubbing

The cardinal feature of clubbing is loss of angle of the nailfold. Other features include increased convex curvature in both a longitudinal and transverse plane, increased fluctuation of the nailbed, and swelling of the terminal phalanx (Fig. 12.2). Remember to look at both hands. Clubbing can rarely be detected in the

Splinter haemorrhages

These are linear red or black streaks under the finger or toenails and (Fig. 12.4) are a feature of a vasculitic process, but the most common cause is mild trauma, and a small number (e.g. about five) is normal.

Nailfold infarcts

Nailfold infarcts (Fig. 12.4) are also a feature of vasculitis, but more specific than splinter haemorrhages. They are often associated with other features of infective endocarditis (see infective endocarditis).

Capillary return

Apart from noting the temperature of the skin, peripheral perfusion may be assessed by capillary return. Light digital pressure to the end of the nail will produce blanching. The speed of capillary return

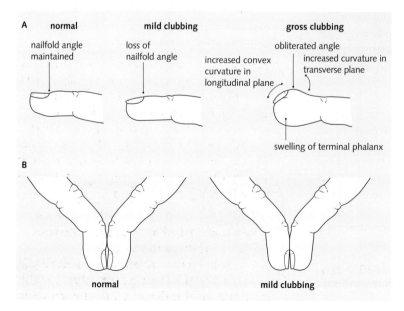

A normal

nailfold angle maintained

mild clubbing

loss of nailfold angle

gross clubbing

obliterated angle

increased convex curvature in longitudinal plane

increased curvature in transverse plane

swelling of terminal phalanx

B

normal

mild clubbing

Fig. 12.2 (A) Features of clubbing. The cardinal sign is loss of angle of the nailfold. (B) If the patient is asked to place his index fingers 'back to back', the diamond-shaped gap normally present is obliterated in early clubbing.

System	Disease associations
	Causes of clubbing
cardiovascular	infective endocarditis* (late sign); congenital cyanotic heart disease; atrial myxoma (very rare)
respiratory	carcinoma of the bronchus*; fibrosing alveolitis*; chronic suppurative lung disease* (empyema, bronchiectasis, pulmonary abscess, cystic fibrosis)
abdominal	Crohn's disease (unusual); cirrhosis
familial	most common cause*

can be visualized. Poor peripheral perfusion can be easily detected. You should press on the nailbed for 5 seconds and the return should take less than 2 seconds. Visible pulsation may be seen in aortic regurgitation.

Nicotine staining
Cigarette staining of the fingertips and nails may counter information given in the history.

Other signs of infective endocarditis
Look for other stigmata of infective endocarditis (rare), for example:
- Osler's nodes (tender nodules on the finger pulps).
- Janeway lesions (see infective endocarditis).

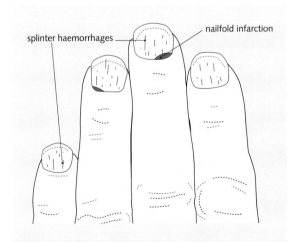

Fig. 12.4 Splinter haemorrhages and nailfold infarcts. If both lesions appear together infective endocarditis or a vasculitic process is highly likely.

splinter haemorrhages

nailfold infarction

Xanthomas
Lipid deposition may occur in tendons, skin, or soft tissues in some hyperlipidaemic states, for example:
- Tendon xanthomas (especially of Achilles tendon, extensor tendons on hands) – type II hyperlipidaemia.
- Palmar xanthomas (skin creases of palms and soles) – type III hyperlipidaemia.

Arterial pulse
The arterial pulse may be palpated at various sites (Fig. 12.5). The pulse has various characteristics, which should be defined in each patient.

Presence and symmetry
Compare the radial pulsations synchronously (e.g. large vessel vasculitis, aortic dissection). Obstruction may delay the pulse. Check for radiofemoral delay, especially in hypertension (e.g. due to coarctation of the aorta). Assess the presence of each pulse, especially if there is embolism or peripheral artery disease.

Rate
Normal pulse rate is 60–100/min. Count for at least 15 seconds at the radial pulse. This may also provide an opportunity for additional visual inspection of the patient. The radial pulse rate may differ from the number of ventricular contractions per minute (e.g. apicoradial deficit in fast atrial fibrillation). Consider the rate within the clinical context (e.g. tachycardia in the presence of fever, hypovolaemia; bradycardia in hypothermia, hypothyroidism).

Rhythm
The normal pulse rhythm is regular sinus rhythm. Any irregularity should be characterized, and if possible confirmed by an electrocardiogram (ECG). Many arrhythmias are characteristic (Fig. 12.6). You should state whether the pulse is regular or irregular.

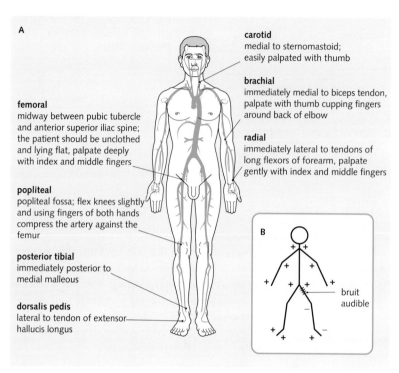

Fig. 12.5 (A) Location of the arterial pulses. (B) Typical notation in the hospital records. (+, pulse present; −, pulse not palpable; bruit audible).

A

carotid
medial to sternomastoid; easily palpated with thumb

brachial
immediately medial to biceps tendon, palpate with thumb cupping fingers around back of elbow

radial
immediately lateral to tendons of long flexors of forearm, palpate gently with index and middle fingers

femoral
midway between pubic tubercle and anterior superior iliac spine; the patient should be unclothed and lying flat, palpate deeply with index and middle fingers

popliteal
popliteal fossa; flex knees slightly and using fingers of both hands compress the artery against the femur

posterior tibial
immediately posterior to medial malleous

dorsalis pedis
lateral to tendon of extensor hallucis longus

B

bruit audible

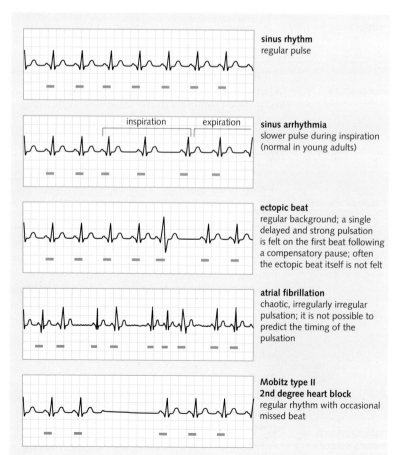

Fig. 12.6 Common arrhythmias. In each recording the upper trace is the ECG and the lower trace illustrates a bar corresponding to each palpable pulsation. It is often possible to elucidate the underlying rhythm disturbance.

sinus rhythm
regular pulse

inspiration   expiration

sinus arrhythmia
slower pulse during inspiration (normal in young adults)

ectopic beat
regular background; a single delayed and strong pulsation is felt on the first beat following a compensatory pause; often the ectopic beat itself is not felt

atrial fibrillation
chaotic, irregularly irregular pulsation; it is not possible to predict the timing of the pulsation

Mobitz type II
2nd degree heart block
regular rhythm with occasional missed beat

And if irregular is it regularly irregular or is it irregularly irregular.

Volume

Pulse volume reflects stroke volume. This is best assessed at the carotid or brachial pulse. There is a wide range of 'normal'. It is important to practice on as many different patients as possible so that you can recognize when abnormal signs are present.

Some of the abnormalities of pulse volume include:

- Pulsus paradoxus. This is detectable in cardiac tamponade or severe asthma. A detectable increase in pulse volume is observed during expiration. Pulsus paradoxus reflects an exaggeration of the normal physiological changes in intrathoracic pressure and the influence of the diaphragm and interventricular septal changes during the respiratory cycle.
- Pulsus alternans. This is a sign of severe left ventricular failure. Alternate pulses are felt as strong or weak due to the presence of bigeminy.
- Coarctation of the aorta. As well as radiofemoral delay (described above), the pulse volume of the femoral pulse is usually noticeably reduced.

Character

With increasing distance from the aorta, particularly in sclerotic vessels, the waveform becomes distorted (Fig. 12.7), so volume and character should be assessed using either the carotid or brachial pulses. A picture of the waveform often correlates with the severity of valvular disorders. This sign requires considerable practice to elicit, so that the range of normality can be appreciated, and abnormalities put into context. Try to become used to the pulse character of the common pathologies (Fig. 12.7).

Blood pressure

Measurement of blood pressure is straightforward, yet it is often performed inadequately, with obvious implications for patient management.

The blood pressure is a vital sign, so should be elicited with great care and given the respect that it deserves! It should be measured to the nearest 2 mmHg.

Description	Waveform	Associations
normal		–
slow rising		aortic stenosis
collapsing (water hammer)		aortic regurgitation persistent ductus arteriosus

Fig. 12.7 Typical arterial waveforms palpated at the carotid pulse in different conditions. The waveform often provides important information about the severity of the underlying pathology.

As with other components of the cardiovascular examination, it is important to adopt a systematic approach, for example as follows:

- Allow the patient to relax – white coat hypertension is a real phenomenon.
- Make sure the cuff is placed centrally over the brachial artery.
- Use a large cuff in obese subjects with an arm circumference over 30 cm – common cause of overestimating blood pressure.
- Deflate the cuff at a steady controlled rate – ideally no more than 2 mm per heartbeat.
- On deflating the cuff, note the point of the first audible sounds (Korotkov I), the point at which sounds become muffled (Korotkov IV), and the point of disappearance of sounds (Korotkov V, which is usually 5–10 mmHg lower than phase IV, but occasionally 0 mmHg). Most observers use phase V as a record of diastolic pressure as this produces less interobserver error.

Occasionally, additional blood pressure readings are indicated:

- Postural – for example if the patient is on antihypertensive medication or has dizziness, or to assess hypovolaemia.
- Comparison of right and left arms – for example for aortic dissection, aortic coarctation.

- Repeated measurements – before diagnosing hypertension, always take readings on a variety of occasions.
- Comparison of the ankle:brachial ratio – for example for aortic coarctation, peripheral vascular disease.

All these can be difficult to get as electronic measuring devices are taking over. You need to have a working knowledge of a manual sphygmomanometer and know where one can be found on the ward.

Neck
Arterial pulse
Follow the usual pattern of:

- Inspection – look at the pulsation (e.g. signs of collapsing pulse).
- Palpation – palpate the carotid artery specifically for volume and character.
- Auscultation – auscultate for the presence of a carotid bruit.

Venous pulse
Assessment of the jugular venous waveform is of fundamental importance to the cardiovascular examination (Fig. 12.8). There are no valves between the right atrium and internal jugular vein, which is readily distensible. Therefore it can act as a manometer reflecting the filling pressure of the right heart. Examine the height of the wave. The jugular venous pressure (JVP) is measured as the vertical height of the column of blood in the internal jugular vein above the sternal angle (Fig. 12.9).

Assessment of the JVP should not be neglected. It is the most direct assessment of the filling pressure of the right heart.

The pulsation should be distinguished from arterial pulsation (Fig. 12.10). If it is not visible, the pressure may be:

- Too low (e.g. in hypovolaemia) – lie the patient flat, test the hepatojugular reflux.
- Too high (e.g. in right ventricular infarction, volume overload) – sit the patient upright.

Note the character of the waveform. A basic appreciation of the normal jugular venous waveform is needed (Fig. 12.10). Assessment of the waveform requires considerable skill and experience. Unfortunately there are no short cuts. Assessment may give clues to pathologies such as tricuspid regurgitation (giant v waves), atrial fibrillation (no atrial systole, so only one component), complete heart block (cannon waves).

Praecordium
Although this is the meat of the cardiovascular examination, clues to underlying pathology should have been derived from the peripheral examination. Follow a strict examination routine. Remember that palpation should precede auscultation.

Characteristics of the jugular venous waveform and arterial pulse in the neck	
Jugular venous pulse	**Carotid pulse**
most prominent deflection is inwards	most prominent deflection is outwards
in sinus rhythm, two deflections for each beat	only one deflection for each beat
height of the wave changes with posture	height is independent of posture
temporary elevation of wave following pressure over the right costal margin (hepatojugular reflux)	constant
can usually be eliminated by light digital pressure over the clavicles	still present after light pressure
not palpable (in absence of tricuspid regurgitation)	palpable

Fig. 12.8 Characteristics of the jugular venous waveform and arterial pulse in the neck.

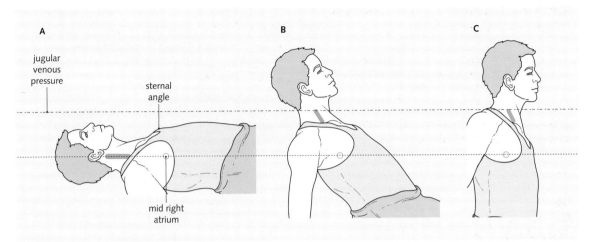

Fig. 12.9 The jugular venous pressure (JVP) is recorded as the vertical height of the visible waveform above the sternal angle. The pressure is fixed, but the anatomical position of the waveform varies according to posture. The jugular venous pressure is usually 2–5 cm.

Apex beat

The apex beat is the most downward and outward position where the cardiac impulse is palpable. Define the following.

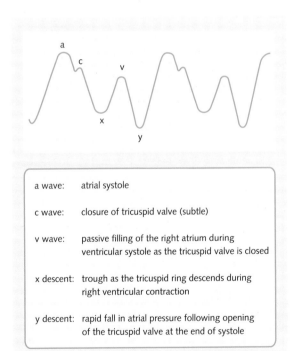

a wave:	atrial systole
c wave:	closure of tricuspid valve (subtle)
v wave:	passive filling of the right atrium during ventricular systole as the tricuspid valve is closed
x descent:	trough as the tricuspid ring descends during right ventricular contraction
y descent:	rapid fall in atrial pressure following opening of the tricuspid valve at the end of systole

Fig. 12.10 The components of the jugular venous waveform. In practice, the c wave is not usually visible. It is only by understanding the normal waveform that pathognomonic signs such as cannon waves and giant v waves can be recognized.

Position. The normal apex beat is within the 5th intercostal space in the midclavicular line (Fig. 12.11). A displaced apex beat usually implies volume overload of the left ventricle.

Character. Check the character of the beat. For example:

- Forceful, 'sustained', 'heaving' – left ventricular hypertrophy.
- Tapping – mitral stenosis.
- Thrusting – volume overload.

Be careful when describing the arterial pulse, apex beat, or heart murmurs, as certain terms often imply specific diagnoses.

Palpate the rest of the praecordium

Note the presence of:

- Heaves – use either the palm or the medial aspect of the hand; right ventricular hypertrophy may cause a left parasternal lifting sensation.
- Thrills – palpable murmurs (especially in aortic stenosis) feel like a fly trapped in one's hands.
- Palpable heart sounds – for example 1st heart sound in mitral stenosis felt as a 'tap' at the apex.

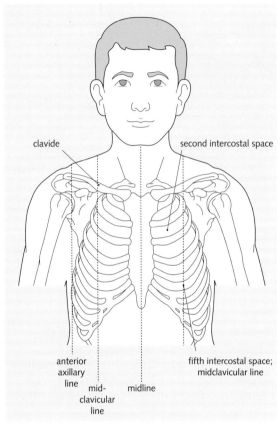

Fig. 12.11 Surface anatomy of the apex beat. It is defined in relation to the intercostal space and imaginary vertical lines related to the clavicle and axilla. The normal apex beat is within the 5th intercostal space in the midclavicular line.

Auscultation

Resist the temptation to auscultate until the rest of the examination routine is completed. It is much easier to auscultate when the sounds can be put into context with the rest of the examination.

An understanding of the cardiac cycle is essential when interpreting findings (Fig. 12.12). To begin with, time what you hear to the patient's pulse, as this helps in determining what you are listening to (Fig. 12.13). You will not pass or fail solely on what you hear. It is only part of the examination. Consider the most useful regions for auscultation (Fig. 12.14).

Listen in a systematic manner. In each region listen for:
- The first heart sound (immediately precedes systole).
- The second heart sound.
- Murmurs during systole.
- 'The absence of silence', usually a murmur, during diastole.
- Any extra sounds (e.g. clicks, snaps).

If a murmur is heard, characterize its features as follows:
- Volume (Fig. 12.15).
- Onset – for example presystolic, early systolic.
- Pattern – for example crescendo–decrescendo pattern of aortic stenosis.

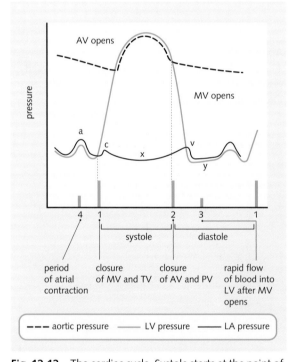

Fig. 12.12 The cardiac cycle. Systole starts at the point of closure of the mitral valve (MV) – first heart sound – when pressure in the left ventricle (LV) exceeds that of the left atrium (LA). There is a period of isovolumetric contraction before the pressure in the LV exceeds that in the aorta at which point the aortic valve (AV) opens and blood starts to flow into the aorta. Following the onset of relaxation of the LV the aortic pressure exceeds that in the LV and the aortic valve closes – 2nd heart sound. The ventricle continues to relax until the pressure falls below that in the filled LA and the MV opens allowing blood to flow rapidly into the LV. Atrial contraction precedes ventricular contraction causing a presystolic accentuation of flow into the LV. (PV, pulmonary valve; TV, tricuspid valve.)

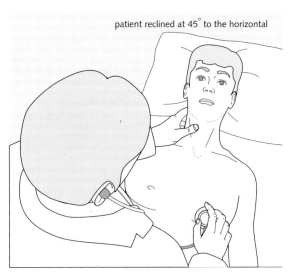

patient reclined at 45° to the horizontal

Fig. 12.13 It is essential to listen to the cardiac sounds while timing their point in the cardiac cycle by palpating the carotid pulse at the same time.

- Termination – compare the early systolic murmur of aortic stenosis and systolic murmur of mitral regurgitation.
- Pitch – for example low-pitched murmur of mitral stenosis.
- Location – where is it heard, and where is it most audible.
- Radiation – for example mitral regurgitation murmur radiating to the axilla.

 Diastolic murmurs are often difficult to hear. Listen specifically for the 'absence of silence' in diastole. Certain manoeuvres (see below) need to be performed to augment the sounds.

To elicit aortic regurgitation, sit the patient forward and listen over the right 2nd intercostal space and left sternal edge (LSE) in fixed expiration using the diaphragm of the stethoscope. To elicit mitral stenosis, role the patient into a left lateral position and listen over the apex in fixed expiration using the bell of the stethoscope. Mild exertion may accentuate the murmur.

The different heart sounds are illustrated in Fig. 12.16.

Figure 12.17 is an illustration of a revision card detailing the order in which to conduct a complete CVS examination and what you are looking to find at each section.

Aortic stenosis

Diagnose the pathology

The features of aortic stenosis are illustrated in Fig. 12.18. The murmur needs to be distinguished from the ejection systolic murmurs associated with:

- Aortic sclerosis – this is common, the patient is usually elderly, and there are no haemodynamic effects.

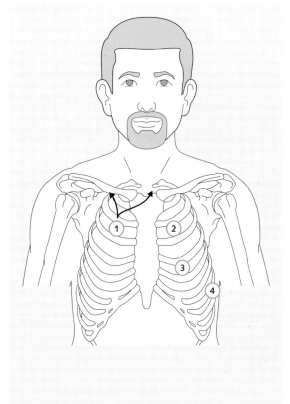

Fig. 12.14 Positions on the chest to auscultate for cardiac sounds. 1. 2nd right intercostal space (aortic area) – mitral murmurs are very rarely audible here; if a murmur is audible, trace it towards the neck. 2. 2nd left intercostal space (pulmonary area) – aortic regurgitation may be louder here. 3. 4th left intercostal space (tricuspid area) – especially for tricuspid regurgitation, but mitral regurgitation and aortic stenosis are often also audible here; aortic regurgitation may be loudest here. 4. Apex (mitral area) – listen specifically for mitral stenosis with the bell of the stethoscope; if a murmur is audible trace it towards the axilla.

Grading of the intensity of a cardiac murmur	
Grade	Intensity
I	just audible under optimal listening conditions
II	quiet
III	moderately loud
IV	loud and associated with a thrill
V	very loud
VI	audible without the aid of a stethoscope

Fig. 12.15 Grading of the intensity of a cardiac murmur. Don't ever be tempted to say a murmur is Grade I or II. You aren't that good ...... yet.!

- Bicuspid aortic valve – this is a common cause of an ejection systolic murmur in an asymptomatic young person.
- Subvalvular aortic stenosis – there is no ejection click.
- Pulmonary stenosis – this is rare and the murmur is loudest in the left 2nd intercostal space.
- Atrial septal defect – here there is a pulmonary flow murmur, fixed splitting of the second heart sound and an associated tricuspid flow murmur.

Assess severity

Features suggestive of significant aortic stenosis include:

- Slow-rising pulse.
- Narrow pulse pressure.
- Displaced apex beat (suggestive of decompensation, unless there is associated aortic regurgitation).

Consider aetiology

The most common causes include:

- Degenerative disease – most common cause.
- Congenital anomaly.
- Rheumatic disease – now less common; look for associated valve pathology.

Aortic regurgitation

Diagnose the pathology

Aortic regurgitation is associated with a diastolic murmur, but there are other clues that indicate the presence of aortic regurgitation (Fig. 12.19).

The murmur of aortic regurgitation is often subtle. A specific attempt should always be made to listen for it. Sit the patient forward and listen with the diaphragm of the stethoscope in fixed expiration. Listen for the 'absence of silence' in diastole.

Significance of different cardiac sounds		
Audible heart sounds	Timing	Cause
first heart sound	immediately presystolic	closure of mitral and tricuspid valves
second heart sound	end of systole	closure of aortic and pulmonary valves
third heart sound	early diastole	corresponds to period of rapid ventricular filling; normal in young fit people; associated with impaired LV function (especially raised end-diastolic pressure) (low-pitched, best heard at apex)
fourth heart sound	immediately presystolic	atrial systole; associated with non-compliant LV (e.g. hypertension); best heard with bell at apex
ejection click	early systole	opening of stenotic aortic valve
opening snap	early diastole	opening of abnormal tricuspid valve and especially mitral valve in mitral stenosis (well-defined short, high-pitched sound best heard with diaphragm at left sternal edge)
pericardial rub	systole and diastole	inflamed pericardium; coarse grating sound (like walking on fresh snow); accentuated by leaning patient forwards; may be very localized

Fig. 12.16 Significance of different cardiac sounds. (LV, left ventricle.)

Cardiovascular examination	
General Inspection:	build, obvious pain/distress, features of Down's/Turner's/Marfan's
Hands:	anaemia, cyanosis (poor peripheral perfusion), capillary refill, xanthomata – clubbing – loss of angle, 'boggy' nail, $\uparrow$longitudinal curvature, 'drumstick' – signs of endocarditis: splinter haemorrhage, Osler's nodes, Janeway lesions
Radial pulse:	rate (55-80 at rest), rhythm Radioradial, radiofemoral delay (co-arc^n) – collapsing pulse (aortic regurg^n), bounding pulse ($\uparrow$HR, CO_2 retention, fever, LVF)
Brachial pulse:	character, volume – slow rising (aortic stenosis), collapsing/waterhammer (aortic regurgitation), – biphasic (aortic stenosis+regurgitation). Small vol (shock, $\uparrow$HR; mitral stenosis)
Eyes:	anaemia, jaundice, arcus, xanthomata, conjunctival haemorrhage
Face:	central cyanosis ($\downarrow SaO_2 \rightarrow$blue mucous membranes) – malar flush (mitral stenosis)
Neck:	carotid pulse – separately – JVP – internal jugular vein – just medial to clavicular head of sternocleidomastoid •height of column above sternal angle. >4 cm if: RV failure, $\uparrow$vol, SVC obstruction a = atrial contraction, c = tricuspid value bulging into atrium, x = atrial relaxation, v = $\uparrow$pressure if atrial filling in ventricular systole, y = tricuspid opening in diastole. •waveform – double impulse No a wave in AF – cannon wave (giant a wave atrial contraction + closed tricuspid) – complete heart block, VT – systolic wave (c and v in ventricular systole) – tricuspid regurgitation
Pericardium	inspect chest deformity, scars, pacemakers, visible pulsations – palpate (i) apex-position (normal 5th ICS, midclavicular), character (tapping/thrusting), LV heave, thrill (MR) (ii) Ⓛ sternal edge–parasternal heave (RVH), thrill of VSD (iii) aortic area–thrill of aortic stenosis, 2nd RICS (iv) trachea - mediastinal shift – auscultate–apex: heart sounds, added sounds, murmurs. Time a carotids – Ⓛ sternal edge, aortic – pulmonary areas, Ⓛ axilla. Carotid bruits – Ⓛ lateral position – mitral stenosis (low pitched diastolic) – sitting forward, breath held in expiration – aortic regurgitation (Ⓛ lower sternal edge)
Lung bases:	pulmonary oedema
Sacral oedema:	ankle oedema
Peripheral:	pulses, femoral bruits
Hepatomegaly, ascites	
BP	
Fundi	– silver wiring, a/v nipping, hard and soft exndates

Fig. 12.17 Revision card for cardiovascular examination.

Features on systemic examination include:
- Pulse – collapsing, high volume.
- Nails – visible capillary pulsation.
- Neck – head nods with each systole; vigorous arterial pulsation in neck.
- Blood pressure – wide pulse pressure.
- Apex – displaced (due to volume overload – bad sign), thrusting.
- Peripheral pulse – diastolic murmur over lightly compressed femoral artery.

Assess severity
Features suggestive of severe disease include evidence of cardiac dilatation and signs of left heart failure.

Consider aetiology
Clues to the underlying pathology may be found as follows:
- Look at posture and arthropathy – ankylosing spondylitis.

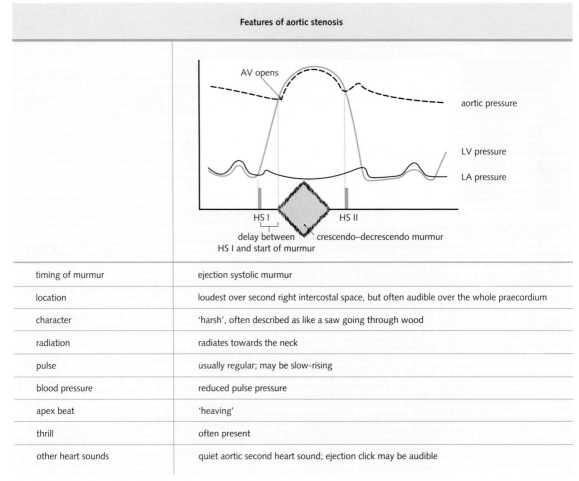

Features of aortic stenosis

timing of murmur	ejection systolic murmur
location	loudest over second right intercostal space, but often audible over the whole praecordium
character	'harsh', often described as like a saw going through wood
radiation	radiates towards the neck
pulse	usually regular; may be slow-rising
blood pressure	reduced pulse pressure
apex beat	'heaving'
thrill	often present
other heart sounds	quiet aortic second heart sound; ejection click may be audible

Fig. 12.18   Features of aortic stenosis.

- Look at eyes – Argyll–Robinson pupils associated with syphilitic aortitis.
- Look for high-arched palate, hypermobility, arachnodactyly – Marfan's syndrome.
- Check for other valve lesions – rheumatic fever, infective endocarditis.

Mitral stenosis

Diagnose the pathology

A particularly high index of suspicion should be raised in a patient with atrial fibrillation. Look for the classical mitral facies (cyanotic discoloration of the cheeks), and a tapping apex beat. The murmur is often very soft and an attempt should always be made to specifically elicit it – lean the patient on the left hand side, and listen with the bell of the stethoscope in fixed expiration. It may be necessary to accentuate the murmur by exercise. The features of the murmur are illustrated in Fig. 12.20.

Assess severity

Look for features of left atrial overload and consequent left heart failure, for example:
- Cyanosis.
- Pulmonary oedema.
- Hypotension (reduced cardiac output).

Look for features of right heart failure (raised JVP, peripheral oedema, left parasternal heave due to right ventricular hypertrophy). Atrial fibrillation occurs later in the natural history of the disease. The opening snap or onset of the murmur is closer to the

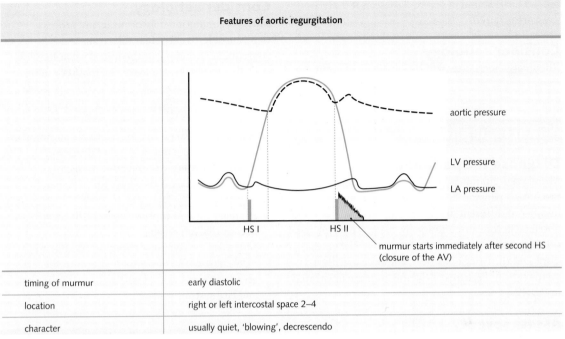

Features of aortic regurgitation

aortic pressure

LV pressure

LA pressure

HS I

HS II

murmur starts immediately after second HS (closure of the AV)

timing of murmur	early diastolic
location	right or left intercostal space 2–4
character	usually quiet, 'blowing', decrescendo

Fig. 12.19 Features of aortic regurgitation.

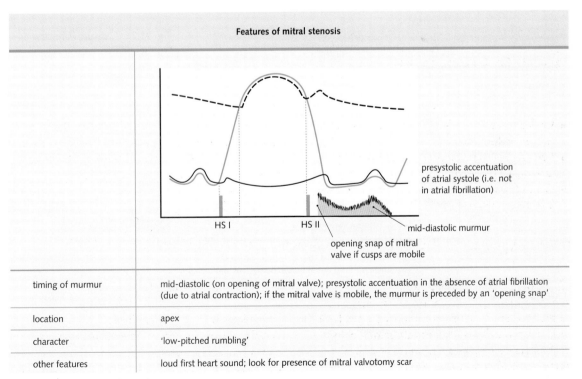

Features of mitral stenosis

presystolic accentuation of atrial systole (i.e. not in atrial fibrillation)

HS I

HS II

mid-diastolic murmur

opening snap of mitral valve if cusps are mobile

timing of murmur	mid-diastolic (on opening of mitral valve); presystolic accentuation in the absence of atrial fibrillation (due to atrial contraction); if the mitral valve is mobile, the murmur is preceded by an 'opening snap'
location	apex
character	'low-pitched rumbling'
other features	loud first heart sound; look for presence of mitral valvotomy scar

Fig. 12.20 Features of mitral stenosis.

second heart sound in severe disease as left atrial pressure is raised.

Consider aetiology

Rheumatic heart disease is by far the most common cause.

Mitral regurgitation

Diagnose the pathology

Mitral regurgitation is commonly heard, and produces a pansystolic murmur. It may be due to a number of different disease processes. Clues may be obtained before auscultation by the presence of atrial fibrillation (common, but less than mitral stenosis), a displaced thrusting apex beat, and occasionally a systolic thrill. Features of the murmur are illustrated in Fig. 12.21.

Assess severity

It is often difficult to assess the severity clinically, but a third heart sound and a mid-diastolic mitral flow murmur may be detected in severe disease. The severity is usually assessed by the symptoms and haemodynamic consequences.

Consider aetiology

Mitral regurgitation may occur in any process that causes left ventricular dilatation and consequent stretching of the mitral valve annulus, as well as valvular pathology. The most common causes are:

- Ischaemic heart disease – by far the most common cause.
- Rheumatic heart disease – relatively common in elderly patients, but now a rare disease in the UK; often associated with mitral stenosis.
- Infective endocarditis – look for peripheral stigmata.
- Papillary muscle rupture – especially after myocardial infarction.
- Mitral valve prolapse – common and due to ballooning of the posterior leaflet into the left atrium; it is associated with a mid-systolic click and late systolic murmur.

Tricuspid regurgitation

Diagnose the pathology

Tricuspid regurgitation can often be recognized from the end of the bed by the observant examiner.

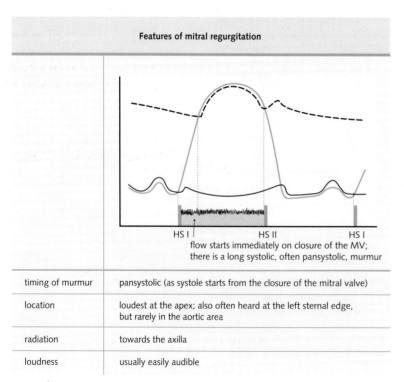

Features of mitral regurgitation

HS I   HS II   HS I
flow starts immediately on closure of the MV;
there is a long systolic, often pansystolic, murmur

timing of murmur	pansystolic (as systole starts from the closure of the mitral valve)
location	loudest at the apex; also often heard at the left sternal edge, but rarely in the aortic area
radiation	towards the axilla
loudness	usually easily audible

Fig. 12.21 Features of mitral regurgitation.

It is usually due to primary left heart disease and secondary right ventricular pressure overload, so the signs may be due to a mixture of pathologies.

The jugular venous waveform shows characteristic giant V waves, and may cause oscillation of the ear lobes if the venous pressure is high enough. The patient often has signs of right heart failure with peripheral oedema and occasionally ascites. If tricuspid regurgitation is suspected, the liver should be palpated for pulsatile hepatomegaly. In addition, the underlying cause should be sought.

The murmur resembles that of mitral regurgitation in many respects (Fig. 12.22).

Assess severity

Look for features of right-sided heart failure.

Consider aetiology

Tricuspid regurgitation usually results from right ventricular overload. The more common conditions predisposing to this are:

- Mitral valve disease.
- Cor pulmonale.
- Right ventricular myocardial infarction.

Primary tricuspid regurgitation may occur in:
- Rheumatic fever – rarely an isolated valve lesion.
- Infective endocarditis – especially in drug addicts (look for needle marks).
- Carcinoid syndrome – look for hepatomegaly, flushing, signs of pulmonary stenosis.

Infective endocarditis

Infective endocarditis may affect any of the heart valves. It often presents in a non-specific manner and should be suspected in all patients with newly diagnosed valvular pathology or those with pre-existing valvular disease who develop pyrexia and malaise or a change in murmur.

Assess valvular pathology and severity

Define the valvular lesions and the haemodynamic consequences by a thorough cardiovascular examination.

Look for peripheral stigmata suggesting endocarditis

A complete systemic examination is essential as manifestations may arise from many systems. Features on systemic examination include the following.

Pyrexia

Fever is almost universal in infective endocarditis. However, it is often low grade and a single temperature reading may be normal. It is very important to follow the progression of fever through the course of the illness as a marker of successful therapy.

Nails (do not forget the toes!)

There are multiple stigmata of infective endocarditis in the hands. Many of these arise from an associated vasculitis. The following signs may be detected in the nails:

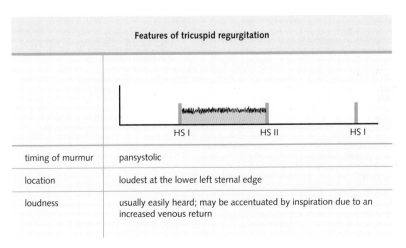

timing of murmur	pansystolic
location	loudest at the lower left sternal edge
loudness	usually easily heard; may be accentuated by inspiration due to an increased venous return

Fig. 12.22 Features of tricuspid regurgitation.

- Splinter haemorrhages. These are a non-specific finding, but common. They are suggestive of a vasculitic process. Although the presence is not specific for vasculitis, the occurrence of new splinter haemorrhages developing in the context of a new murmur and fever is highly suggestive.
- Nailfold infarcts. These are also suggestive of a vasculitic process. They are more specific, but less common than splinter haemorrhages.
- Clubbing. A late sign and hopefully not present!

Hands

Vasculitic signs may also be detected in the hands:

- Osler's nodes. Do not forget the four Ps (painful, purple, papules on the pulps) of the fingers – this is rare, but enjoyed by examiners!
- Janeway lesions. These are rare transient macular patches on the palms.

Eyes

Fundoscopy is essential (especially in the exam setting). Look for Roth's spots, which are characteristic flame-shaped haemorrhages on the retina with white centres.

Splenomegaly

Splenomegaly is usually barely palpable if at all. There is little correlation with the duration or severity of the disease.

Haematuria

An immune complex nephritis is a common feature. Remember that urinalysis is part of the examination. Haematuria usually clears with successful antibiotic therapy. Occasionally confusion may arise as the long-term antibiotic therapy may precipitate

interstitial nephritis (e.g. penicillins) or be nephrotoxic (e.g. gentamicin).

Neurological signs

Endocarditis may present with neurological signs due to septic emboli in the brain. The elderly may present non-specifically with confusion.

Consider aetiology

Risk factors for infection may be elicited from the examination:

- Right-sided valve lesions – especially in intravenous drug abusers (*Staphylococcus aureus* and fungal disease more likely).
- Underlying valve lesion – usually present; *Streptococcus viridans* is the most common agent; the most common predisposing valvular lesions are mitral and aortic valve disease, ventricular septal defect (VSD), patent ductus arteriosus (PDS), and coarctation of the aorta.
- Prosthetic valve.
- Dental hygiene – often the mouth is primary portal of entry.

Heart failure

A diagnosis simply of 'heart failure' is inadequate. An attempt must be made to assess its severity, functional impact, and aetiology.

Establish the diagnosis and differentiate the features of right and left heart failure

Clues from the systemic examination are shown in Fig. 12.23. High output cardiac failure may also occur (Fig. 12.24). Not all of the features may be

Signs of right and left heart failure	
Right heart failure	**Left heart failure**
raised jugular venous pressure	third heart sound
peripheral oedema	displaced apex beat (if volume overload)
ascites	pulmonary oedema
hepatomegaly	tachycardia
left parasternal heave	cyanosis
cyanosis	cool, sweaty, pale skin (low output state)
tricuspid regurgitation	mitral regurgitation (due to volume overload of left ventricle)

Fig. 12.23 Features of right and left heart failure.

present and they depend upon the severity and underlying cause. Often the two conditions coexist.

Assessment of severity is usually dependent upon the history and the functional limitation imposed on the patient.

Consider aetiology

The principal causes are:

- Impaired myocardial contractility.
- Arrhythmia.
- Volume overload.
- Pressure overload.
- Impaired filling.

Features of these conditions are illustrated in Fig. 12.24.

Myocardial infarction

Often, there are no specific physical signs following a myocardial infarction (MI), but the physical examination can reveal complications and guide management, both in the acute setting and in the ensuing period.

Inspection

A quick visual inspection may reveal signs of pain or discomfort, necessitating better analgesic control. Assess peripheral perfusion – a cold, sweaty, cyanosed, pale patient suggests shock.

Look specifically for complications

Always check for the presence of complications such as left or right heart failure and the presence of arrhythmias.

Left heart failure

Look for features of left heart failure such as:

- Signs of poor peripheral perfusion (impaired cardiac output).
- Low-volume pulse.
- Inspiratory crepitations at the lung bases.
- Gallop rhythm with third heart sound.
- Dyspnoea.

These signs may indicate that the patient will not tolerate β-blockade or may benefit from diuretics and angiotensin-converting enzyme (ACE) inhibitors.

Features of different types of heart failure on systemic examination	
Cause of heart failure	**Features**
impaired myocardial contractility ischaemic heart disease	most common cause; may present as right, left or biventricular failure; look for features to suggest other vascular disease (e.g. carotid bruits, signs of hypertension, etc.)
cardiomyopathy	look for systemic disease (e.g. amyloid, etc.)
myocarditis	look for signs of systemic infection; tachycardia is often a prominent feature; listen for associated pericardial rub
arrhythmia	common; often exacerbates underlying heart disease; may be able to detect arrhythmia from the pulse; aim to distinguish a primary arrhythmia from one resulting from poor myocardial perfusion
volume overload aortic regurgitation mitral regurgitation tricuspid regurgitation	look for signs of an underlying valvular defect; for left-sided lesions, identify a displaced apex beat
pressure overload hypertension aortic stenosis pulmonary embolus	slow-rising pulse; narrow pulse pressure; sustained apex beat right-sided signs associated with hypotension
impaired ventricular filling mitral stenosis cardiac tamponade restrictive cardiomyopathy	right heart failure; pulsus paradoxus; note jugular waveform

Fig. 12.24 Features of different types of heart failure on systemic examination.

Right heart failure

It is very important to recognize the patient with a right ventricular infarction. A disproportionately raised JVP in association with very poor peripheral perfusion, hypotension, and ECG signs are characteristic. Fluid balance in these patients is critical and demands central monitoring to assess left atrial filling pressure.

 In the presence of shock and signs of right heart failure, always consider the presence of a posterior infarct, which may be subtle on the ECG.

Arrhythmia

Check the pulse carefully. Usually there is a mild tachycardia. The presence of a bradycardia suggests an inferior wall MI. The pulse may give clues to an underlying rhythm disturbance, for example:

- Heart block – especially following anterior wall MI.
- Atrial fibrillation – common.
- Ventricular extrasystoles.

These should be confirmed as the patient will have continuous ECG recording.

Subsequent examination

Once patients are on the ward, they should be examined at least daily. Particular features to assess include:

- Pulse rate (β-blocker, primary cardiac rhythm disturbance).
- Blood pressure (e.g. cardiogenic shock, primary hypertension, new therapy with β-blocker or ACE inhibitor).
- Signs of heart failure.
- Murmurs – especially that of mitral regurgitation due to papillary muscle rupture and the long systolic murmur of ventricular septal defect.
- Pericardial rub.
- Psychological rehabilitation – often, the greatest morbidity on discharge from hospital is psychological; this should be recognized by eliciting the patient's concerns, and treated early by appropriate education and reassurance.
- Signs of deep vein thrombosis – especially if there has been prolonged bed rest.

Examination routine

Patient exposure and position

The patient should be exposed to the waist in a similar fashion to exposure for the cardiovascular examination and seated comfortably on a couch, inclined at 45° to the horizontal in a well-lit room.

Remember inspection, palpation, percussion, auscultation

General inspection

This should be performed systematically. As with other systems, think about which features you are looking for from the history before inspection. It is convenient to look first at the patient generally, and then to inspect specific features from the head downwards. This process need only take a few seconds.

General features

Note the following features:
- Age and sex of the patient.
- General health and body habitus.
- Comfort at rest. For example how easily can the patient climb onto the examination couch?
- Respiratory rate. It is imperative that you have counted the respiratory rate. Don't make it obvious you are observing the patient's breathing as this may influence the rate, especially in anxious patients.
- General environment. For example in a hospital, look on the bedside cabinet for sputum pots, nebulizers, inhalers, peak flow charts.

Head

Look for evidence of:
- Central.
- Plethora (e.g. due to secondary polycythaemia due to chronic hypoxia).
- Cigarette staining of hair and smell of cigarettes.

Chest

Note the presence of :
- Scars (Fig. 13.1).
- Breathing pattern (e.g. shallow or pursed lip and use of accessory muscles – sternomastoid, intercostals, abdominal, etc.)
- Chest wall deformity (e.g. pectus excavatus).
- Asymmetry (e.g. due to previous tuberculosis causing upper lobe fibrosis; kyphoscolisosis causing constrictive problems).
- Obvious tracheal deviation.

Specific examination

A more detailed systematic examination can now begin.

Hands

In particular look for the presence of:
- Clubbing.
- Peripheral cyanosis – if present, check for central cyanosis.
- Tremor – to demonstrate, ask patient to hold out their hands with the wrists cocked back and to close their eyes then look for a tremor. The tremor of carbon dioxide retention is classically flapping in nature. If a patient can see their hands they can more easily control any tremor.
- Cigarette staining of nails and fingers.
- Painful swelling of the wrists (and ankles) is suggestive of hypertrophic arthroplasty due to squamous cell cancer of the lung.

Blood pressure and arterial pulse

A quick assessment of the pulse rate and blood pressure is useful. A hyperdynamic circulation may occur in carbon dioxide retention.

Head

An assessment should include specific inspection of:
- Eyes – to reveal for example Horner's syndrome (due to carcinoma of bronchus), jaundice, conjunctival pallor.
- Mouth – for example tongue and mucous membranes may be cyanosed.

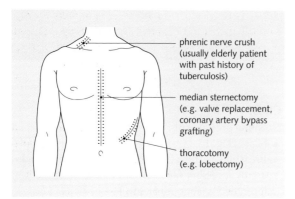

Fig. 13.1 Scars related to the respiratory system.

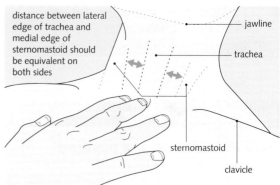

Fig. 13.2 Examination technique for assessing tracheal position. Place two fingers on either side of the trachea and judge the distance between the fingers and the sternomastoid tendons.

Neck
Lymphadenopathy
Examine the cervical and supraclavicular lymph nodes. It may be easier to defer this part of the examination until the patient is sitting forward so that palpation can be performed from the rear.

Tracheal position
Remember that this part of the examination is slightly uncomfortable (Fig. 13.2). The trachea may be shifted by pathology outside the chest (e.g. thyroid enlargement). Mediastinal position can also be assessed by determining the position of the apex beat.

The tracheal position is often neglected by students, but this sign is of fundamental importance as it indicates the presence of a focal chest expanding (e.g. tension pneumothorax, massive pleural effusion) or constricting process (fibrosis, lung collapse).

Chest
When examining the chest remember that there are anterior, lateral and posterior aspects to examine. The routine for chest examination is straightforward, but the interpretation of signs requires experience as very often they reflect only a 'qualitative' difference from the normal state. An appreciation of the range of normality demands practice! It is invaluable to have a more experienced observer who can provide constructive criticism of your approach and

interpretation of signs with you while you are examining the patient.

Very few chest pathologies are manifest as a single abnormal sign. Rather, a constellation of signs needs to be interpreted in context and then integrated. The competent student doctor will be constantly analysing the elicited signs and refining a differential diagnosis, anticipating how the next sign may modify the assessment. This highlights the importance of adopting an active approach to the examination. Inspiration rarely comes at the end of the examination!

It is a matter of preference whether the whole process is performed on the front of the chest and then the back, or whether each component of the examination is completed for the whole chest in turn, but the former is more comfortable for the patient and is preferred.

Inspection
If tracheal shift is noted, look more closely for asymmetry, especially scalloping below the clavicles suggestive of loss of volume of the upper lobe.

Palpation
There are three main components to this section:
- Assessment of mediastinal position.
- Assessment of chest expansion.
- Tactile vocal fremitus (TVF). (Vocal resonance will also be discussed in this section for ease of explanation.)

Assessment of mediastinal position. If the trachea is deviated, the position of the lower mediastinum can be assessed by determining the position of the apex beat.

Chest expansion. Assess the degree and symmetry of chest expansion. Expansion should be assessed in the infraclavicular, costal margin, and lower rib region posteriorly (Fig. 13.3).

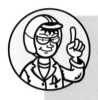

If there is unilateral chest pathology, the side of the chest with reduced expansion always indicates the side of the pathology.

Tactile vocal fremitus. Place the medial aspect of the hand on the chest wall and ask the patient to make a resonant sound (e.g. say 'ninety nine'). The sound waves are transmitted as low-frequency vibrations, which are palpable. Different regions of the chest should be examined systematically, in particular comparing symmetry of the two sides. Make an attempt to define abnormalities in the upper, middle, and lower lobes. This requires an awareness of the surface markings of these lobes.

Vocal resonance. This is included here as it is complementary to TVF. Place the stethoscope on the chest wall and ask the patient to whisper 'one, two,

three'. The distinct sounds are not normally heard, but a resonant sound as the sound waves are altered by transmission through the airways and chest wall. Once again, different regions should be examined systematically, comparing symmetry. Increased vocal resonance is termed 'whispering pectoriloquy'.

The degree of TVF or vocal resonance is dependent upon the transmission of sound waves to the chest wall from the large bronchi. It is therefore dependent upon the volume of sound generated and the conductivity of the lungs, which is dependent upon how close the stethoscope is to a large bronchus. It is:
- Increased in consolidation or lung collapse with a patent airway.
- Decreased in pleural effusion, pneumothorax, or collapse with an obstructed bronchus.

In practice, it is easier to detect decreased or absent tactile vocal fremitus and increased vocal resonance from the normal state. Hence, the two signs complement each other.

Percussion

Percussion is performed by placing the middle or index finger of one hand on the chest wall and hyperexpanding the proximal and distal interphalangeal joints so that the middle phalanx is closely opposed to the chest wall, and tapping it with the opposite index finger. This action should come from the wrist, rather than being a hammering action, and be just heavy enough to detect resonance. The percussing finger should be rapidly withdrawn after striking. Resonance is felt, just as much as it is heard. Percussion should be performed systematically as for TVF. Findings may include:
- Hyperresonance of the percussion note. This is often difficult to elicit, but is present if there is more air in the chest cavity (e.g. pneumothorax, emphysema).
- A dull percussion note. This occurs if the lung tissue is replaced by solid material (e.g. consolidation) or if solid material is present between the chest wall and the lung (e.g. pleural effusion, pleural thickening). When this is classical, the note is said to be stony dull.

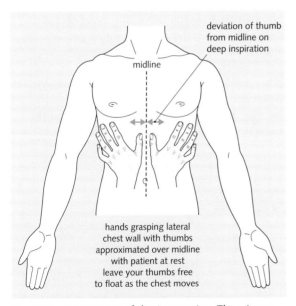

Fig. 13.3 Examination of chest expansion. The primary objective is to assess symmetry. Assess expansion in the upper, lower, and middle regions of the chest. Place hands around the lateral chest wall and approximate the thumbs in the midline (but not resting on the chest). Ask the patient to take a deep breath and observe the displacement of the thumbs from the midline.

Auscultation

Breath sounds are produced by turbulent airflow, and transmitted through the airways, lung parenchyma, pleurae, and chest wall. Changes in any of these structures can alter the sounds heard.

Auscultation is usually performed with the bell of the stethoscope as the patient breathes fairly deeply. Once again, it is important to compare findings on the two sides.

The aim of auscultation is to define:
- The quality of the breath sounds (Fig. 13.4).
- The presence of added sounds – as with cardiac murmurs, characterize the quality, volume, and timing.
- Vocal resonance (see above).

Added sounds should be characterized systematically. Note the presence of the following.

Crackles (crepitations). These may be caused by secretions in the larger airways (e.g. in bronchitis, pneumonia, bronchiectasis). They are usually present throughout inspiration and may clear on coughing. Alternatively, reopening of occluded small airways during the later part of inspiration occurs in parenchymal disease (e.g. fibrosis, interstitial oedema) where they tend to have a finer quality. Coughing will then have no effect.

Wheezes (rhonchi). These have a musical quality and usually result from narrowing of the bronchi due to oedema, spasm, tumour or secretions. They occur in:
- Asthma – polyphonic, mainly expiratory, diffuse.
- Bronchitis – may clear on coughing, may have an inspiratory component.

- Fixed obstruction – monophonic (e.g. due to bronchial carcinoma).

Pleural rub. This sound is due to friction between the visceral and parietal pleurae in inflammatory conditions (pleurisy). It is often described as the sound of walking on crisp, newly fallen snow.

Other tests

Patients may have their own peak flow meter with them or one may be available. Ask them to perform this, watch and assess their technique. Ask the patient what their peak flow is normally, compare this to today's reading and then against what their predicted peak flow would be. Many wards and examination settings will have spirometry available. Get the patient to do this as well. With both of these tests always get the patient to have three attempts so that the best can be recorded.

Summary

At the end of the respiratory examination, it is important to take time to reflect on your findings. Remember that few lung pathologies have a single pathognomonic feature and that abnormalities are often a matter of qualitative judgement of deviation from normality rather than the simple presence or absence of a sign. The key to a successful examination is to be attentive and open to differential diagnoses from the start, so that physical signs can be anticipated rather than taking you by surprise. Figure 13.5 shows a revision card for the respiratory system.

Description of quality of breath sounds		
Breath sounds	**Features**	**Examples**
vesicular breathing	progressively louder during inspiration, merging into expiratory phase with rapid fading in intensity	normal pattern
bronchial breathing	laryngeal sounds transmitted efficiently to chest wall if lung substance becomes uniform and more solid—blowing quality; pause between inspiratory and expiratory phases; expiratory phase as long as inspiratory phase	consolidation; collapse with patent bronchus; fibrosis
diminished volume	impaired conduction due to increased pleural/chest wall thickness or increased air acting as poor conductor	pleural effusion; pleural thickening; obesity; emphysema; pneumothorax

Fig. 13.4 Description of the quality of breath sounds.

Respiratory examination

Undress to waist, sit on edge of bed. Look around–O_2, nebulizer, sputum pot, inhalers, spacer, etc.

General appearance	cachexia, respiratory distress, cyanosis/pallor/plethoric etc. Sputum, temperature chart
Hands	clubbing, peripheral cyanosis, nicotine stains, asterixis (CO_2 retention trap)
Pulse, RR Face	central cyanosis, pallor, nasal flaring, cervical lymphadenopathy, jugular veins
Inspection of chest	RR, pattern of breathing, chest wall deformities, scars, chest wall movements
Palpation of chest	position of trachea, cricosternal distance, supraclavicular lymph nodes, RV heave
Chest expansion Vocal fremitus	assess upper and lower chest movement palpate chest wall as patient repeats '99
Percussion	compare both sides, including clavicles, supraclavicular, axillae hyper-resonant/resonant or normal/dull/stony dull
Auscultation	breathe in and out thro' mouth. intensity–nature (vesicular/bronchial), air entry – bronchial breath sounds–high–pitched blowing, pause between insp and exp, consolidation/collapse – wheeze (rhonchi–high/low pitch, insp/exp, monophonic/polyphonic effect of coughing – crackles (crepitations) -loud coase/fine and high pitched. Early insp–diffuse airways destruction (eg. COPD) Late insp–diffuse fibrosis, pulmonary oedema, bronchiectasis, consolidation – pleural rub–friction betwn pleura →localized creating, e.g. pleurisy, pulmonary infarction, pneumonia – vocal resonance–auscultate as patient says '99'. Assess volume and clarity, whispering pectoriloquy.
Relevant CVS examination	e.g. heart sounds, JV, hepatomegaly, ankle oedema

	Chest movement	Mediastinum	Percussion	Breath sounds	Visual resonance	Added sounds
Consolidation	↓ affected side	–	Dull	Bronchial	↑	Fine crackles
Collapse	↓ affected side	shift → lesion	Dull	↓ Vesicular	↓	–
Localized fibrosis	↓ affected side	shift → lesion	Dull	Bronchial	↑	Coarse crackles
CFA	↓ both sides	–	Normal	Vesicular	↑	Fine crackles
Pleural effusion	↓ affected side	shift away	Stony dull	↓ Vesicular	↓	–
Pneumothorax	↓ affected side	shift away	Hyper-resonant	↓ Vesicular	↓	–
Asthma	↓ both sides	–	Normal	Prolonged exp	Normal	Exp polyphonic wheeze
COPD	↓ both sides	–	Normal	Prolonged exp	Normal	Exp wheeze, crackles

Overinflation	high shoulders, ↑ant–post. chest diameter, using accessory muscles of resp^n, limited chest expansion and caediac absent hepatic caraiac dullness on percussion
Diffuse airways obstruction	wheeze, muffed cough, overinflation, costal margin moves in on inspiration, prolonged, expiration, early insp crackles, ↑forced expiration time

Fig. 13.5 Revision card for respiratory examination.

Pleural effusion

Diagnose the pathology

The physical signs can be anticipated from a basic appreciation of the pathology (Fig. 13.6).

Assess severity

Analyse the significance of physical signs:

- How high up the chest can percussion be demonstrated to be stony dull?
- Define the level of decreased breath sounds and reduced TVF.

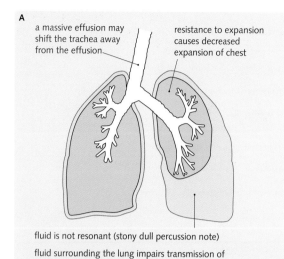

A

a massive effusion may shift the trachea away from the effusion

resistance to expansion causes decreased expansion of chest

fluid is not resonant (stony dull percussion note)

fluid surrounding the lung impairs transmission of soundwaves from the airways to the chest wall (causing ↓ TVF, vocal resonance and ↓↓ breath sounds)

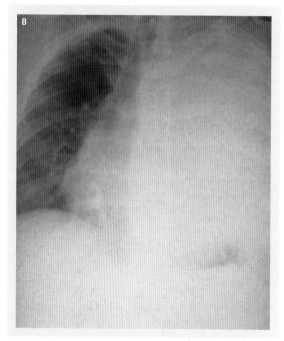

B

Fig. 13.6 (A) Physical signs of a pleural effusion. (B) Radiograph of a massive left pleural effusion. Note the tracheal deviation to the right. TVF, tactile vocal fremitus.

- How short of breath is the patient? (This may be altered by coexisting pathology and speed of onset.)
- Is the trachea shifted away from the effusion?

Consider aetiology

Look for clues in the systemic examination:
- Palpable supraclavicular and/or axillary lymphadenopathy – malignancy.

- Hepatomegaly – secondary malignancy.
- Peripheral oedema – hypoalbuminaemia, heart failure.
- Third heart sound – left heart failure.

Consider the more common causes of pleural effusion (Fig. 13.7).

Pneumothorax

Diagnose the pathology

A small pneumothorax can be hard to identify, but index of suspicion should be high in tall thin young adults with sudden-onset pleuritic chest pain and dyspnoea. The basic clinical signs can be elucidated from basic principles (Fig. 13.8).

Assess severity

Most pneumothoraces do not cause haemodynamic compromise, but it is important to recognize a tension pneumothorax.

A tension pneumothorax is a medical emergency and should be identified and treated before requesting a radiograph. Treatment is immediate decompression with a 14G needle placed in the second intercostal space in the midclavicular line.

Consider aetiology

Most spontaneous pneumothoraces occur in previously fit young adults and are idiopathic. Look for underlying lung disease that may have precipitated the event. Consider the three major groups of precipitating pathologies, which are:
- Underlying medical disease (e.g. asthma or emphysema with bullae, carcinoma, tuberculosis).
- Iatrogenic (e.g. after central venous line insertion, especially subclavian line, intubated patient with positive pressure ventilation, after pleural aspiration or biopsy).
- Trauma (e.g. fractured ribs, ?surgical emphysema).

Common causes of a pleural effusion	
Transudates	**Exudates**
fluid which has passed through a membrane	fluid containing proteins and white cells
left heart failure*	infection* (pneumonia, tuberculosis, empyema, etc.)
hypoalbuminuric states* (e.g. nephrotic syndrome, liver failure)	malignancy* (primary bronchial or metastatic)
fluid overload in renal failure	pulmonary infarction*
hypothyroidism	subphrenic abscess
	pancreatitis
Meigs's syndrome (right pleural effusion association with ovarian fibroma)	collagen vascular disease (e.g. rheumatoid arthritis)
	haemothorax

Fig. 13.7 Common causes of a pleural effusion. The more common causes are marked with an asterisk.

Lung collapse

Diagnose the pathology

Lung collapse may occur with a patent or occluded bronchus. The physical signs will differ and may depend upon severity and underlying cause (Figs 13.9 and 13.10).

Consider aetiology

Consider the more common causes of collapse.

Extrinsic compression

The most common cause is lymph node compression due to tumour or tuberculosis.

Intrinsic obstruction

Intraluminal obstruction may occlude the airway and cause distal collapse. The more common causes include:

- Tumours – look for clubbing.
- Retained secretions – postoperative, debilitated patients.
- Inhaled foreign body – usually apparent from history, especially right lower lobe – a medical emergency!
- Bronchial cast or plug – for example, due to aspergillosis, blood clot.

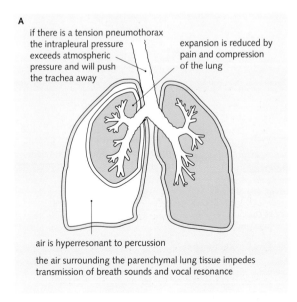

A

if there is a tension pneumothorax the intrapleural pressure exceeds atmospheric pressure and will push the trachea away

expansion is reduced by pain and compression of the lung

air is hyperresonant to percussion

the air surrounding the parenchymal lung tissue impedes transmission of breath sounds and vocal resonance

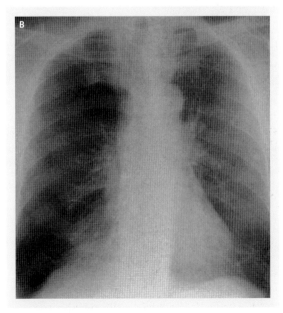

B

Fig. 13.8 (A) Physical signs of pneumothorax. (B) Radiograph of a right pneumothorax.

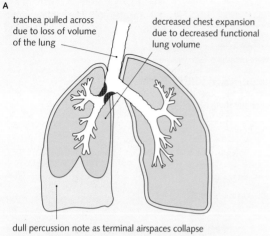

A

trachea pulled across due to loss of volume of the lung

decreased chest expansion due to decreased functional lung volume

dull percussion note as terminal airspaces collapse

If the upper airway is occluded, breath sounds and vocal resonance cannot be transmitted efficiently to the chest wall; if the airway is patent, the denser lung parenchyma transmits sounds more efficiently and bronchial breathing with whispering pectoriloquy may be present.

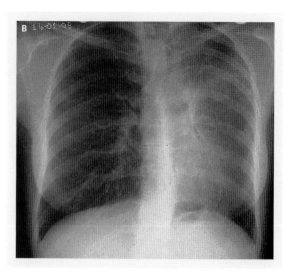

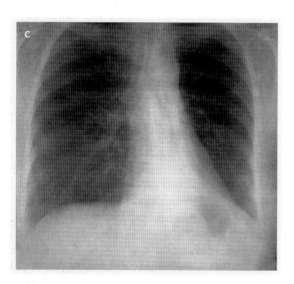

Fig. 13.9 (A) Radiographic features and physical signs of lung collapse with and without patent upper airways. (B) Radiograph of left upper lobe collapse: loss of lung volume is indicated by deviation of the trachea to the left, mediastinal shift to the left, and loss of volume of the left lung; in addition, note the classic veil-like opacification over the left lung. (C) Radiograph of left lower lobe collapse: note the raised left hemidiaphragm, mediastinal shift to the left, loss of volume and hypertranslucency of the left lung, and depressed left hilum indicating loss of lung volume, in association with a change in density behind the heart shadow.

Physical signs of lung collapse with and without patent upper airways

Sign	Patent upper airway	Obstructed bronchus
expansion	always reduced on side of lesion	always reduced on side of lesion
trachea	deviated to side of collapse, especially upper lobe collapse	deviated to side of collapse, especially upper lobe collapse
percussion	dull	dull
TVF	usually normal or increased	decreased or absent
vocal resonance	whispering pectoriloquy	—
breath sounds	increased; bronchial breathing	absent or decreased

Fig. 13.10 Physical signs of lung collapse with and without patent upper airways. TVF, tactile vocal fremitus.

Consolidation

Diagnose the pathology

Consolidation implies replacement of air in the acini with fluid or solid material. The lung parenchyma is heavy and stiff, but transmits sound waves to the chest wall more efficiently. In addition, the lower airways often collapse during expiration, but may open explosively during inspiration when negative intrathoracic pressure is generated, producing crepitations (Fig. 13.11).

Consider aetiology

The important causes of consolidation include:

- Pneumonia – most common cause, especially if in classical lobar distribution.
- Pulmonary oedema – may be cardiogenic or non-cardiogenic.
- Pulmonary haemorrhage – for example due to pulmonary vasculitis.
- Aspiration.
- Neoplasms – for example alveolar cell carcinoma.

Look for systemic clues of the aetiology:

- Fever, green sputum in sputum pot – pneumonia.
- Third heart sound, mitral murmurs, peripheral oedema – cardiogenic.
- Nailfold infarcts, livedo reticularis, splinter haemorrhages – vasculitis.
- Clubbing – underlying primary bronchial carcinoma.

Differential diagnosis

Clinically, the main differential diagnosis is between pneumonia and pulmonary oedema. This is usually apparent from the clinical setting. It is more likely to be pneumonia if the consolidation is in a lobar distribution or unilateral (especially right-sided). In addition, a pleural effusion, raised jugular venous pressure, and peripheral oedema are more common in pulmonary oedema, but not diagnostic.

Lung fibrosis

Pulmonary fibrosis results in lungs that are rigid and resistant to expansion. The fibrotic disease often shrinks the lung, resulting in a constrictive process. The thicker parenchyma will, however, transmit sound waves more efficiently to the chest wall. As with other

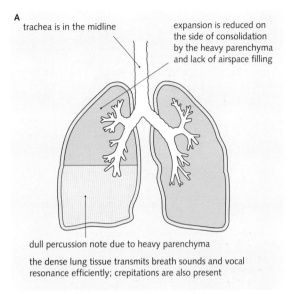

A

trachea is in the midline

expansion is reduced on the side of consolidation by the heavy parenchyma and lack of airspace filling

dull percussion note due to heavy parenchyma

the dense lung tissue transmits breath sounds and vocal resonance efficiently; crepitations are also present

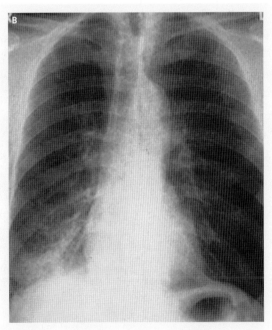

Fig. 13.11 (A) Physical signs of consolidation. (B) Radiograph of right lower lobe pneumonia.

parenchymal processes, the small airways may open explosively in inspiration causing crepitations. The disease may be unilateral (e.g. tuberculosis) or bilateral (e.g. cryptogenic fibrosing alveolitis).

Diagnose the pathology

Distinguish between unilateral and bilateral disease. The tracheal position is most useful as often there is coexisting pathology (Fig. 13.12).

115

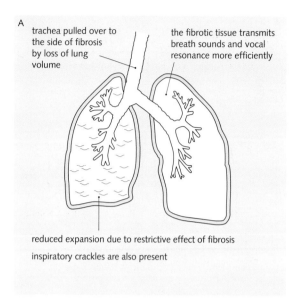

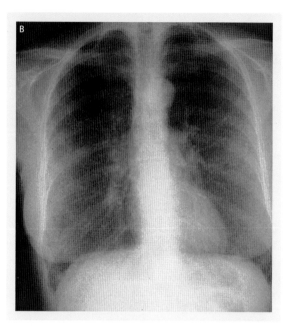

A — trachea pulled over to the side of fibrosis by loss of lung volume

the fibrotic tissue transmits breath sounds and vocal resonance more efficiently

reduced expansion due to restrictive effect of fibrosis

inspiratory crackles are also present

Fig. 13.12 (A) Physical signs of pulmonary fibrosis. (B) Radiograph of bilateral mid and lower zone pulmonary fibrosis.

Fig. 13.13 Causes of pulmonary fibrosis. The more common causes are marked with an asterisk.

Causes of pulmonary fibrosis	
Cause	Examples and signs
infection*	tuberculosis (typically upper lobe)
collagen disorder	rheumatoid lung (usually basal); scleroderma
extrinsic allergic alveolitis*	especially upper lobes
sarcoidosis*	look for erythema nodosum and other stigmata
radiation	look for radiation burns
drugs	busulphan, bleomycin; etc.
cryptogenic fibrosing alveolitis	rare; begins in lower lobes; look for clubbing
asbestosis	—
ankylosing spondylitis	upper lobes; rigid back; peripheral arthritis; aortic regurgitation; etc.

Consider aetiology

The more common causes of pulmonary fibrosis are illustrated in Fig. 13.13.

Integrating physical signs to diagnose pathology

Figure 13.14 illustrates how the different physical signs elicited in the respiratory system can be integrated so that the basic underlying pathological cause can be identified. Remember that this is only part of the examination process. It is important to assess the severity of the pathology and its underlying cause so that specific therapy can be offered.

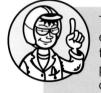

The importance of assessing expansion (to reveal the side of the pathology) and tracheal position (for expanding or constricting lesion) cannot be overemphasized.

Examination findings in the basic lung pathologies					
Lung pathology	Tracheal position	Percussion note	TVF/vocal resonance	Volume of breath sounds	Added sounds
pneumothorax	normal (deviated away in tension pneumothorax)	hyperresonant (often subtle)	decreased (or absent)	decreased or absent	—
consolidation	normal	dull	increased	increased (bronchial breathing)	inspiratory crackles
fibrosis	pulled towards	slightly dull	increased	increased	inspiratory crackles
pleural effusion	normal (deviated away if massive)	stony dull	reduced or absent	decreased or absent	often crackles immediately above effusion
lobar collapse (patent airway)	pulled towards	dull	increased	increased (bronchial breathing)	—
lobar collapse (occluded bronchus)	pulled towards	dull	decreased	decreased	—

Fig. 13.14 Examination findings for the basic lung pathologies. Note that this refers to unilateral lesions. The expansion is always reduced on the side of the lung pathology. TVF, tactile vocal fremitus.

Asthma

A diagnosis of asthma is usually apparent from the history. The aim of the examination is to assess severity, look for complications, and to consider precipitating factors.

Assess severity

This is assessed by talking to the patient. If the patient cannot finish a sentence they are having a severe attack and urgent help should be summoned. Use objective reproducible measures of severity and classify the attack as mild, moderate, or severe. Remember that not all of the features need to be present in a severe attack (Fig. 13.15). The essential parameters to assess are pulse rate, respiratory rate, peak flow rate, and (in hospitals) arterial blood gas estimate.

Other features of a serious or life-threatening attack include:

- Difficulty speaking.
- Bradycardia or hypotension.
- Exhaustion.
- Silent chest.
- Cyanosis.

Look for complications

Examine for the presence of a pneumothorax. This is the main reason for radiography in hospitalized patients.

Assessment of severity of an acute asthma attack			
Feature	Mild	Moderate	Severe
pulse rate (/min)	<100	100–110	>110
respiratory rate (/min)	<20	20–30	>30
peak flow rate	>75% predicted	50–75% predicted	<50% predicted
arterial blood gases	PaO_2 high/normal; $PaCO_2$ low	PaO_2 normal; $PaCO_2$ low or low normal (<5 kPa)	PaO_2 <8 kPa; $PaCO_2$ high normal or high (>5 kPa)

Fig. 13.15 Assessment of severity of an acute asthma attack. In the hospital setting, arterial blood gases (ABG) form part of the routine assessment. Pulsus paradoxus, if easy to elicit, is useful, but often it is difficult – it is a waste of time making an inaccurate 'best guess'.

Consider aetiology

Look for signs of a chest infection, which is common. In older patients with new-onset asthma, look for nasal polyps, which are also associated with aspirin sensitivity. Also inspect for features of atopy, especially in younger patients (e.g. eczema, dry skin, thinning of lateral half of eyebrows from rubbing).

Asthma is potentially fatal. A rapid and objective assessment is essential.

Lung cancer

Lung cancer is the most common fatal malignancy in men and its incidence in women is on the increase. It can present in many ways and show many features on examination.

Inspection

Look for clues such as:
- Cachexia (common).
- Cigarette staining in hair.
- Scar from lobectomy.
- Radiotherapy burn on chest wall.

Hands

There are often signs in the hands as follows:
- Clubbing – may predate clinical diagnosis.
- Clues to smoking history – nicotine staining on nails.
- Hypertrophic pulmonary osteoarthropathy (HPOA) – pain and swelling of the wrists, especially with small cell carcinoma.

Face

Horner's syndrome (small pupil, partial ptosis, enophthalmos, anhidrosis) due to invasion of the sympathetic ganglion T1 by direct spread) may be a feature of upper lobe disease.

Neck

Palpate for a supraclavicular lymph node. Look for features of superior vena cava obstruction (swollen face and neck, plethora, dilated veins over trunk).

Chest

Look for features of:
- Pleural effusion (common).
- Loss of lung volume due to lobar or lung collapse.

Evidence of spread

Direct spread

Examine specifically for other features of direct spread:
- Pancoast's tumour – apical tumour invading the lower brachial plexus (especially C8, T1, T2) causing sensory loss, wasting, and weakness of the small muscles of the hand.
- Phrenic nerve – diaphragmatic palsy.
- Pericardium – effusion (look for features to suggest tamponade).

Metastatic spread

Examine for features of metastatic spread, for example:
- Hepatomegaly.
- Focal neurological signs due to cerebral metastases.
- Localized bony tenderness.

14. Abdominal Examination

Examination routine

A thorough abdominal examination is fundamental to both surgical and medical clerking, but the emphasis clearly changes according to the presenting complaint.

Patient exposure and position

Ensure good lighting. Patients should be undressed so that a view of the whole abdomen (from nipple to knees) can be obtained. Provide a blanket for warmth and modesty. Lie the patient flat on the couch with a single pillow behind their head (though this may not always be possible if, for example, the patient has orthopnoea or musculoskeletal abnormalities), with arms by their side. If patients are unable to fully relax their abdomen, ask them to flex their hips to 45° and knees to 90° (Fig. 14.1).

The key is to have a relaxed patient. You will be able to elicit signs more easily if the patient is comfortable.

General inspection

Observe the general appearance of the patient. Time spent at this stage is invaluable. Take at least 10 seconds, making a mental checklist, for example:

- Is the patient comfortable or distressed at rest?
- Is there any obvious pain?
- Is there any cachexia, pallor, jaundice, abnormal skin pigmentation, distension, etc.

A rapid but systematic survey of the patient should ensue.

Hands

Careful examination of the hands is fundamental to the abdominal examination and may yield vital clues of underlying abdominal disease.

If asked to examine the abdominal system in an examination, always start by looking at the hands.

Note the presence of:

- Metabolic flap (asterixis). This may indicate hepatic encephalopathy (or carbon dioxide retention and uraemia).
- Signs of chronic liver disease. Inspect and palpate both hands for the presence of Dupuytren's contracture, palmar erythema, leuconychia (white nails), spider naevi, and clubbing.
- Anaemia. If the patient is profoundly anaemic, palmar skin creases may be pale. Koilonychia (spoon-shaped nails) suggests iron deficiency anaemia.

Eyes

Inspect the sclerae for jaundice, and the lower eyelid for anaemia.

Jaundice is easily overlooked. It is harder to detect in artificial lighting.

Face

Note abnormal pigmentation around the lips, or angular stomatitis, which occurs in many medical conditions, especially iron deficiency anaemia, malabsorption and oral infections.

Oral cavity

Inspect the oral cavity and tongue for:

- Ulceration (e.g. due to inflammatory bowel disease, chemotherapy).
- Inflammation.
- Oral candidiasis (e.g. due to antibiotic therapy, immunodeficiency, diabetes mellitus).
- Halitosis (e.g. due to infection, poor hygiene, hepatic fetor, uraemia, diabetes mellitus).
- Pigmentation (e.g. Addison's disease)

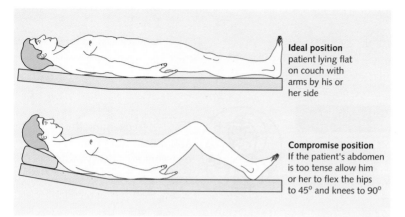

Fig. 14.1   Ideal position for examination of the abdomen.

Ideal position
patient lying flat on couch with arms by his or her side

Compromise position
If the patient's abdomen is too tense allow him or her to flex the hips to 45° and knees to 90°

Chest wall

Note the presence of gynaecomastia and spider naevi. The presence of more than five spider naevi is considered to be suggestive of liver disease. These characteristically blanche if the central arteriole is pressed.

Supraclavicular lymphadenopathy

Pay particular attention to the left side and look for Virchow's node (Fig. 14.2). If present is this Troisier's sign?

Exposure of the abdomen

Following general inspection, the abdomen should be exposed from the nipples to symphysis pubis. Follow the usual routine of inspection, palpation, percussion, auscultation.

Inspection

Stand at the end of the bed and inspect the abdomen for:

- Symmetry (e.g. massive splenomegaly produces a bulge on the left side).
- Abnormal pulsation (e.g. due to abdominal aortic aneurysm).
- Shape (e.g. distension).

Remember the five Fs from Chapter 5.
Return to right-hand side of the abdomen and actively inspect for the presence of:
- Scars (Fig. 14.3).
- Sinuses (e.g. due to retained suture material).

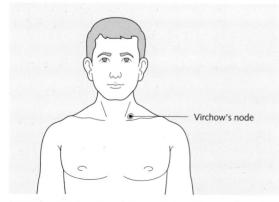

Fig. 14.2   Virchow's node is a palpable left supraclavicular lymph node. Troisier's sign refers to the presence of a palpable left supraclavicular node in association with gastric carcinoma. This node is easiest to palpate from behind.

Virchow's node

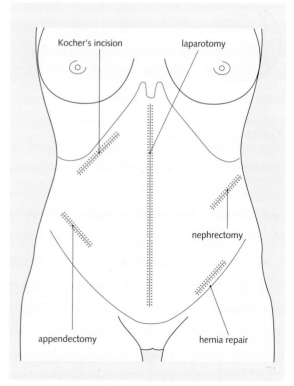

Kocher's incision   laparotomy

nephrectomy

appendectomy   hernia repair

Fig. 14.3   Surgical scars on the abdominal wall.

- Fistulas (e.g. due to Crohn's disease).
- Visible peristalsis (e.g. due to intestinal obstruction).
- Distended veins.
- Flank haemorrhages (e.g. due to pancreatitis).

Ask patients whether they are aware of any abnormal lumps or areas of tenderness. This may give a clue to the area of pathology. Ask patients to cough, observing pain (peritoneal irritation) and also the hernial orifices.

Palpation

Before palpating, ask the patient where the pain is. Warn the patient that you are going to lay your hand on their abdomen. Lay your hand on the point furthest from the pain and work towards it. The three stages to abdominal palpation are:
- Light palpation.
- Deep palpation.
- Specific palpation of the intra-abdominal organs.

Light palpation

Commence palpation at a site remote from the area of pain. All areas of the abdomen must be palpated systematically. Picture the abdomen in nine regions (Fig. 14.4). (Some people refer to abdominal quadrants as shown in Fig. 14.5.) This helps you to

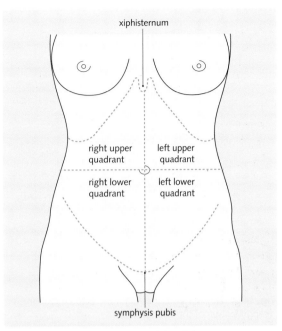

Fig. 14.5 The four quadrants of the abdomen.

adopt a systematic approach to the examination and when presenting your findings.

Light palpation is performed to elicit any tenderness or guarding. Lie the hands and fingers flat upon the abdomen and press very gently. It is often useful to kneel down beside the bed. It is essential to be as gentle as possible:
- To gain the patient's confidence.
- To prevent voluntary guarding (tensing of the abdominal wall musculature as light pressure is applied), which will mask pathological signs.

Deep palpation

Warn the patient that you will be pressing more firmly and feel for any obvious masses (Fig. 14.6) or tenderness in the nine regions. If a mass is identified, determine its characteristics systematically.

Specific palpation of the intra-abdominal organs

Liver. Always start in the right iliac fossa when examining the liver or the spleen as both expand towards this region. Place your hand flat with fingers pointing towards the patient's head, (or alternatively to the left flank), and palpate deeply while asking the patient to breathe in and out deeply. Keep your hands still while the patient is breathing in as the liver edge moves downwards on inspiration. If nothing is felt, repeat the process with the hand slightly higher up the abdomen, advancing a few centimetres at a time until the costal margin is reached.

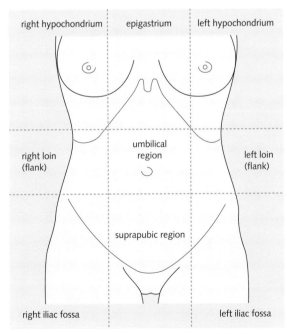

Fig. 14.4 The regions of the abdomen. It is helpful to be aware of these regions when palpating or presenting physical findings as this helps in the differential diagnosis.

121

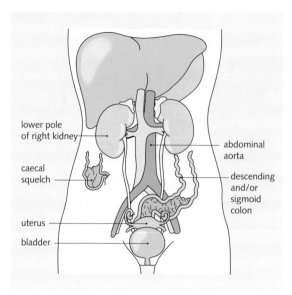

Fig. 14.6   Normal structures that may be palpable on deep palpation of the abdomen.

The liver may be palpated in normal subjects, especially if they are thin or if there is chest hyperinflation (Fig. 14.7). If the liver edge is palpable, describe:

- The size of the liver (express as finger breadths below the costal margin).
- Its contour (regular or irregular).
- Its texture (smooth, nodular).
- Any tenderness (see hepatomegaly, p. 124).

After this percuss out the superior and inferior borders of the liver.

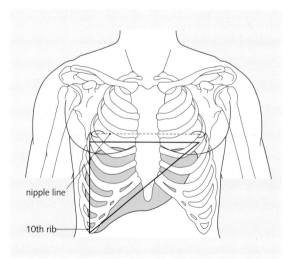

Fig. 14.7   Surface anatomy of the liver.

Spleen.   The spleen is examined by a similar process as for the liver. Start in the right iliac fossa with fingers pointing towards the left costal margin and ask the patient to breathe in and out while advancing towards the left costal margin. If there is no obvious splenomegaly, ask the patient to roll onto the right side, place your left hand around the lower left costal margin and lift forwards as the patient inspires, while palpating with your right hand (Fig. 14.8).

A normal spleen is not palpable.

Kidneys.   The kidneys are examined bimanually by the technique of ballottement. The left kidney is felt by placing your left hand in the left loin below the 12th rib lateral to the erector spinae muscles and above the iliac crest with the right hand placed anteriorly just above the anterior superior iliac spine.

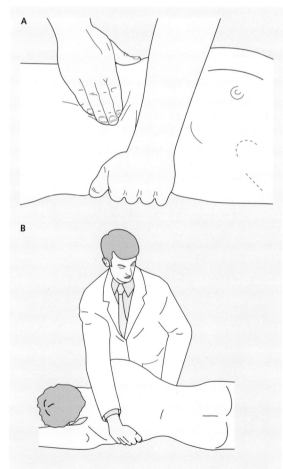

Fig. 14.8   Palpation of the spleen. (A) Initial examination. (B) If the examination is difficult, the patient should be asked to roll onto the right side, push the spleen forwards with your left hand and palpate with your right hand.

During inspiration, the left hand is then lifted gently upwards towards the right hand (Fig. 14.9).

The kidney may be palpable in thin normal individuals. The right kidney is examined with the right hand posteriorly and the left hand anteriorly.

In normal individuals, the right kidney lies lower than the left (due to downward displacement by the liver) and is more likely to be palpable (Fig. 14.10).

Abdominal aorta. Palpate specifically for an abdominal aortic aneurysm (AAA). This is performed by placing the palmar surfaces of both hands laterally and with the fingertips positioned in the midline a few centimetres below the xiphisternum (Fig. 14.11).

- An AAA is both pulsatile and expansile (fingertips will be pushed outwards).
- A non-aneurysmal abdominal aorta is only pulsatile (fingertips pushed upwards, but not outwards) (Fig. 14.12).

Percussion
Percuss over the whole abdomen and particularly over masses. This is also a sensitive method for eliciting peritonitis. Specifically percuss for ascites by testing for shifting dullness. Percuss from the midline to the flank. If ascites is present, the initially resonant note will become dull. Note the point of transition on the skin, ask the patient to roll away from that side, wait a few seconds, and percuss over that area. If ascites is present the initially dull note will become resonant (Figs 14.13 and 14.14).

Auscultation
Listen specifically for bowel sounds. The presence or absence of bowel sounds is important. Listen for 30 seconds before concluding that bowel sounds are absent. Much mythology has been generated about the quality of these sounds, but this should be interpreted with caution. Listen specifically for bruits over the aorta and renal arteries.

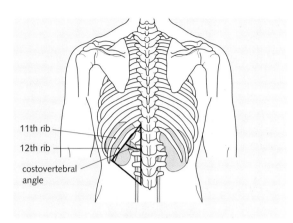

Fig. 14.10   Surface anatomy of the kidneys.

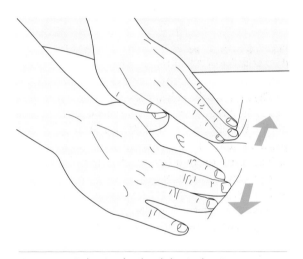

Fig. 14.11   Palpation for the abdominal aorta.

A complete abdominal examination includes assessment of:
- The hernial orifices. See Chapter 16.
- External genitalia. See Chapter 16.
- A rectal examination.

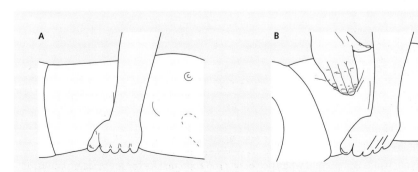

Fig. 14.9
Palpation of the kidneys.

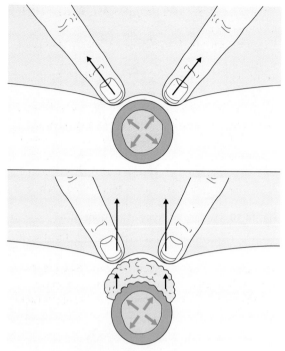

Fig. 14.12 Distinction between aortic pulsation and movement of an overlying structure. True pulsatility is indicated by outward displacement of the palpating hands.

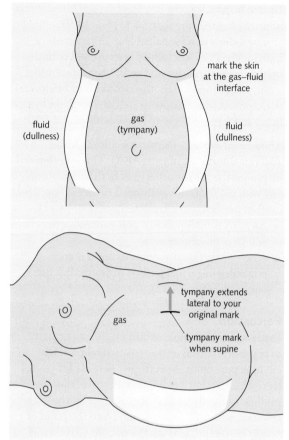

mark the skin at the gas–fluid interface

fluid (dullness)

gas (tympany)

fluid (dullness)

tympany extends lateral to your original mark

gas

tympany mark when supine

Fig. 14.13 Shifting dullness is a key sign of ascites.

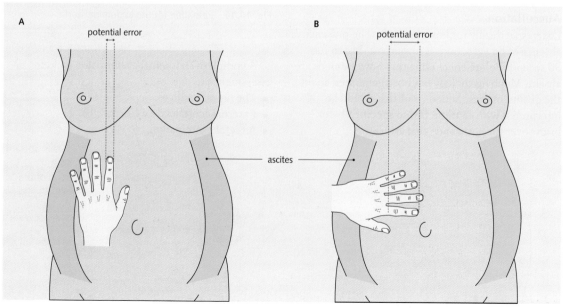

A

potential error

B

potential error

ascites

Fig. 14.14 Correct orientation of your hands is important when percussing the abdomen for the presence of ascites. (A) Correct positioning of the hand. (B) Incorrect positioning of the hand.

Rectal examination

The rectal examination is usually performed with the patient in the left lateral position, with both hips and knees fully flexed (Fig. 14.15). It is essential to explain the procedure to the patient and to be gentle! It is usually possible to palpate lesions up to 6–8 cm from the anal verge. Before performing a digital examination:

- Inspect the anus, its margins, and surrounding skin.
- Look for skin tags, excoriation, prolapsed or thrombosed haemorrhoids, fistulas, fissures, abscesses, or ulceration due to an anal carcinoma.
- Ask the patient to bear down or strain. This may reveal the presence of a rectal prolapse or occasionally a polyp.

While performing a digital rectal examination, the sphincter tone should be assessed and any tenderness elicited.

Structures palpable during a normal digital rectal examination

Palpate anteriorly, laterally, and posteriorly. Note the following:

- Posteriorly – the tip of the coccyx and sacrum are palpable.
- Laterally – ischial spines and ischiorectal fossa.
- Anteriorly in males – prostate (smooth lateral lobes separated by the median sulcus); a prostatic carcinoma may be differentiated from benign prostatic hypertrophy by the loss of the median sulcus and possibly the presence of a palpable hard, craggy, irregular mass.
- Anteriorly in females – cervix through the vaginal wall and occasionally the body of the uterus.

The normal rectum may contain some faeces. Always look at the glove after examination for blood or mucus. Melaena stool has the appearance

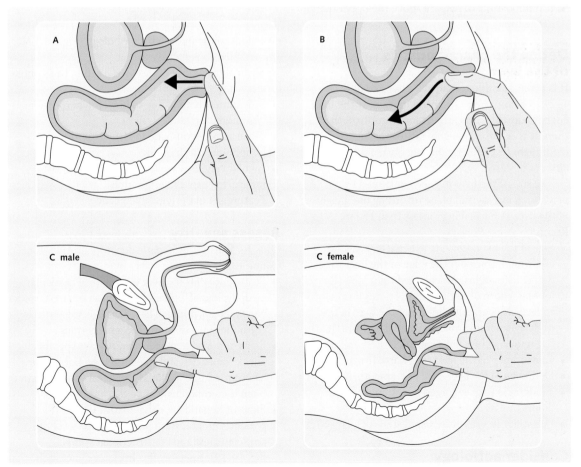

Fig. 14.15   The rectal examination. (A) Insert the tip of your index finger into the anal canal. (B) Follow the curve of the sacrum. (C) Sweep the finger around the pelvis, noting any irregularities, masses, or tenderness. Examine the glove on withdrawal of your finger.

of sticky tar and an offensive characteristic smell. A rectal carcinoma may be palpable as a shelf-like lesion associated with blood on the glove.

Always wipe the patient after examination and offer further tissues.

Hepatomegaly

Identify the mass as the liver

The liver is palpable in the right upper quadrant. Hepatomegaly is not usually confused with other organomegaly, but the liver should be distinguished from an enlarged right kidney. The features of hepatomegaly include:

- Palpable below the right costal margin (in gross hepatomegaly, it may extend to the left costal margin).
- Downward movement on inspiration.
- Dullness to percussion.
- It is impossible to palpate above the upper margin of the liver.

Define the characteristics of the liver

It is often possible to palpate a liver edge 1–2 cm below the right costal margin. If the liver edge is palpable, it is important to confirm that there is true hepatomegaly rather than a low diaphragm (e.g. due to chronic obstructive airways disease).

The size of the liver may be confirmed by percussion in a sagittal plane recording the 'height' of the liver. A normal liver is less than 15 cm. Record:

- Size of the liver. Once true hepatomegaly is confirmed, trace out the edge of the liver to define its margins. An enlarged right lobe (Riedel's lobe) is a normal finding. In the notes it is helpful to record accurately the size of the liver in the midclavicular line, midline, and if appropriate the left midclavicular line (Fig. 14.16).
- Consistency of the liver (e.g. hard, firm).
- Definition of the liver edge (e.g. smooth, knobbly).
- Tenderness (e.g. engorged liver in right heart failure).
- Pulsatility (e.g. as in tricuspid stenosis).

Consider aetiology

It is important to look for other features on systemic examination if hepatomegaly is found as they may

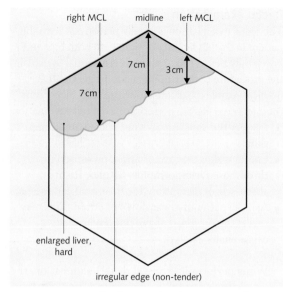

Fig. 14.16 Example of a record in the case notes for hepatomegaly. MCL, midclavicular line.

give clues to the underlying pathology (Fig. 14.17). In particular look for:

- Signs of chronic liver disease (e.g. due to alcoholic cirrhosis).
- Splenomegaly (e.g. due to portal hypertension, lymphoma).
- Generalized lymphadenopathy (e.g. due to lymphoma, carcinoma).
- Jugular venous wave (e.g. due to right heart failure, tricuspid regurgitation).
- Features of underlying malignancy.

Assess severity

Look for features of hepatic decompensation, for example:

- Features of chronic liver disease (e.g. testicular atrophy, loss of axillary hair, gynaecomastia, spider naevi, leuconychia). These features suggest that the underlying disease process is chronic.
- Signs of portal hypertension. Always specifically check for ascites and splenomegaly. Look for a 'caput medusae' (dilated collateral veins radiating from the umbilicus).
- Signs of hepatic encephalopathy. Check the patient's mental state (especially for level of consciousness and constructional apraxia, Fig. 14.18). Specifically check for a metabolic flap (asterixis) and fetor hepaticus.
- Jaundice.

Causes of hepatomegaly	
Causes*	Features on examination
cirrhosis	features of chronic liver disease; features of portal hypertension; hard irregular, knobbly liver common
alcoholic	common; look for evidence of alcoholic toxicity in other systems (e.g. neuropathy)
primary biliary	usually middle-aged female; pruritus common (look for excoriation); xanthelasma
haemochromatosis	skin pigmentation; gonadal atrophy; more common in men
α-1-antitrypsin deficiency	signs of chronic obstructive airways disease
secondary carcinoma*	hard irregular knobbly liver edge; systemic features of malignancy (e.g. cachexia, etc.); lymphadenopathy; signs of primary (e.g. palpable breast lump, etc.)
congestive cardiac failure*	raised jugular venous pressure; peripheral oedema prominent; third heart sound; look for features of tricuspid regurgitation
infections (hepatitis A, B, C—rarely; glandular fever; cytomegalovirus; leptospirosis; hydatid; amoebic)	features are usually apparent from the history, but look for generalized lymphadenopathy
lymphoproliferative disorder (lymphoma; leukaemia; polycythaemia)	splenomegaly; generalized lymphadenopathy; anaemia or plethora; petechiae; etc.
miscellaneous amyloid polycystic fatty liver	splenomegaly; waxy skin; chronic disease; palpable kidneys; signs of uraemia

Fig. 14.17 Causes of hepatomegaly. The most common causes are cirrhosis, secondary carcinoma, and congestive cardiac failure.

Splenomegaly

Identify the mass as the spleen

A mass in the left upper quadrant is usually a spleen. It is not normal to be able to palpate the spleen. It must be enlarged 2–3-fold before it becomes palpable. It must be distinguished from the left kidney.

The characteristics of the spleen on physical examination include:

- Presence in the left upper quadrant.
- Upper edge not palpable.
- Expansion towards the right lower quadrant.
- On inspiration, movement towards the right lower quadrant.
- A notch may be palpable.
- Dullness to percussion. The dullness extends above the costal margin.
- Not ballottable.

Assess spleen size

In a manner analogous to assessing the degree of hepatomegaly, it is important to measure the descent of the spleen from the left costal margin (Fig. 14.19).

Consider aetiology

The more common causes of splenomegaly are illustrated in Fig. 14.20. In particular, note the presence of:

- Hepatomegaly – portal hypertension, lymphoproliferative disorder.
- Generalized lymphadenopathy – lymphoproliferative disorder.
- Size of spleen – massive splenomegaly is usually due to chronic malaria, myelofibrosis, or chronic myeloid leukaemia (CML); a barely palpable spleen has a much wider differential diagnosis.

Figure provided by doctor	Attempt at copying by encephalopathic patient

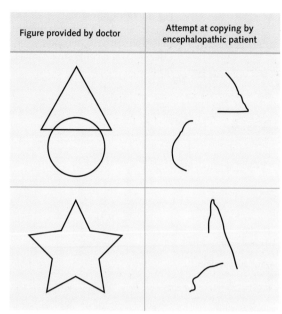

Fig. 14.18 Hepatic encephalopathy is associated with constructional apraxia. Ask the patient to copy a simple figure such as a five-pointed star or simple overlapping geometric shapes.

Fig 14.21 is an outline of the approach to the abdominal examination.

Anaemia

The causes of anaemia are widespread. Remember the section in Chapter 5. The diagnosis is largely made from detailed laboratory testing and imaging investigations. However, it is essential that the investigation is focused and this relies upon a systematic assessment during the history and examination.

Anaemia is usually detected clinically if the haemoglobin concentration is less than 10 g/dl. The signs of anaemia include:

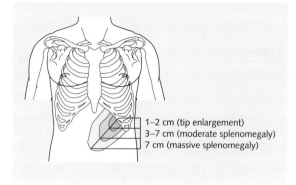

1–2 cm (tip enlargement)
3–7 cm (moderate splenomegaly)
7 cm (massive splenomegaly)

Fig. 14.19 Different degrees of splenomegaly.

- Conjunctival or mucosal pallor.
- Loss of colour in the palmar skin creases.

The more common causes of anaemia are:
- Iron deficiency anaemia.
- Folate deficiency.
- Vitamin B_{12} deficiency.
- Haemolytic anaemia.

However, these diagnoses are insufficient as an underlying cause still needs to be identified in order to provide suitable treatment and prognostic information.

Attempt to define the cause of anaemia

A thorough systematic examination is essential. Clues may be found by considering the following.

General inspection

Inspect the face carefully. Look at the general health of the patient (e.g. cachexia suggests chronic disease), and note specifically any obvious disorders (e.g. rheumatoid arthritis). Some clues to iron deficiency and megaloblastic anaemia are illustrated in Fig. 14.22.

Fig. 14.20 Causes of splenomegaly.

Causes of splenomegaly		
Large (past umbilicus)	**Moderate (to umbilicus)**	**Mild (just palpable)**
Myelofibrosis	Chronic lymphatic leukaemia	Portal hypertension
Chronic myeloid leukaemia	Lymphoma	Lymphoma
Malaria	Portal hypertension	Rheumatoid arthritis (Felty's syndrome)
		Chronic lymphatic leukaemia

Gastrointestinal examination	
General	lie patient flat with arms at side wasting, scars, liver flap (asterixis), cock wrists – Hands–clubbing, leuconychia, spider naevi, palmar erythema, Dupuytren's – Head–jaundice, anaemia, purpura – Mouth–telangiectasia, pigmentation, ulceration, tongue, hepatic fetor (sweet smell) – Supraclavicular node. (Virchow's Ⓛ: Troisier's sign.) – Chest wall-gynaecomastia, spider naevi, bruising/purpura, muscle wasting
Observe abdomen	– breathe in deeply, cough – areas of fullness, masses, ascites – visible pulsation (aneurysm) – scars, striae – peristalsis – distended veins, direction of flow – hernias – everted umbilicus (ascites)
Palpate abdomen	– ask if tender, watch patient's face, kneel down – gentle palpation in each quadrant, for masses, tenderness – deep palpation – palpate liver from Ⓡiliac fossa, with inspiration, size, border smoothness, tenderness – palpate spleen from Ⓡiliac fossa with inspiration (confused with kidney–cannot get above spleen, dull to percussion, moves with resp, can't ballot). Turn onto Ⓡ feel under Ⓛcostal margin – palpate kidneys–bimanually, ballot – palpate for aortic aneurysm
Percussion	– liver spleen – shifting dullness – centre of abdomen to flank, mark point, roll patient to side, back towards umbilicus – fluid thrill – examiner's hand on midline, flick one side, detect on other
Auscultate	– bowel sounds – bruits aorta, hepatic, renal
Hernial orifices	– cough
Genitalia	
PR	
Urinalysis	

Fig. 14.21 A summary of the abdominal examination.

Note racial origin, for example:
- Mediterranean – thalassaemia.
- Afro-Caribbean – sickle cell anaemia.
- Northern European – hereditary spherocytosis.

Look for causes of blood loss

A systematic survey for a potential source of blood loss should be performed, for example:
- Abdominal scars.

Fig. 14.22 Features on general inspection of a patient with anaemia. Asterisks indicate the more common causes.

Features on general inspection in an anaemic patient	
Cause	Features
iron deficiency*	koilonychia (spoon-shaped nails); painless glossitis; angular stomatitis
hereditary haemorrhagic telangiectasia	visible telangiectasia on face and mouth
Peutz–Jegher's syndrome	pigmented macules around the lips and mouth
megaloblastic anaemia*	mild jaundice (lemon–yellow tinge) due to ineffective erythropoiesis; beefy red swollen tongue; angular stomatitis
pernicious anaemia	usually middle-aged or elderly female; look for features of other autoimmune disease (e.g. vitiligo)

- Gastrointestinal (GI) bleeding – look for abdominal masses; a rectal examination is mandatory.
- Genito-urinary source – look for a palpable bladder or kidneys, perform urinalysis.

Look for features of a chronic disease

Look for features of chronic disease such as:
- Infections (e.g. tuberculosis, osteomyelitis, infective endocarditis).
- Connective tissue disease.
- Crohn's disease.
- Malignancy.

Exclude pregnancy

Pregnancy may be associated with folate and iron deficiency.

Perform a thorough abdominal examination

Pathology of the GI tract may cause anaemia, for example:
- GI bleeding, malabsorption (e.g. due to coeliac disease) – iron deficiency anaemia.
- Gastrectomy, blind loop syndrome, Crohn's disease – anaemia due to folate or vitamin B_{12} deficiency.

In addition an intra-abdominal malignancy may be detected.

Organomegaly is associated with different types of anaemia:
- Liver disease is associated with macrocytic anaemia.
- Splenomegaly may be responsible for haemolytic anaemia.
- A large uterus may be due to pregnancy or be a cause for blood loss.
- Polycystic kidneys may be a cause of chronic renal failure and consequent anaemia.

Look for signs of haemolysis

Splenomegaly or mild jaundice may indicate that the underlying cause is haemolysis.

Assess severity of anaemia

Try to make an assessment of the functional consequences of the anaemia. It is often hard to correlate the degree of pallor with the haemoglobin level. The functional impact of anaemia depends upon the underlying condition, the age and fitness of the patient, and the speed of onset. Look for signs of decompensation, for example:

- Hypotension – rapid blood loss may result in hypovolaemia and hypotension; postural blood pressure is the most sensitive indicator.
- Tachycardia – this develops early as a means of increasing oxygen delivery to the peripheral tissues in anaemia.
- Dyspnoea – note the exercise tolerance of a patient (e.g. short of breath at rest or on climbing onto the examination couch).
- Heart failure – especially in the elderly.

Acute gastrointestinal bleed

Assess the functional impact

This is a medical emergency. Do not struggle on your own trying to sort this out. It is a team effort, which requires senior support and involvement. If you come across a patient with a significant GI bleed, as a student get help. Chapter X has a section on the approach to the unwell patient. The initial examination should follow the standard routine of Airway, Breathing & Circulation (ABC). When a problem is identified it must be treated before moving on. It is important to recognize which patients are in danger of exsanguination. The process of assessment and emergency treatment should run in parallel.

Determine the site of bleeding

It is often clear that the bleeding is from the upper or lower GI tract. The vast majority of patients presenting with an acute GI bleed have a lesion at the level of the duodenum or above. Features to suggest an upper GI tract source of bleeding include:
- Haematemesis. Exclude haemoptysis or epistaxis with swallowing and subsequent vomiting of blood.
- Frank blood or 'coffee ground' material in the nasogastric (NG) aspirate.
- Absence of a bilious NG aspirate.
- Melaena. It is essential to perform a rectal examination. A melaena stool indicates bleeding proximal to the right colon and bleeding of usually more than 500 ml in the previous 24 hours. Note that the presence of blood per rectum does not always indicate a lower GI bleed as a very brisk upper GI bleed can result in apparently fresh blood per rectum.

Features of a lower GI bleed include the passage of bright red blood per rectum (haematochezia). This is not pathognomonic (see above), but if the bleeding is from the upper GI tract, the patient will invariably be profoundly hypovolaemic. Common causes of a lower GI bleed are haemorrhoids and diverticular disease.

Perform a detailed abdominal examination

A systematic abdominal system examination may provide further clues to the cause, for example:

- Abdominal masses (tumours, diverticular masses, abdominal aortic aneutysm (AAA)).
- Signs of liver disease. GI bleeding is common in liver failure, particularly of an alcoholic aetiology.
- Surgical scars. May indicate previous peptic ulcer disease for example.
- Rectal examination findings. Note stool colour. This may indicate the location of the bleeding point as well as the speed of bleeding.

 The examination is aimed at assessing the degree of hypovolaemia, rate of blood loss, source of bleeding, and urgency of resuscitation. The initial haemoglobin estimate may be misleading, so the requirement for blood transfusion relies upon thorough clinical assessment.

Acute abdominal pain

Acute abdominal pain is one of the most common causes of presentation to a casualty department. The differential diagnosis is vast, ranging from trivial conditions to life-threatening surgical emergencies. It is important to adopt a systematic approach to the examination. Consider the differential diagnosis throughout the examination (see Fig. 5.2) so that further management strategies can be instituted efficiently. The main aims of the examination are:

- To establish the cause of pain.
- To assess whether the patient would benefit from admission to hospital.
- To assess whether the patient requires surgical intervention.

General inspection

Before specifically examining the abdomen, look at the patient as a whole. It is helpful to ask the following questions.

Does the patient look unwell?

Patients with acute peritonitis usually look obviously unwell. They are disinterested in their surroundings and lie still so as not to aggravate the pain. Patients with renal colic may also appear distressed, but tend to be restless and in obvious pain. Conversely, patients who are laughing, smiling, or eating are most unlikely to have any significant acute surgical disease.

How old is the patient?

Different diseases are more common in different age groups. For example:

- Acute diverticulitis or AAA is much more common with increasing age.
- Acute appendicitis is commonest in young children and adolescents, but occurs in all age groups.
- Ectopic pregnancy is only going to occur in women of childbearing age.

What sex is the patient?

In women the differential diagnosis needs to be broadened to include gynaecological conditions. The other causes of intra-abdominal pain can occur in either sex, but some have a tendency to be more common in one sex. For example:

- Gallstones are more common in women.
- Peptic ulceration is more common in men.

Specific inspection

Perform a more specific inspection starting at the head and working down to the feet, noting the following.

General appearance

Cachexia may be due to chronic illness or malignancy.

Jaundice

The presence of jaundice should alert the doctor to:

- Gallstones – obstruction of the common bile duct, cholecystitis, pancreatitis.
- Chronic liver disease – associated with gastritis, acute alcoholic hepatitis, and pancreatitis as well as oesophageal varices.

Conjunctival pallor

In the context of acute abdominal pain, it may be hard to assess skin coloration as the patient often appears pale, grey and sweaty. However, conjunctival pallor may suggest the presence of a chronic bleeding lesion, for example:

- Peptic ulcer.
- Colonic tumour with subsequent obstruction or intussusception.

Stigmata of chronic liver disease

See explanation of jaundice above.

Fever

The presence of fever suggests that an active inflammatory process is present.

Left supraclavicular lymphadenopathy

This is suggestive of intra-abdominal malignancy.

Check vital signs

It is essential to check the vital signs as a baseline and to determine the urgency of therapy. Check the following.

Oral temperature

Even in the presence of peritonitis and active infection the patient may not have a fever, especially if shocked. However, the presence of pyrexia indicates that organic pathology is almost invariably present.

Pulse rate

It is unusual to have a tachycardia in the absence of active pathology. However, a very anxious patient may have tachycardia. The sequential recording of pulse rate is an accurate indicator of systemic disturbance if there is a progressive tachycardia. Equally, a completely normal pulse in the presence of severe acute abdominal pathology is unusual. However, beware reliance on the pulse if the patient is on β-blockers.

Blood pressure

Check supine blood pressure. If the patient is able to cooperate, it is useful to check postural blood pressure. If the patient has shock or hypovolaemia there will be a drop in blood pressure on standing.

Assess fluid status

If the jugular venous waveform is easily visible, the jugular venous pressure provides a useful marker of fluid status.

Abdominal examination
Inspection

Inspect the abdomen noting:

- Visible peristalsis – suggestive of obstruction.
- Abdominal distension – may be due to obstruction.
- Rigidity – a tense, boardlike abdomen occurs in the presence of peritonitis.
- Any skin discoloration – pancreatitis may be associated with a bluish discoloration in the loins due to extravasation of bloodstained pancreatic juice into the retroperitoneum.
- Obvious hernias.
- Abdominal scars – their presence raises the possibility of obstruction due to adhesions.
- Obvious organomegaly – for example massive polycystic kidneys may cause bulging in the flank. Bleeding into a cyst may be the cause for the pain.

Note the site of the pain

Ask the patient to show you exactly where the pain is on the abdomen. The location of the pain is the key to the underlying cause (see Fig. 5.2).

Examine the abdomen in detail

Perform a detailed abdominal examination as described at the start of this chapter. In particular, note:

- Presence or absence of signs of peritonitis.
- Presence of any abdominal masses.
- Location of the tenderness.

Signs of peritonitis

The presence of unexplained peritonitis is an indication for surgical intervention. The features of peritonitis are:

- Signs of shock (tachycardia, hypotension, which becomes progressive on serial observation; Fig. 14.23).
- Tenderness.
- Guarding (a sign of severe tenderness).
- Rebound tenderness. This is a useful discriminatory sign as many anxious patients have involuntary guarding upon palpation, but do not expect tenderness on withdrawal of the palpating hand. The tenderness may be distant to the site of palpation. Watch the patient's face for signs of rebound tenderness.
- Localized pain distant to the site of palpation.
- Absent bowel sounds.

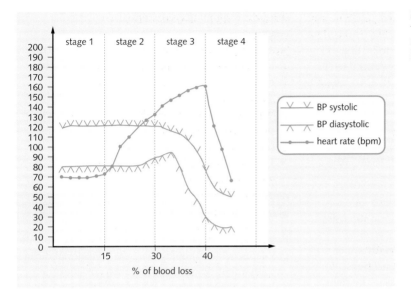

Fig. 14.23 This figure shows the four stages of shock. Note how much blood you have to lose before your blood pressure drops.

Presence of an abdominal mass

Examination of palpable liver, spleen, and kidney is discussed on pp. 121 and 122. In the context of acute abdominal pain, a mass in the right or left iliac fossa is most relevant.

Mass in the right iliac fossa

The most common causes are an appendix mass or carcinoma of the caecum. The differential diagnosis is shown in Fig. 14.24.

Mass in the left iliac fossa

The same diseases as shown in Fig 14.23 may cause a left iliac fossa mass, except for carcinoma of the caecum, Crohn's disease and tuberculosis. Diverticulitis is common and may cause a mass. Carcinoma of the colon usually presents with weight loss or a change in bowel habit, but occasionally presents as a left iliac fossa mass especially if it is causing obstruction.

Fig. 14.24 Causes of a right iliac fossa mass.

Causes of a right iliac fossa mass	
Causes	**Features**
appendix mass	preceding history of central abdominal pain moving to the right iliac fossa; anorexia; tender mass; persistent fever and tachycardia; tender per rectum(PR)
carcinoma of the caecum	firm distinct mass; often non-mobile; usually non-tender; patient does not look acutely unwell
tuberculosis	more common in patients from the Indian subcontinent or Africa
Crohn's disease	patient may appear hypovolaemic owing to diarrhoea; oral aphthous ulcers; skin tags; mass usually mobile and of rubbery consistency; tender mass
psoas abscess	ill-defined mass; lumbar tenderness
iliac lymph nodes	
iliac artery aneurysm	

Location of the pain
Generalized
Generalized abdominal pain is likely to be due to generalized peritonitis. The history is central to the diagnosis.

Epigastric
The most common causes of epigastric pain are:
- Peptic ulcer.
- A biliary cause (biliary colic or cholecystitis).
- Pancreatitis.

Peptic ulcer usually produces no signs unless perforation has occurred, though pyloric stenosis may result in visible peristalsis.

Biliary pain is more usually in the right upper quadrant. Often there are no abdominal signs, though there is commonly tenderness in the right upper quadrant upon inspiration.

Pancreatitis often produces surprisingly few abdominal signs for the degree of shock.

The conditions that cause abdominal pain, shock and a soft abdomen are:
- Pancreatitis.
- Bowel infarction.
- Dissection of an AAA.
- Referred pain from a myocardial infarction.

Loin pain
The main causes of loin pain are:
- Renal colic.
- Pyelonephritis.
- Musculoskeletal pain.

Right iliac fossa pain
The most important cause of right iliac fossa pain is acute appendicitis, although this is relatively rare. However, the differential diagnosis is wide. Other causes include:
- Gastroenteritis.
- Mesenteric adenitis.
- Ruptured ovarian cyst.
- Acute salpingitis.
- Perforated peptic ulcer.
- Acute cholecystitis.
- Crohn's disease.
- Acute diverticulitis (rarely on the right).
- Renal colic.
- Ectopic pregnancy.

Medical conditions
It is important to remember that medical conditions may present with acute abdominal pain, so a detailed systemic examination is essential. In particular, examine:
- The cardiovascular system. Inferior myocardial infarction or angina occasionally present with predominantly upper abdominal pain.
- The respiratory system. Pneumonia (especially with lower lobar disease) may cause right or left upper quadrant pain. Look for signs of consolidation.
- Diabetic ketoacidosis.

Chronic renal failure

Patients with chronic renal failure often have specific problems, which should always be considered during an assessment. For dialysis patients, consider the following points.

Assess dialysis access
Haemodialysis
Note the presence of the arteriovenous fistula (AVF), its site (e.g. radial, brachial), and the palpable thrill. Look for access sites used and other possible access sites; include goretex graft, shunts, or central venous catheters.

Look specifically for signs of infection (especially with venous catheters).

Peritoneal dialysis
Look at the exit site of the peritoneal dialysis catheter for evidence of tunnel infection or exit site infection. If the patient has reported abdominal symptoms, it is important to inspect the dialysis fluid for turbidity, blood, or cloudiness suggestive of peritonitis.

Assess fluid balance
Fluid overload is a common problem in anuric patients.

Measure the patient's weight at every visit. This is the most sensitive guide to changes in fluid balance on a day to day basis.

Look for other signs of fluid overload such as:
- Raised JVP.
- Peripheral oedema – if the patient has a normal plasma albumin, peripheral oedema usually indicates a fluid overload of approximately 3 kg.

- Uncontrolled hypertension.
- Pulmonary oedema – often a combination of fluid overload and cardiac failure.

Some patients develop symptoms such as lightheadedness, fainting, or malaise towards the end of dialysis. Look for signs of dehydration such as:
- Dry mucous membranes.
- Postural hypotension.

Check lying and standing blood pressure

Most dialysis patients have hypertension and pristine blood pressure control is central to reducing long-term morbidity from cardiac disease. Postural blood pressure assessment is useful for determining fluid balance. Erythropoietin therapy may exacerbate hypertension.

Look for activity of underlying disease

It is important to remember the underlying cause of renal failure as this may cause special problems in management. For example:
- The diabetic patient has a particularly high risk of cardiovascular disease.
- A patient with a vasculitic illness may develop recurrent vasculitis with extrarenal complications (e.g. pulmonary haemorrhage).
- Amyloidosis may progress causing systemic complications.

Perform a full systemic examination

 Do not forget the original disease causing the renal failure!

Renal failure is a multisystem disease, and a full assessment is essential.

Palpable kidneys

It is unusual to be able to palpate normal kidneys in any but very lean patients. If a kidney is palpable, it is necessary to:
- Identify the mass as a kidney.
- Consider the underlying cause.

Identify the mass as a kidney

The right kidney is often palpable in a thin subject; the left is palpable less often. Features of an enlarged palpable kidney include:
- Location in the loin (paracolic gutter).
- It is usually only possible to palpate the lower pole.
- Downward movement on inspiration (the spleen tends to move towards the right iliac fossa).
- Usually resonant to percussion (see spleen or liver, p. 000; it is overlaid by the colon).
- It can be ballotted (almost a pathognomonic sign).
- It may be possible to 'get above' the mass (compare directly with the liver or spleen.

A palpable kidney is rarely confused with any other organ, but it should be clearly differentiated from the spleen on the left and the liver on the right (Fig. 14.25).

Define the characteristics of the kidney

Once the organ has been identified as kidney, define the size, consistency, and shape. Listen over the organ for a bruit, which may be present if there is renal artery stenosis or a tumour.

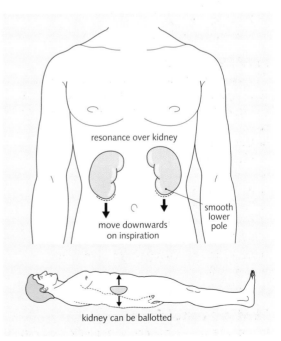

resonance over kidney

smooth lower pole

move downwards on inspiration

kidney can be ballotted

Fig. 14.25 Features of a palpable kidney.

Consider aetiology
Bilateral palpable kidneys
The most common causes of bilaterally palpable kidneys are:
- Polycystic kidneys (the most common cause). The kidneys may be massive. Most other causes result in smooth hemiovoid masses, but occasionally individual cysts may be palpable. Look for an associated polycystic liver, signs of uraemia, or an arteriovenous fistula.
- Bilateral hydronephrosis.
- Amyloidosis. The patient may have a typical facies, hepatosplenomegaly, peripheral neuropathy, or obvious underlying inflammatory disease (e.g. rheumatoid arthritis, chronic osteomyelitis).

Other causes are shown in Fig. 14.26.

Unilateral palpable kidney
The most common causes are similar, but in order of frequency include:
1. Polycystic kidneys.
2. Renal cell carcinoma.
3. Hydronephrosis.
4. Hypertrophy of a single functioning kidney (kidney only just palpable).

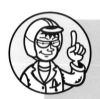

Do not forget to check the urinalysis.
Transplanted kidneys are normally placed in the right iliac fossa.

Fig. 14.26 Causes of single or bilaterally enlarged kidneys.

Causes of enlarged kidneys, single or bilateral	
Causes	**Features**
polycystic kidneys	usually bilateral; large cysts may be individually detected; check blood pressure; note uraemic complications; may detect hepatomegaly
hydronephrosis	unilateral or bilateral; may be tender if acute; check prostate and palpable bladder

malignancy
  Wilms' tumour (child)
  Renal cell carcinoma (hypernephroma)
	look for systemic features of malignancy

miscellaneous
  pyonephrosis
  single cyst
  amyloid
	tender
	usually incidental finding
	rare; look for underlying disease

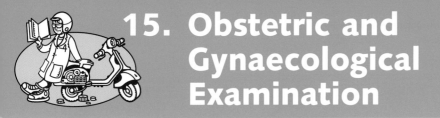
Taking an obstetrics or gynaecology history does not differ from the standard history format outlined in Chapter 2. However, there are some specialist questions that need to asked. It is important to remember that this is a sensitive area for many women who many not feel comfortable discussing this area with medical students, especially male medical students.

The gynaecological history

This should include:

Menstrual history
- Ask about the menarche, and if appropriate the menopause.
- When was the first day of the last menstrual cycle?
- The pattern of bleeding and the length of time between cycles. It is important to remember that the menstrual cycle is from the first day of bleeding to the next first day of bleeding. Try to establish the pattern of bleeding. How many days does this last for, what kind of protection is used, how often does it need to be changed, does the woman ever flood through her protection and does she ever pass clots?
- Ask the patient about menstrual pain: e.g. is the pain before menstruation starts and relieved by it or is menstruation itself painful? Try to determine the severity and what functional impact this has on her life. What analgesics does she use and for how long for? Does she have any other associated cyclical symptoms?

Try and remember at all times what is happening to your patient's hormone level throughout the normal menstrual cycle (Fig. 15.1).

Contraception and sexual history
A contraceptive history should be taken. This should include which methods have been tried and how suitable the women felt they were for her.

If appropriate, you may need to ask about the woman's sexual history. Is she sexually active? Do not make assumptions about her sexuality or sexual orientation. This is a very sensitive area and great care should be taken when asking about sexual history. It is often a good idea to leave this until the end of the interview when you have had the most amount of time to build up a rapport. This should include the number of partners she has had over the past year and the sex of the partners. How often has she had intercourse, and if appropriate whether or not she had dyspareunia. You should also ask if she has had any sexually transmitted diseases.

Smear tests
You should also ask when the patient's last smear test was. Has she been attending a clinic and has she had any abnormal smears? What treatment did she require for these.

Vaginal discharge and continence
Symptoms of any vaginal discharge should be recorded. When does it occur (when during the cycle, post coital or post menopausal), how much is there and its nature (consistency, colour, smell and is there any blood)?

Urinary abnormalities should be asked about: e.g. frequency, nocturia and dysuria. Are there any symptoms of stress incontinence (usually a consequence of lax pelvic muscluature following childbirth) or urge incontinence (usually due to detrusor instability)?

The obstetric history

This is usually a happy time for people, but remember, there may also be a lot of anxiety especially if previous pregnancies have been lost. You should find out about the current pregnancy first.

Ask about the last menstrual period, and then use the wheel to calculate her expected due date.

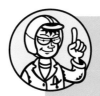

A favourite OSCE question involves working out a woman's date for delivery using the gestational calendar. Find one and practise with it.

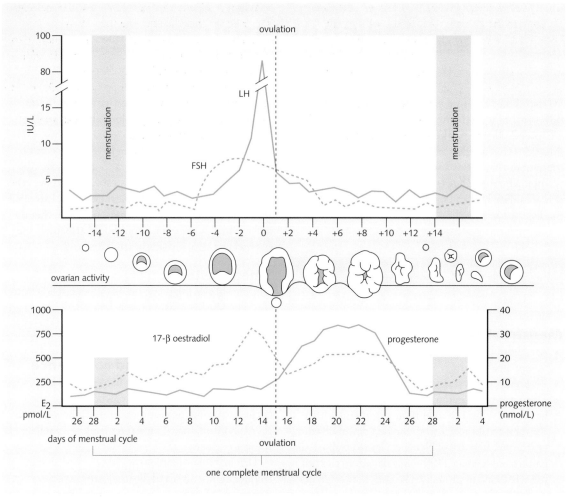

Fig. 15.1 Hormone levels in the normal menstrual cycle. Considerable variations can be found that are still compatible with normal menstrual function.

Was there any difficulty in getting pregnant? Ask if she has had any of the symptoms of pregnancy, e.g. early morning sickness. You may ask about any cravings. Has the mother felt any fetal activity yet?

Previous obstetric history

- How many times has she been pregnant and how many children does she have? This is a delicate way of starting to find out about miscarriages and abortions.
- Are all the children to one father? If not, clarify the paternities.
- When the children were born what was their gestation and did any of them have to go to a special care baby unit?

- Have there been any fetal abnormalities or any postnatal complications?
- During her previous pregnancies has she had any medical problems, e.g. pre-eclampsia or diabetes?
- Were her previous labours difficult (what did she use for analgesia and was this satisfactory)?
- Did she require instrumental deliveries or caesarian sections?
- Has she had any postnatal psychological problems, e.g. postnatal depression.

You should also take a gynaecological history as outlined above.

When asking about medications she is on ask whether or not she is taking folic acid.

It is important to take a family and a social history. Particular attention should be paid to any inherited diseases that run in the family, e.g. cystic fibrosis. It is also useful to know if there is a history of twins in the family. Ask the mother about her marital status. Ask if she is employed how long does she intend to work while pregnant. Is the home suitable for children or will she need to be re-housed? Does she still drink alcohol? If so, how much. Does she smoke? Again, if so how much. The mother should be encouraged to stop or at least cut down smoking and drinking. This is also a good opportunity to find out if the woman is considering breast feeding.

When dealing with pregnant mothers remember that pregnancy is not a disease state. Most pregnancies are uncomplicated and don't require to be medicalized. At times we can become biased in our views of pregnancy because we see and remember the problematic patients. You will need to decide for yourself what you feel about medical interventions in pregnancy and what an appropriate level of medical involvement is.

16. Surgical Examination

Surgery is a rich hunting ground for the OSCE question setter! There are lots of different examinations that you need to be proficient at. Hopefully your course handbooks or study guide will detail which lumps and bumps you should be able to examine. Be aware, not all surgical units will have a full range of surgical specialities so the onus is on you to find a willing middle grade who will help you perfect your examination routine on patients. This chapter details how to examine some surgical pathologies. It should be used in conjunction with hands on bedside teaching.

 Practice makes perfect. In an exam you should look as if you've done this a thousand times before. Practise them with and on your friends.

Lumps in the groin

This is one method that will take you through how to examine a lump in the groin that covers all the salient special tests you will be expected to perform.

First, expose the patient's abdomen. The standard teaching is nipples to knees but umbilicus to knees will normally suffice.

- Look at the patient lying down.
- Can you see any obvious swelling? Where is it, is it superior or inferior to the inguinal ligament, or is it in the scrotum? What colour is it, e.g. is it erythematous.
- Are there any scars from previous surgery?
- If nothing can be seen, then ask the patient to stand. Can you see anything now?

 Remember, God gave us two of most things for easy comparison. Don't forget to check for contralateral pathology in the heat of the moment.

Next define the swelling. Lumps have three dimensions so measure the length, breadth and depth. There is likely to be a measuring tape located at the bedside, so use it. Now you have its size define the shape of it.

- Is the lump fluctuant and can you transilluminate it? When you feel it, does it extend beyond the obvious skin markings?
- Test the lump for a cough impulse. Place your hand over the swelling and ask patient to cough. Does the swelling get worse?

Ask the patient to reduce the swelling themselves. Put pressure over the deep inguinal ring (half way between the pubic tubercle and the anterior superior iliac spine) and ask the patient to cough. If a swelling appears medial to the pressure then it's a direct hernia. Release the pressure and ask the patient to cough again if the hernia appears now, it is an indirect hernia (Fig. 16.1).

Next check the other side for any similar defects.

Ask the examiner if you may now proceed to examine the abdomen and scrotum. You will probably be told you've done enough, so cover the patient up and wash your hands!

Differential diagnosis of groin swellings
Above the inguinal ligament

- Sebaceous cyst, lipoma.
- Direct/Indirect inguinal hernia.
- Imperfectly descended testis.

Below the inguinal ligament

- Sebaceous cyst, lipoma, lymph nodes.
- Femoral hernia.
- Saphena varix (dilation of the saphenous vein at the confluence with the femoral vein).
- Femoral aneurysm (expansile pulsation, bruit, not compressable with no cough impulse).
- Imperfectly descended testis.
- Psoas abscess (rare).

Alternatively think of the mass in terms of structure as in Fig. 16.2

incorrect

correct

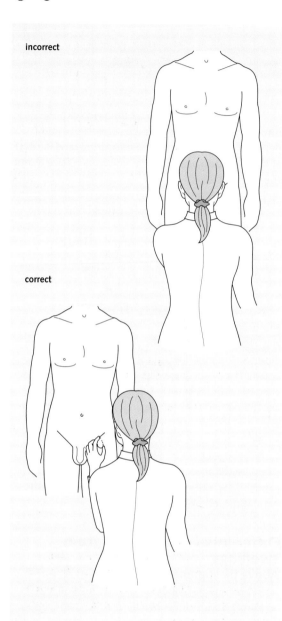

Fig. 16.1 Examination of a hernia. If examining a swelling stand at the patient's side. Try to imagine what it will look as if you're doing if you don't!

Differential diagnoses of lumps in the groin	
hernias	inguinal/femoral
vascular	saphena varix/femoral aneurysm
lymph nodes	lymphadenopathy (infection/neoplasm/lymphoma)
muscles	psoas abscess
testicular	ectopic testes
skin/subcutaneous	lipoma/sebaceous cyst

Fig. 16.2 Differential diagnoses of lumps in the groin

Examination

Observe the swelling from the anterior and posterior aspects of the scrotum. Define its size, shape and note the skin colour.

Gently palpate the swelling. This is best achieved by rolling the testes between the thumb and finger. Find and feel the epididymis and feel the spermatic cord.

Try to assess the swelling. What is its size, shape, fluctuance and does it transilluminate? There ought

It is hoped this will avoid the situation where a female student asked a registrar how to do this and the reply was 'Just do what you normally do'.

to be a light at the bed side of these patients. Can the upper edge of the mass be felt (e.g. can you get above it) and is it separate from the testes?

Your differential should run along these lines:

- Cystic, testicular and not usually tender: hydrocele (Fig. 16.3A).
- Cystic, separate and not usually tender: epididymal cyst (Fig. 16.3B).
- Solid and testicular: tumour, orchitis (very tender), granuloma, gumma (Fig. 16.3C).
- Solid, separate and usually tender: chronic epididymitis (Fig. 16.3D).

Scrotal swellings

You are unlikely to be able to practise this on your friends! However, a sock, two kiwi fruits and a banana make a passable scrotum for practice purposes.

Peripheral vascular disease

Arteriopaths are challenging patients to examine. They will have multiple medical problems all of

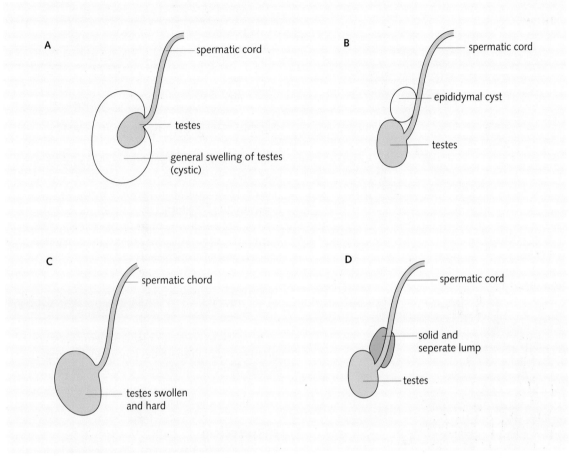

Fig. 16.3 Differential diagnoses of scrotal swellings.

which will need to be investigated. This is an approach to examing their limbs.

Expose both legs completely, whilst preserving the patient's dignity, this includes taking their socks off. If they have a dressing on this should be taken down and the underlying wound inspected. You should have a nurse along to help you if this needs to be done.

Inspect both legs and feet for:

- The colour of the skin. Is it white, red or black? Each is associated with differing degrees of vascular insufficiency.
- Trophic changes, e.g. is the skin smooth and shiny, is there loss of hair (note where this occurs) or wasting of subcutaneous tissue. Careful note should be made of any ulcers. If there is an ulcer present this should be examined. Please see p. 145 for how to do this.
- Look specifically at the pressure points in the limb for ulcers. Pay special attention to the lateral

aspect of the foot, the head of the 1st metatarsophalangeal, the heel and malleoli.
- Finally, inspect the tips of the toes and between the toes. Patients are often immobile and will be unable to care for their feet. A small lesion here can rapidly progress.

Palpate both legs for:

- Feel both legs for a difference in temperature. Note the level of any temperature change.
- Count the capillary refill time in both feet or stumps (to do this press on the nail bed for 5 seconds and count. The capillary refill should be less than 2 seconds).
- Feel for all the pulses in the legs (femoral, popliteal, dorsalis pedis and posterior tibial). Classify the pulse as normal, diminished or absent. Figure 16.4 shows the arterial tree of the lower limb (this is much loved of examiners).

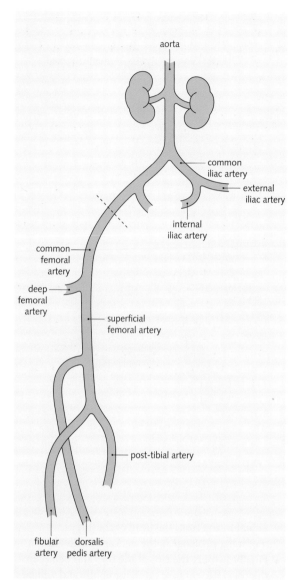

Fig. 16.4 The arterial tree of the lower limb.

Ascultate and listen along the major vessels for arterial bruits.

Special tests

Elevate the leg to 15° and look for venous guttering. Keep elevating the leg until it becomes white (ischaemic) and note the angle. This is known as Buerger's angle and is normally >90°. From this elevated position lower the leg over the side of the bed and look for reactive hyperaemia (this is Buerger's test).

There will often be a Doppler ultrasound probe around (especially in examinations). This is used to measure the ankle/brachial pressure index. Take a

ABPI	Significance
1–1.2	Normal
0.8	Claudication pain
0.4	Rest pain
<0.4	Ulceration and gangrene

Fig. 16.5 Ankle/brachial pressure index (ABPI).

blood pressure in the ankle with the Doppler probe and a brachial blood pressure with the Doppler probe. Divide the ankle pressure by the brachial pressure to give a ratio (Fig. 16.5).

You should also examine the patient's cardiovascular system for other signs of arterial disease and an aortic aneurysm.

Varicose veins

Varicose veins are a common problem. They are often found in outpatient clinics and day surgery wards. They are often good examination candidates as well. When asked to examine a patient's varicose veins follow the usual pattern.

Inspection

Keep the patient decent and expose both legs with the patient standing up. Observe the patient's legs and the distribution of the varicose veins. Note the nutritional state of the patient's legs (especially the area superior to the medial malleolus) you should also look for any eczematous changes, pigmentation and varicose ulcers.

Palpation

Palpate and compare both legs. Is there a difference in temperature? Is the patient tender over the medial aspect of the lower leg? You should specifically palpate the ankle for dermatoliposclerosis. Is there ankle oedema? These signs give an indication of the chronicity of the problem.

Specific tests

There are some special tests that you should perform when examining someone's varicose veins.

Feel the saphenofemoral junction (4 cm inferior and lateral to the pubic tubercule – NB, remember Fig 16.2). Is there a swelling here? If so, it is likely to be a saphena varix. With your fingers on the saphenofemoral junction ask the patient to cough, if you feel an impulse it is suggestive of venous incompetence. Last, perform the percussion test. Tap the top of the vein and feel below for an impulse, if one is present it is suggestive of superficial veinous incompetence.

You should now ask the patient to lie down and elevate the leg to empty the veins. Place two fingers on the saphenofemoral junction and ask the patient to stand. As you are doing this carefully observe the leg. If the veins rapidly fill then the lower leg perforators are incompetent. Now release your fingers. If there is rapid filling of the leg then there is an incompetent saphenofemoral valve.

The school of perfection says that you should auscultate over the veins for bruits in case there is an AV malformation.

To conclude your examination you should examine the abdomen for any masses. If you are suspicious of an obstruction a per rectum should be done. It is rare to do this in practice.

Examination of an ulcer

An ulcer is a break in the continuity of an epithelial surface. Ulcers are associated with a number of conditions, some of which have been discussed above. At some point in your career someone will present you with an ulcer and ask your opinion about it. It helps to have a system to help you describe it.

Inspection

Take off all of the dressing and gently clean off any topical applications. Expose the whole ulcer completely. Inspect the ulcer noting:

- Its position, size and shape.
- The base (colour, penetration of underlying structures e.g. tendon/bone).
- Any discharge from the ulcer (blood, pus or serous fluid).
- Measure the depth of the ulcer in mm.
- Inspect the edge (Fig 16.6).
- Feel the surrounding tissues for any tenderness or temperature changes.
- Note the nutrition of surrounding tissue and check for regional lymph nodes.
- You should also make an assessment of the neurovascular supply to the area, e.g. sensation and muscle power.

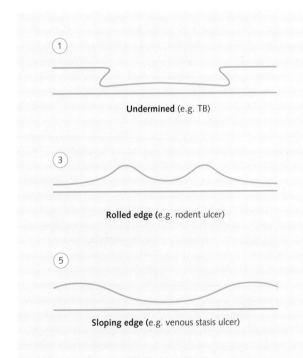

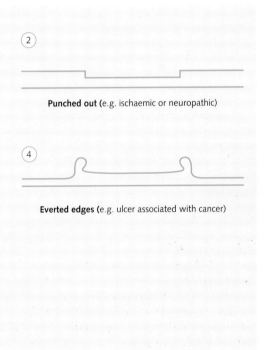

Fig. 16.6 Classification of an ulcer.

17. Neurological Examination

Examination routine

The neurological examination is often considered to be the most difficult part of the examination by students and is most commonly omitted or performed badly. In a full routine assessment, it is essential to perform at least a basic neurological assessment. This need not take more than a few minutes, but provides essential information.

More than in any other system, it is vital to be systematic, objective, and methodical, and to be aware of the pathological significance of any elicited sign. It is essential to record exactly what has been assessed rather than putting meaningless phrases (e.g. 'CNS – tick'). Interpretation of neurological conditions often relies on changes of neurological signs with time, highlighting the need to ensure accuracy when writing up the medical record.

Cranial nerves

It is important to understand the basic anatomy and function of the individual cranial nerves when interpreting physical findings. For each cranial nerve, function, anatomy, examination routine, and interpretation of the physical signs will be considered.

Olfactory nerve (cranial nerve I)
Function
The olfactory nerve is a sensory nerve conveying the sense of smell.

Anatomy
Nerve fibres pass from sensory receptors in the nasal cavity through the cribriform plate to the olfactory bulb, where they synapse, and then pass towards the anterior perforated substance.

Examination
Ask patients whether they have noticed any change in their sense of smell. Test smell in each nostril separately using a sniff test. Use common, easily recognizable, non-irritant substances (e.g. vanilla, orange, coffee).

Interpretation
It is relatively unusual to detect lesions of the olfactory nerve on physical examination. Formal testing is rarely needed unless a lesion of the anterior cranial fossa is suspected. If a lesion is detected, note the following:
- Anosmia is usually due to nasal rather than neurological disease.
- The olfactory nerve is vulnerable as it passes through the cribriform plate, especially if there is a head injury. Also consider frontal lobe tumours and meningitis (infective or neoplastic).

Optic nerve (cranial nerve II)
Function
The optic nerve is a sensory nerve conveying the sense of vision from the retina.

Anatomy
The optic nerve leaves the eye via the optic foramen, partially decussates at the optic chiasm, and synapses at the lateral geniculate nucleus. Secondary fibres pass to the occipital cortex via the optic radiation (see 'Interpretation' below).

Examination
Visual acuity. Assess distant and near vision formally using Snellen and Jaeger charts allowing patients to wear their spectacles, or crudely at the bedside (e.g. count fingers from 2 metres or read newsprint) for each eye.

Visual fields. Test by confrontation. Sit opposite the patient so that you are approximately 1 metre apart at the same level. Both of you then cover one eye, and you bring a test object (traditionally a white hat pin, but in the clinic other objects may need to be substituted, e.g. a pen top) into the field of vision from each quadrant midway between yourself and the patient. The patient states when he or she first sees the object, and you can then compare the patient's visual field directly with yours.

Pupillary reflexes. These are discussed under oculomotor nerve (see p. 148).

Fundoscopy. See Chapter 22, p. 201 for detail.

Interpretation
Visual field defects should be correlated with the anatomical site of the lesion. It is helpful to understand the visual pathway (Fig. 17.1).

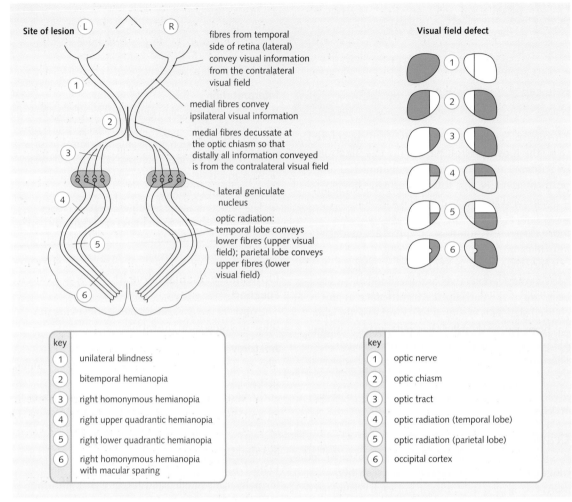

Site of lesion   L   R

fibres from temporal
side of retina (lateral)
convey visual information
from the contralateral
visual field

medial fibres convey
ipsilateral visual information

medial fibres decussate at
the optic chiasm so that
distally all information conveyed
is from the contralateral visual field

lateral geniculate
nucleus

optic radiation:
temporal lobe conveys
lower fibres (upper visual
field); parietal lobe conveys
upper fibres (lower
visual field)

Visual field defect

key	
1	unilateral blindness
2	bitemporal hemianopia
3	right homonymous hemianopia
4	right upper quadrantic hemianopia
5	right lower quadrantic hemianopia
6	right homonymous hemianopia with macular sparing

key	
1	optic nerve
2	optic chiasm
3	optic tract
4	optic radiation (temporal lobe)
5	optic radiation (parietal lobe)
6	occipital cortex

Fig. 17.1   The visual pathway. Lesions at different parts of the pathway produce characteristic field defects.

Oculomotor, trochlear, and abducens nerves (cranial nerves III, IV, VI)

Function

The oculomotor, trochlear and abducens nerves are considered together as they supply the extraocular muscles (Fig. 17.2). The oculomotor nerve also supplies levator palpebrae superioris, which opens the upper eyelid. In addition, it also has parasympathetic fibres supplying the sphincter pupillae (constricts the pupil) and the ciliary muscle of lens.

Anatomy

The oculomotor nucleus lies in the midbrain. It passes close to the posterior communicating artery before entering the lateral wall of the cavernous sinus on the way to the orbit.

The trochlear nucleus lies lower in the midbrain. Fibres pass dorsally, decussate, pass around the

Nerve supply and movement produced by the extraocular muscles

Nerve	Muscle	Movement
oculomotor	medial rectus	adduction
	inferior rectus	inferior movement (especially when eye abducted)
	superior rectus	superior movement
	inferior oblique	superior movement (especially when eye adducted)
trochlear	superior oblique	inferior movement (especially when eye adducted)
abducens	lateral rectus	abduction

Fig. 17.2   Nerve supply and movement produced by the extraocular muscles.

midbrain, and enter the lateral wall of the cavernous sinus.

The abducens nerve originates close to the facial nerve in the pons, emerges in the cerebellopontine angle and has a very long intracranial course, passing over the petrous temporal bone on the way to the cavernous sinus.

Examination

Inspection. Look at the eyelids for ptosis, and symmetry.

Pupils. Look at pupil size and symmetry. Test the pupillary reflex by shining light on the pupil from the side, looking at both the direct and consensual response.

Ocular movements. Observe the patient following a target up, down, to either side, and for convergence. Note diplopia or nystagmus.

Interpretation

When interpreting physical signs, note the following:
- Ptosis (Fig. 17.3).
- Abnormal pupillary reflexes. The afferent limb is from the optic nerve, the efferent pathway is via the oculomotor nerve. An intact consensual reflex with an absent direct reflex implies a lesion of the IIIrd nerve. Conversely, pupil constriction only when light is shone into the opposite eye implies a sensory deficit.
- Holmes–Adie pupil. This is common in normal women. The pupil is large with an absent light reflex and delayed accommodation reflex, which is sustained. It is often associated with absent ankle reflexes.
- Nystagmus. This may be due to visual disturbances or lesions of the labyrinth, cerebellum, brainstem, or central vestibular connections. See Nystagmus section.
- VIth nerve palsy (loss of eye abduction). This is often a false localizing sign. The VIth nerve has a very long intracranial course and is vulnerable to compression as it passes over the petrous temporal bone. Any pathology causing raised intracranial pressure may result in a VIth nerve palsy.
- VIth nerve lesions may be due to a lesion in the pons or cerebellopontine angle. This often occurs in association with a VIIth (or VIIIth) nerve palsy and may result in contralateral pyramidal tract signs.
- IVth nerve palsy. This rarely occurs in isolation. Orbital trauma often damages the tendon causing muscular weakness.

Nystagmus

Nystagmus often causes anxiety in the exam candidate, however, it is relatively simple to describe. It is caused by posterior fossa disease or ear pathology.

First, which eye is the nystagmus most obvious in? Second, is the nystagmus greater when looking to the affected side (e.g. present in the right eye and worse when looking right). This is the most common situation. Nystagmus is caused by:
- Contralateral vestibular lesion (associated with vertigo and deafness).
- Multiple sclerosis.
- Middle ear surgery.
- Meniere's disease.

Fig. 17.3 Causes of ptosis. CVA, cerebrovascular accident.

Causes of ptosis	
Cause	**Examples**
third nerve palsy complete ptosis, associated with widely dilated pupil, and eye paralysed with outward and downward deviation	posterior communicating artery aneurysm 'coning' of the temporal lobe mononeuritis multiplex (e.g. due to diabetes mellitus, vasculitis) midbrain lesion
Horner's syndrome loss of sympathetic supply to eye, partial ptosis, pupillary constriction, enophthalmos and decreased sweating on affected side	brain lesion (e.g. CVA lateral medullary syndrome); cervical cord lesion (e.g. syringomyelia) T1 root lesion (e.g. apical lung cancer, cervical rib) sympathetic chain lesion (e.g. neoplasia)
neuromuscular disease	myasthenia gravis botulism
myogenic	senile degenerative changes dystrophia myotonica

- Ipsilateral cerebellar lesion (associated with other cerebellar signs).
- Neoplasia.
- Cerebrovascular accident (CVA).
- Ipsilateral brainstem lesion. These can be infective, vascular (the most likely), neoplastic or demyelinating in origin.

If the patient has vertical nystagmus this implies a central lesion. If it is down gaze consider pathologies around the foramen magnum. If it is up gaze the lesion will be around the superior colliculus.

 Sixth nerve palsy is commonly a false localizing sign and results from raised intracranial pressure.

Trigeminal nerve (cranial nerve V)
Function
The trigeminal nerve conveys sensory and motor nerve fibres. The main functions are:
- Sensory – somatic sensation to the face.
- Motor – muscles of mastication (masseters, temporalis, pterygoids).

Anatomy
The trigeminal nerve is split into the following three divisions (Fig. 17.4):
- Ophthalmic.
- Maxillary.
- Mandibular.

The trigeminal ganglion lies near the pons. The nerve fibres pass near the medial lemniscus to the thalamus.

Examination
Sensory. Test modalities of sensation over the three distributions of the nerve (e.g. forehead, cheeks, chin) bilaterally.

Corneal reflex. Lightly touch the cornea with cotton wool, approaching from the side, and observe a brisk contraction of orbicularis oris (blinking).

Motor. Inspect for wasting of temporalis and masseter. Test jaw opening against resistance (unilateral pterygoid weakness will cause the jaw to deviate to the side of the weakness).

Jaw jerk. This is often difficult to interpret.

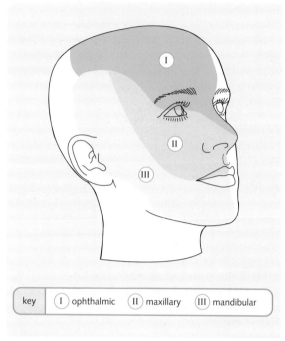

key (I) ophthalmic (II) maxillary (III) mandibular

Fig. 17.4 Dermatomes of the three divisions of the trigeminal nerve.

Interpretation
When examining the Vth nerve, note the following points:
- An absent corneal reflex may be the first sign of ophthalmic herpes. Lesions of the Vth and VIIth nerves can be distinguished by comparing the contralateral responses. The afferent limb is from the Vth nerve, the efferent limb is provided by the facial nerve, and is usually bilateral.
- Central lesions are often associated with other localizing signs (e.g. first division in association with IIIrd, IVth and VIth nerve in the cavernous sinus; cerebellopontine angle lesions).
- Sensory lesions are much more common than motor lesions.

Facial nerve (cranial nerve VII)
Function
The facial nerve is primarily a motor nerve, but conveys fibres of three different modalities:
- Motor – to muscles of facial expression.
- Parasympathetic – to lacrimal, submaxillary, and sublingual glands.
- Sensory – taste for the anterior two-thirds of the tongue and an insignificant part of the external ear.

Anatomy

The motor nucleus lies in the pons close to the VIth nerve. It emerges in the cerebellopontine angle and enters the internal auditory meatus with the VIIIth nerve, giving off the nerve to stapedius and chorda tympani (taste) before emerging through the stylomastoid foramen and passing peripherally through the parotid gland, giving off various branches.

Examination

Inspection. Inspect the face for:
- Asymmetry (e.g. loss of nasolabial fold, drooping and dribbling from corner of mouth, weak smile).
- Facial expression.
- Involuntary movements.

Muscle strength. Examine the individual muscles. The lower face may be assessed by smiling, whistling, pursing lips; the upper face by closure of eyes, elevation of eyebrows, frowning.

Taste. Taste is rarely formally tested.

Interpretation

By far the most important component of the facial nerve is motor. Upper motor neuron (UMN) lesions often result in relative preservation of movements of the upper face due to crossed innervation (Fig. 17.5). In addition, emotional expression may be preserved. Lower motor neuron (LMN) VIIth nerve lesions do not spare the muscles around the eyes. The site of the lesion can often be localized, for example to the:
- Pons – for example due to a CVA; associated with VIth nerve lesion and contralateral pyramidal tract signs.
- Cerebellopontine angle – for example due to an acoustic neuroma; associated with lesions of the VIth, VIIth, and VIIIth nerves as well as cerebellar ataxia.
- Facial canal – for example due to Bell's palsy, herpes zoster; associated with loss of taste and hyperacusis as well as muscles of facial expression.
- Parotid gland – for example due to sarcoidosis, parotid tumour; individual facial muscles may be affected.

Vestibulocochlear nerve (cranial nerve VIII)
Function

The vestibulocochlear nerve is a sensory nerve. It has two primary functions:
- Auditory – sense of hearing.
- Labyrinthine – sense of balance.

Anatomy

Auditory. Sensory fibres from the cochlea enter the cerebellopontine angle in association with the facial nerve, synapse in the lower pons, and ascend in the lateral lemnisci.

Vestibular. Fibres pass with the auditory division, but synapse in the vestibular nucleus in the medulla, from which there are connections to the cerebellum, extraocular muscles, and higher centres.

Examination

Auditory. Crude assessment can be made for each ear (e.g. 'can hear whispered voice'). If a defect is found, conductive or sensory deficits may be identified using tuning fork tests (Fig. 17.6) as follows:
- Rinne's test – using a 256 Hz tuning fork, compare subjective loudness when it is

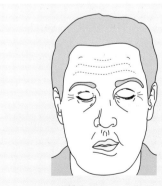
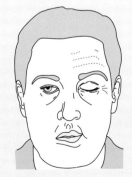
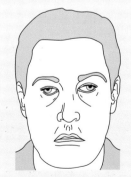

Right UMN weakness **Right LMN weakness** **Bilateral LMN weakness**

Fig. 17.5 Facial weakness. Patients are asked to close their eyes and purse their lips. Note the failed eye closure in lower motor neuron (LMN) lesions and the nasolabial fold with drooping mouth in both upper motor neuron (UMN) and LMN lesions.

151

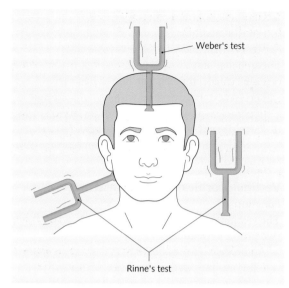

Fig. 17.6 Tuning fork tests. The tuning fork is placed on the vertex of the head in Weber's test. In Rinne's test a tuning fork is struck and placed close to the external ear or rested on the mastoid process.

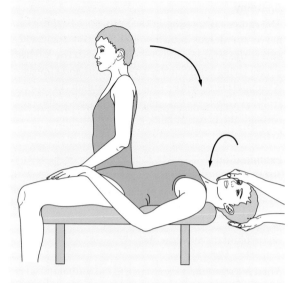

Fig. 17.7 Hallpike's manoeuvre for testing positional nystagmus.

presented close to the external auditory meatus and when the base is applied to the mastoid – a positive test (normal) occurs if the former appears louder.

- Weber's test – apply the base of the tuning fork to the middle of the forehead and ask the patient whether he or she hears the sound in the midline or to one side – the test is abnormal if the sound is lateralized.

Vestibular. This function is not routinely tested. Positional nystagmus can be observed by holding the patient's head over the end of the examination couch and then fully extending and turning it with the eyes open. This test is called Hallpike's manoeuvre (Fig. 17.7).

Interpretation

If hearing loss is identified, try to identify the underlying cause. Note that:

- Tuning fork tests are useful for identifying the hearing deficit as primarily conductive or sensory in origin (Fig. 17.8).
- Deafness is commonly conductive (e.g. due to otitis media, ear wax).
- Sensory deafness can be further defined by formal audiometry to ascertain the frequency of loss.

Vertigo is most commonly peripheral. Central lesions (e.g. cerebellar lesions) are not associated with deafness or tinnitus, but are often associated with pronounced ataxia between the episodes of vertigo and persistent nystagmus.

Glossopharyngeal nerve (cranial nerve IX)
Function

The glossopharyngeal nerve has three functions:
- Sensory – taste for the posterior two-thirds of tongue, most of oropharynx, and soft palate.
- Parasympathetic.
- Motor – to stylopharyngeus.

Fig. 17.8 Assessment of tuning fork tests.

Assessment of tuning fork tests			
Condition	Rinne's (left ear)	Rinne's (right ear)	Weber's
normal hearing	positive	positive	heard in midline
conductive deficit in right ear	positive	negative	heard on right side
sensory deficit in right ear	positive	positive	heard on left side

Anatomy

The motor and sensory nuclei lie in the medulla. The nerve leaves the skull with the Xth and XIth nerves at the jugular foramen.

Examination

Gag reflex. Ask the patient to say 'aah' with his or her mouth open and observe palatal movement. Touch the posterior wall of the oropharynx with an orange stick. This elicits constriction and elevation. If there is no response, ask the patient whether he or she felt the stimulus. The presence or absence of the gag reflex does not correlate with whether a patient has a safe swallow reflex after a CVA.

Interpretation

The gag reflex is unpleasant, and should only be performed if a lesion of the IXth or Xth nerves is suspected.

The afferent limb is via the IXth nerve, the efferent from the Xth.

Vagus nerve (cranial nerve X)
Function

The vagus nerve supplies innervation to the viscera in the thorax and foregut as well as having smaller motor and sensory functions. The main functions are:

- Parasympathetic – visceral innervation to heart, lungs, foregut.
- Motor – to larynx, soft palate, pharynx.
- Sensory – for dura mater of the posterior cranial fossa, small part of the external ear.

Anatomy
The nucleus lies in the medulla.

Examination
Speech. Listen for dysphonia or a bovine cough associated with recurrent laryngeal nerve palsy.

Soft palate. Observe the uvula. In a unilateral lesion, it will droop away from the lesion.

Gag reflex. See above for glossopharyngeal nerve.

Interpretation
In the presence of dysphonia, the vocal cords should be examined.

Accessory (spinal accessory) nerve (cranial nerve XI)
Function
The spinal accessory nerve is a motor nerve supplying the sternomastoid and trapezius muscles.

Anatomy
The anterior horn cells of the cervical cord innervate these muscles, but fibres pass up to the medulla before descending again through the jugular foramen.

Examination
Test the bulk and power of sternomastoid. Ask patients to:
- Force their chin downwards against the resistance of your hand (bilateral).
- Turn chin to one side against resistance (unilateral weakness affects turning to the opposite side).

The power of trapezius can be tested by asking patients to shrug their shoulders against resistance.

Hypoglossal nerve (cranial nerve XII)
Function
The hypoglossal nerve is a motor nerve supplying innervation to the muscles of the tongue.

Anatomy
The nucleus is in the medulla.

Examination
Inspection. Look at the tongue for wasting and fasciculation.

Protrusion. Ask patients to protrude their tongue. If there is a unilateral lesion, the tongue will deviate towards the side of the lesion.

Motor system

When examining the motor system, the aim is to:
- Identify any lesions.
- Ascertain whether the lesion is an UMN or LMN lesion.
- Locate the anatomical site of the lesion.
- Consider the differential diagnosis of lesions at that site.

The fundamental distinction is between UMN (above the anterior horn cells) and LMN lesions (Fig. 17.9).

The examination should follow a strict routine of:
- Inspection.
- Palpation.

Features of UMN and LMN lesions	
UMN	**LMN**
no muscle wasting (but there may be disuse atrophy)	wasting
increased tone ('clasp-knife')	flaccid
weakness of characteristic distribution	marked weakness
hyperreflexia	depressed or absent reflex
abnormal plantar response	normal plantar response
no fasciculation	fasciculation

Fig. 17.9 Features of upper motor neuron (UMN) and lower motor neuron (LMN) lesions.

- Assessment of muscular tone.
- Assessment of power.
- Assessment of tendon reflexes.
- Assessment of coordination.
- Assessment of gait.

Inspection

Inspection should begin as the patient enters the examination room. Note posture, gait, coordination, abnormal movements, etc. The patient should be fully exposed on the examination couch so that individual muscle groups can be observed. Inspect specifically for:

- Wasting – note symmetry; look specifically for distribution (e.g. proximal wasting).
- Fasciculation (spontaneous contraction of small groups of muscle fibres) – usually implies a LMN lesion (e.g. motor neuron disease).
- Tremors – note whether coarse and whether a resting tremor or an intention tremor.

Palpation

Palpate the muscle groups, specifically noting:
- Muscle bulk.
- Tenderness (e.g. myositis).

Assessment of muscular tone

Normally, there is a limited resistance through the range of movement.

 When assessing muscular tone it is essential that the patient is properly relaxed and lying in a neutral position.

If increased tone is suspected, attempt to elicit clonus (Fig. 17.10). Assessment of tone is subjective and requires experience, but specifically consider:

- Hypertonia – for example 'clasp-knife' (high resistance to initial movement and then sudden release; characteristic of UMN lesions), 'lead-pipe rigidity' (resistance through the range of movement; in Parkinson's disease this in combination with the tremor produces 'cogwheel rigidity').
- Hypotonia – for example due to LMN and cerebellar lesions.

Assessment of power

Individual muscle groups should be tested to assess power. When testing, patients should be at a slight mechanical advantage so that if they have normal power, they can just overcome the resistance of the examiner. Muscle strength can be classified according to the Medical Research Council (MRC) grade (Fig. 17.11).

It is usually sufficient to test:
- Movements of the neck.
- Shoulder abduction and adduction.
- Movements of the elbows, wrists, and hands.
- Movements of the hips, knees, and ankle.

When detecting a weakness, it should be categorized as either UMN or LMN. If classified as LMN, the physical signs should be integrated to identify the lesion anatomically (Fig. 17.12).

When testing each muscle group, always consider:
- The myotome.
- The peripheral nerve supplying the muscles.

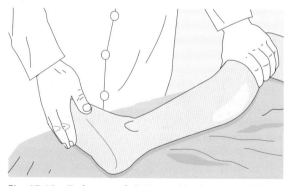

Fig. 17.10 Technique of eliciting ankle clonus. Bend the patient's knee slightly, supporting it with one hand. Grasp the forefoot with the other hand and suddenly dorsiflex the foot. Clonus is made up of regular oscillations of the foot. Sustained (>4 beats) clonus indicates an upper motor neuron (UMN) lesion. One or two beats is normal.

MRC Classification of muscle power	
Grade	MRC grade of muscle strength
0	no movement
1	flicker of movement visible
2	movement possible with gravity eliminated
3	movement possible against gravity, but not resistance
4	movement possible against resistance, but weakened (often subdivided to 4–, 4, 4+)
5	normal power

Fig. 17.11 Medical Research Council (MRC) classification of muscle power.

The major movements in the upper and lower limb are illustrated in Figs 17.13 and 17.14. It is essential to be systematic if a weakness is identified, so that the pattern of involvement can be recognized as corresponding to a nerve root, peripheral nerve, or an individual muscle group (Fig. 17.15). This can be correlated with the other features of the examination of the peripheral nervous system.

Specific tests for the more common peripheral neuropathies are considered later.

Assessment of tendon reflexes

The reflexes should be elicited using a tendon hammer. Compare the relative responses, both against normality and with each side. Make a note of the response – whether it appears normal, brisk, or reduced. If no response is obtained, try methods to reinforce the reflex. For example ask patients to clench their teeth or hook their fingers around each other and try to separate their hands without disentangling their fingers (Fig. 17.16). The nerve roots of the more commonly elicited reflexes are listed in Fig. 17.17 and the reflex arc is shown in Fig. 17.18.

Disruption of the reflex may be due to a lesion at the level of the:

- Peripheral nerves (peripheral neuropathy). Typically the reflex is depressed early in the course of the pathology.
- Spinal cord.
- Neuromuscular junction.
- Muscle (myopathy). The reflex is usually retained until late in the natural history of the disease.

Assessment of coordination

Coordination in the upper limb is tested by the finger–nose test. Hold a finger at arm's length from patients and then ask them to rapidly touch the tip of their nose, and then the tip of your finger with their index finger. The smoothness and accuracy of the movements should be interpreted and put into context with any muscle weakness.

Fig. 17.12 It is usually possible to localize a lower motor neuron (LMN) lesion as originating in the spinal cord, nerve root, peripheral nerve, neuromuscular junction, or muscle.

Features of LMN lesions originating in the spinal cord, nerve root, peripheral nerve, neuromuscular junction, and muscle		
Location of lesion	Examples	Features
anterior horn cells	motor neuron disease; polio	usually symmetrical; no myotome/nerve root distribution; often distal initially; no sensory involvement
nerve root (radiculopathy)	nerve root compression	distribution of affected muscles according to myotome; may have associated dermatomal sensory loss
peripheral nerve (neuropathy)	carpal tunnel	weakness according to nerve supply of affected nerve; usually associated sensory loss; early loss of reflexes
neuromuscular junction	myasthenia gravis	loss of power fluctuating in severity; not in distribution of peripheral nerve or myotome
muscle (myopathy)	n.a.	often has characteristic distribution of a particular disease; reflexes may be preserved early in disease; no sensory loss

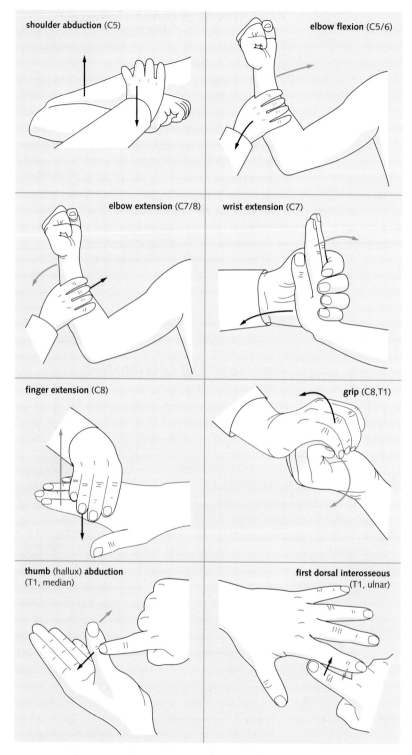

shoulder abduction (C5)

elbow flexion (C5/6)

elbow extension (C7/8)

wrist extension (C7)

finger extension (C8)

grip (C8,T1)

thumb (hallux) abduction
(T1, median)

first dorsal interosseous
(T1, ulnar)

Fig. 17.13 The major muscle groups tested in an assessment of power in the upper limb. Patients should be at a slight mechanical advantage so that they can just overcome the resistance offered by the examiner.

The lower limbs may be assessed by the heel–shin test. Ask patients to place their right heel on their left shin and to slide it down and up the shin, and then to repeat the test using the left heel.

If there is an intention tremor or dysmetria (irregular error in the distance and force of limb movements), cerebellar pathologies can be investigated by looking for dysdiadochokinesis. Ask patients to rapidly slap one palm with the other

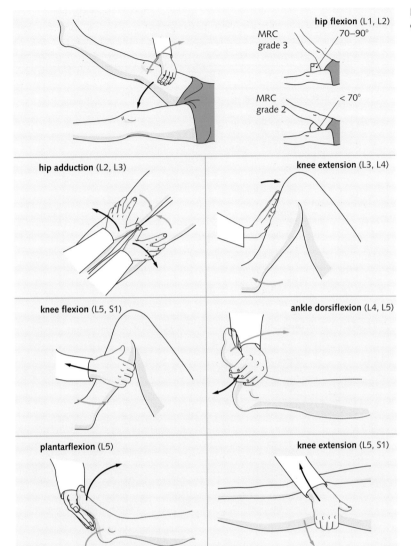

Fig. 17.14 Testing muscle groups of the lower limb.

hand alternating between the palm and back of the hand.

Assessment of gait

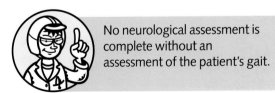

No neurological assessment is complete without an assessment of the patient's gait.

At a basic level, gait should be assessed as the patient walks into the examination room. Certain gaits are characteristic of certain pathologies. For example:

- Spastic gait – the extensor muscles are stiff and the foot is plantarflexed so patients have a stiff gait and avoid catching their toes on the ground by circumducting the leg at the hips.
- Ataxia – the gait is wide-based and there is also marked clumsiness when patients are asked to walk in a straight line placing their heel immediately in front of the toe of the opposite foot (e.g. in cerebellar ataxia).
- High-stepping gait – in patients with foot drop, the foot is lifted high off the ground and then slapped back down.
- Parkinsonism – the gait is slow and shuffling and there is no associated arm swinging; patients often find it difficult to stop and turn around.

Nerve roots, peripheral nerves, and muscles responsible for each movement			
Movement	**Myotome**	**Peripheral nerve**	**Main muscle groups**
shoulder abduction	C5,6	axillary	deltoid
shoulder adduction	C5,6,7,8	lateral pectoral, thoracodorsal	pectoralis major, latissimus dorsi
elbow flexion	C5,6	musculocutaneous	biceps
elbow extension	C6,7,8	radial	triceps
wrist extension	C7,8	radial	long extensors
wrist flexion	C8	ulnar and median	long flexors
pronation	C6,7	median	pronator teres, pronator quadratus
supination	C6,7	musculocutaneous, radial	biceps, supinator
finger abduction	T1	ulnar	dorsal interossei
finger adduction	T1	ulnar	
opposition of thumb	T1	median	opponens pollicis
extension of thumb at the interphalangeal joint	T1	radial	extensor pollicis longus
hip extension	L4,5	inferior gluteal	glutei
hip flexion	L2,3	femoral	iliopsoas
knee flexion	L5, S1	sciatic	hamstrings
knee extension	L2,3,4	femoral	quadriceps
dorsiflexion of foot	L4,5	peroneal	tibialis anterior, long extensors, peroneus, extensor digitorum brevis
plantar flexion of foot	S1,2	tibial	gastrocnemius, tibialis posterior
inversion of ankle	L4	peroneal, tibial	tibialis anterior, tibialis posterior
eversion of ankle	S1	peroneal	peronei, long extensors, extensor digitorum brevis
extension of great toe	L4,5, S1	deep peroneal	extensor hallucis longus

Fig. 17.15 Nerve root, peripheral nerve, and muscle responsible for each movement. By integrating the pattern of weakness, it should be possible to recognize a pattern corresponding to these anatomical subdivisions.

- Waddling gait – for example due to proximal myopathy.

Sensory system

Patients are usually aware of numbness, paraesthesiae, or altered sensation indicating a sensory pathology, but examination of the sensory system forms part of a routine assessment. Attempt to identify the modality of sensory loss and its distribution (e.g. correlating with a dermatome, peripheral nerve). A knowledge of the dermatomes is essential (Fig. 17.19).

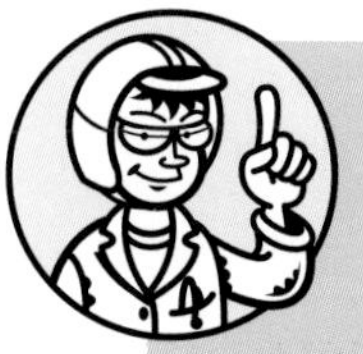

Useful dermatomes to remember are: C5, deltoid; C6 thumb; C7, middle finger; C8, little finger; T4, nipple; T8, xiphisternum; T10, umbilicus; T12, symphysis pubis; L4, medial leg; L5, between great and second toe; S1, lateral border of foot.

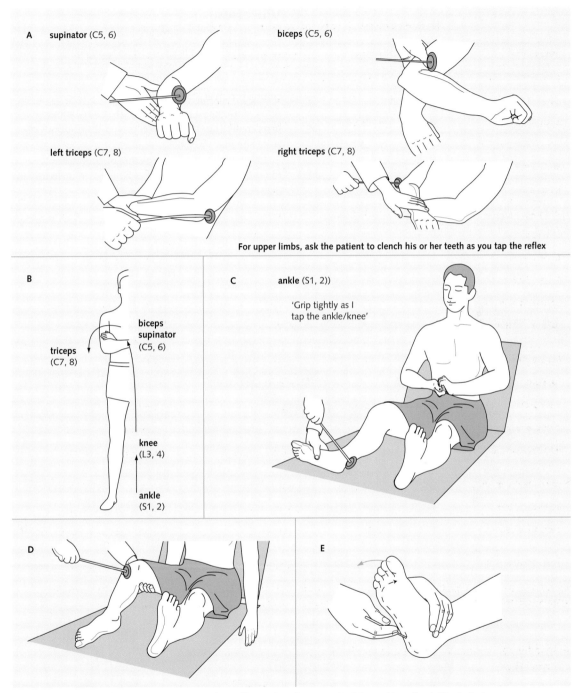

Fig. 17.16 Eliciting the more common tendon reflexes. Reinforcement of the ankle reflex is illustrated.

Light touch

Dab (do not stroke) the skin lightly with a small wisp of cotton wool. If there is decreased sensation, this should be mapped out. Start from the area of decreased sensation and move outwards as this is more sensitive.

Pin prick

Use a disposable pin or needle gently and check that the patient can identify the stimulus as sharp. Temperature sensation is also conveyed in the spinothalamic tracts, so is not usually routinely assessed.

Nerve roots supplying the major reflexes	
Reflex	Nerve root
biceps	C5*, C6
brachioradialis	C6*, C7
triceps	C6, C7*, C8
knee	L2, 3*, 4*
ankle	S1, S2
anal	S2, 3, 4

Fig. 17.17 Nerve roots supplying the major reflexes. Asterisks indicate the major nerve root supplying each reflex.

Vibration

Place the base of a vibrating 128 Hz tuning fork on the distal phalanx of the great toe. Patients should be aware of a buzzing sensation. Ask patients to close their eyes and to indicate when they think that the tuning fork has stopped vibrating. Usually vibration sense is impaired peripherally. If absent, move proximally (i.e. from lateral malleolus to upper tibia and then iliac crest).

Loss of vibration sense is one of the earlier physical signs indicative of peripheral neuropathy in diabetes mellitus.

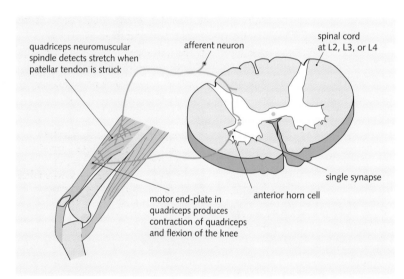

Fig. 17.18 Neurological pathway for the knee jerk.

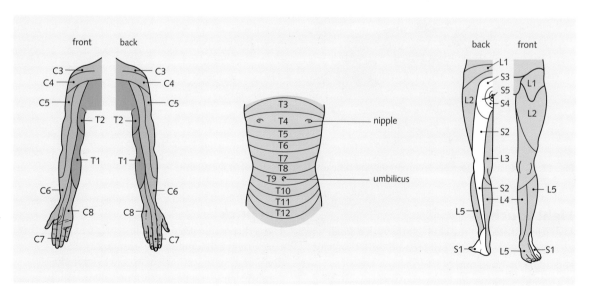

Fig. 17.19 Distribution of the dermatomes on the surface of the body.

Joint position sense

Start distally. Move the great toe passively either extending or flexing, and observe whether the patient can identify the direction of movement. Be careful not to contact the second toe with your hand as this may give additional sensation to the patient. When you hold the toe, hold it by the side, this prevents the patient feeling the increase in pressure when moving the toe up or down. If there is impairment, test the ankle and knee.

Romberg's test

Romberg's test may be positive if there is impaired position sense. Patients are asked to stand upright with their eyes closed. Marked swaying when patients close their eyes is 'Rombergism' (Fig. 17.20).

Higher functions

There are many sophisticated tests of mental function. A crude screening test is the mini-mental test. This may reveal the presence of dementia and is an essential part of any examination of an elderly person. Furthermore, a change in mental functioning may be identified over a period of time.

Other tests should include:
- State of consciousness.
- Emotional state.
- Speech (e.g. to reveal receptive or expressive dysphasia).

If a cortical lesion is suspected, attempt to localize it (Fig. 17.21).

Patterns of neurological damage

It is helpful when assessing neurological lesions to be aware of common patterns of deficits so that the anatomical site of the lesion can be determined (e.g. myopathy, peripheral neuropathy, nerve root, cortical). Some of the more important lesions are described below.

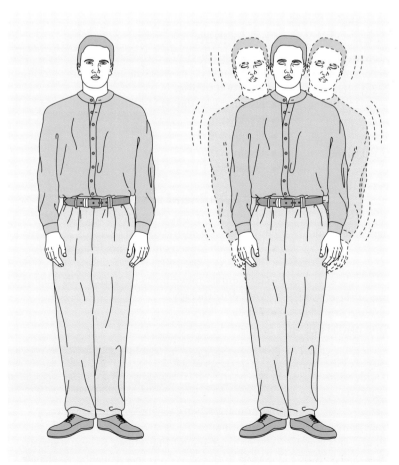

Fig. 17.20 Romberg's test. A positive test indicates impaired position sense. Patients can maintain a good posture when their eyes are open, but sway when asked to close their eyes.

Typical features of localized cortical lesions	
Lobe affected	**Features**
frontal lobe	predominant mood and behavioural changes; disinhibition; motor cortex may be involved; pout reflex
temporal lobe	dominant: sensory dysphasia, alexia (agraphia); non-dominant: may cause visuospatial deficits
parietal lobe (dominant)	aphasia; dysgraphia; dyslexia; right–left disorientation
parietal lobe (non-dominant)	neglect of contralateral sensation; altered body image; dressing apraxia; constructional apraxia

Fig. 17.21 Typical features of localized cortical lesions.

Myopathy

Weakness and wasting of muscles occurs in a distribution that is characteristic of the particular type of myopathy (e.g. facioscapulohumeral muscular dystrophy, Duchenne muscular dystrophy). Reflexes are preserved until the disease is advanced.

Peripheral nerves

Radial nerve

Damage to the radial nerve may cause wrist drop. Test sensation over the first dorsal interosseous muscle. Test extension of the interphalangeal joint of the thumb (e.g. compression neuropathy after sleeping with arm over a chair).

Median nerve

Damage to the median nerve (e.g. carpal tunnel syndrome) characteristically produces:
- Sensory loss over the palmar aspect of the lateral three and a half fingers.
- Wasting of the thenar eminence.
- Weakness of opposition, flexion, and abduction of the thumb.

Ulnar nerve

Ulnar nerve lesions (e.g. due to trauma at the elbow) result in:
- Sensory loss over the little finger and medial half of the ring finger.
- Wasting of the hypothenar eminence.
- Weakness of finger abduction and adduction.

Lateral popliteal nerve

The lateral popliteal nerve is sometimes damaged during a fracture to the head of the fibula. This may result in:

- Impaired sensation of the lateral calf.
- Foot drop.
- Weakness of dorsiflexion and eversion of the foot.

Peripheral neuropathy

Generalized neuropathy is usually in a 'stocking and glove' distribution. Tendon reflexes are lost early in the cause of disease.

Cerebellum

The main features of cerebellar pathology are:
- Gait ataxia (wide-based).
- Intention tremor.
- Dysdiadochokinesis.
- Nystagmus.
- Hypotonia.
- Dysmetria.
- Dysarthria ('staccato speech').

Extrapyramidal system

There is a wide range of extrapyramidal syndromes. They tend to be characterized by:
- Decreased movement (e.g. bradykinesia in Parkinson's disease).
- Involuntary movements (e.g. tardive dyskinesia with drug therapy).
- Rigidity.

Summary of neurological examination

In summary, when carrying out a neurological examination:
- It is of paramount importance to be systematic. Most of the signs represent a qualitative change

from normality. This can only be recognized with practice.

- Identifying a lesion is the easy part. A given lesion may be due to multiple pathologies at various locations in the nervous system. The next stage is to prepare a list of all the elicited signs and consider whether a single pathological lesion could account for them. If so, identify its anatomical site.
- Remember that lesions produce characteristic patterns of physical signs. For example if a weakness is identified consider whether the pattern fits into an UMN or LMN pattern. If it is LMN, look for features that identify the site of the lesion (i.e. at the muscle itself, the neuromuscular junction, a peripheral nerve, a nerve root, or anterior horn cells). If the lesion is UMN in pattern, there are usually other localizing signs that allow identification of the anatomical point of pathology.
- Once the anatomical location of the lesion has been identified, prepare a differential diagnosis of possible pathologies that could produce a lesion at that site. Consider collateral information from the history or systemic examination to narrow down the differential diagnosis.

Stroke

Usually a diagnosis of stroke is apparent from the history, but the examination is crucial to confirm the presence of a focal neurological deficit, document baseline function objectively, and to consider aetiological factors.

Assess level of consciousness
See section on the unconscious patient (p. 165).

Define the neurological deficit
A full neurological assessment is essential to ascertain the degree of damage. It is often possible to identify the vascular territory affected. Occasionally, the lesion produces a more subtle lesion such as impaired cognition. The anatomical site of damage may offer prognostic information.

Consider aetiology
The systemic examination may offer clues to the underlying cause.

Pulse
Arrhythmias, especially atrial fibrillation, predispose to emboli. Consider the possibility of a recent

myocardial infarction, which may have caused a watershed infarct or been complicated by transient arrhythmias.

Blood pressure
Hypertension is one of the major risk factors for stroke. In the acute setting, it should be interpreted with caution and treated even more cautiously as an abrupt drop in blood pressure may cause further ischaemia as autoregulation will be impaired.

Eyes
Argyll Robertson pupils may suggest syphilis (now a rare cause of stroke in the UK) or diabetes mellitus.

Fundoscopy
Look for evidence of hypertensive and diabetic retinopathy.

Face
The facial appearance may suggest an underlying pathology, for example plethora (polycythaemia), mitral facies.

Neck
Listen carefully for a carotid bruit as a source of embolus. Have a low threshold for considering a Doppler scan of the carotid vessels as a patient with over 70% stenosis of the internal carotid artery may benefit from subsequent endarterectomy. Although detection of carotid bruits is not particularly sensitive, it is highly specific for the probability of significant stenosis.

Heart
Listen for any murmurs. Mitral stenosis (especially in association with atrial fibrillation) is a potent risk factor for left atrial thrombus and subsequent embolus. Consider the possibility of endocarditis (especially if there is a murmur). If there is fixed splitting of the second heart sound in association with a flow murmur, look for sources of paradoxical embolus from the venous circulation.

Epileptiform seizure

The diagnosis of epilepsy usually relies upon an objective eyewitness account. The doctor rarely sees a fit in an individual patient.

Acute seizure

The priority is to ensure that patients do not harm themselves, and then to assess and if necessary provide specific therapy for the seizure. One should:

- Protect the airway.
- Ensure that the patient will not harm him or herself.
- Observe the nature of the seizure activity (e.g. tonic–clonic, focal, absence attack).
- Check pulse rate and if possible blood pressure.
- Check blood sugar (BM), obtain blood for electrolytes (toxins).
- If seizure is prolonged undertake measures for status epilepticus.

Post-ictal

Usually the patient is seen in the post-ictal period, having been brought to hospital after collapsing. The history is central to the diagnosis (see 'Presenting complaints'), and very often the examination is unremarkable. The examination may be useful when considering the differential diagnosis or for assessing the aetiology and functional consequences of the seizure (Fig. 17.22). Remember, any neurological symptoms may be observed after a seizure but they should be monitored and seen to resolve.

Perform detailed neurological assessment

In particular, focus on:

- Level of consciousness. Check the Glasgow Coma Score (Fig. 17.23) until a normal level of consciousness is achieved as seizure may be the presentation of head injury or intracranial bleed.
- Paralysis. A post-ictal focal weakness (Todd's paralysis) may be present for 24 hours following a seizure, but consider the presence of an acute

Glasgow coma score	
Eyes (E)	
open spontaneously (with blinking)	4
open to command of speech	3
open in response to pain (applied to limbs or sternum)	2
not opening	1
Motor function (M)	
obeys commands	6
localizes to pain	5
withdraws from pain	4
flexor response to pain (decorticate)	3
extensor response to pain (decerebrate)	2
no response to pain	1
Vocalization (V)	
appropriate speech	5
confused speech	4
inappropriate words	3
groans only	2
no speech	1

Fig. 17.23 The Glasgow Coma Score.

CVA or intracranial space-occupying lesion if neurological signs are present.

- Eyes. Check pupillary responses and fundoscopy to exclude papilloedema.

Perform systemic examination to identify precipitating cause

It is particularly important to perform a detailed systemic examination to try to identify an underlying cause for the epileptic seizure so that specific therapy may be offered. Consider:

- Alcohol withdrawal – signs of chronic liver disease, smell of alcohol on breath, unkempt condition, common.
- Trauma.
- Pyrexia – infants.
- Encephalitis – fever, level of consciousness, focal neurological signs, herpetic ulcer.

Fig. 17.22 Assessment of a patient during a seizure may reveal the presence of a condition other than typical epilepsy.

Assessment of a patient during a seizure to reveal conditions other than typical epilepsy	
Cause of collapse	Discriminatory features
syncope	usually apparent from prodromal history; check pulse rate (e.g. tachyarrhythmia, Stokes–Adams attack); check postural blood pressure; pallor during episode
narcolepsy	no convulsions; patient rousable
hysteria	often many atypical features; usually only occur when there is an audience; no urinary incontinence/tongue biting

- Malignancy – look for signs of primary bronchial, breast, colonic, or kidney tumour.
- Degenerative brain disease (e.g. dementia).

Unconscious patient

Assessment of the unconscious patient provides a great challenge for the diagnostic and management skills of the doctor. The first priority is to ensure that the patient is stable before performing a detailed assessment. This all needs to be practised until it is second nature. You can't learn the skills from a book as they are practical procedures but you can learn the framework. You are likely to be required to demonstrate you are competent at the management of the unconscious patient (e.g. an OSCE question). The Trust Resuscitation Officer is a great source of experience and will be able to help you become proficient at this.

Adopt a SAFE approach
- S – Shout for help
- A – Approach with care
- F – Free the patient from danger
- E – Evaluate the patients ABC (see below)

The SAFE approach is designed to ensure that you do not become a casualty yourself. While approaching a patient in A&E may not present any danger, stopping to help at a road traffic accident will. If the patient is in harm's way either remove the harm or remove the patient from the harm. Only when both you and the patient are safe can you start to assess the patient.

Keep it simple. You are only aiming for two things:
1 Air goes in and out
2 Blood goes round and round

The best way to achieve this is with the ABC principles
- *Airway*. Check that it is patent, this includes looking in the mouth to remove any obstructions, e.g. false teeth or debris. Can the patient maintain their own airway? If they cannot you will need to help with this (e.g. triple airway manoeuvre with or without a Guedel Airway).
- *Breathing*. Now that the airway is patent is the patient breathing? If not you need to breath for them, either mouth-to-mouth or with a bag and mask, depending on where you are. The patient needs to be on 100% oxygen in this situation. Look at the chest: does it rise and fall equally? If it doesn't, do they need a chest drain?
- *Circulation*. Does the patient have a pulse? If they've got a pulse do they have a blood pressure. If there is no pulse CPR needs to be started and an ECG attached. The guidelines for the management of a cardiac arrest are under constant revision, so look up the Resuscitation Council web site at www.resus.org.uk for the latest algorithm. If the patient is shocked (e.g. remember the section on GI bleeding) then they need a fluid challenge. In the adult this is 2 l of Hartmann's solution, in children it is 20 mg/kg of a colloid of your choice. The patient needs two large intravenous cannulae. If you haven't got access after two attempts stop wasting time trying. In adults do a venous cut down, in children under age 6 place an intraosseous needle. When you get blood or marrow do a BM and cross match.

Remember you do not move from A to B until you have dealt with A, etc. Resuscitation is a team effort. This is why you shouted for help right at the beginning. Practise the practical things on mannikins so you know what you are trying to do. When you are presented with a major trauma or a cardiac arrest it is frightening. You *are* allowed to be scared – I still am. Afterwards sit down and have a cup of tea with everyone involved and share your feelings and appraise what happened. There are always things you have done well and things to remember for next time.

Assess level of consciousness

The Glasgow coma score (GCS) is widely used to provide a simple reproducible objective assessment of conscious level. This is based on the best responses obtained (Fig. 17.23). If you don't have time to assess the GCS use the AVPU scoring system: is the patient A alert, V responds to voice, P responds to pain, or U unresponsive.

The Glasgow coma score is particularly useful if repeated observations are made so that a rapid and unambiguous diagnosis of a deteriorating level of consciousness can be made.

Perform full neurological examination

Look for any localizing signs. Pay particular attention to:

- Pupil size and response to light (Fig. 17.24) (including symmetry) – some drugs (e.g. opiates) constrict pupils; other drugs (e.g. phenothiazines, amphetamines) dilate pupils; 'coning' results in a single fixed dilated pupil; pontine lesion results in pinpoint pupils; brain death results in fixed dilated pupils.
- Fundi (especially for papilloedema).
- Gag and corneal reflexes.
- Motor responses.
- Tendon reflexes.
- Abnormal tone.

Perform detailed systemic examination

The six traumatic things that kill you quickly and can be treated are best remembered as ATOM FC.

A   Airways obstruction
T   Tension pneumothorax
O   Open pneumothorax
M   Massive haemothorax
F   Flailed chest
C   Cardiac tamponade.

Coma may be due to metabolic, infective, cardiovascular pathology, etc. In particular note:

- Evidence of trauma or head injury (look for otorrhoea or cerebrospinal fluid leaking from the nose).
- Temperature (e.g. hypothyroidism, infection).
- Evidence of needle marks (indicating diabetes mellitus or drug addiction).
- Jaundice or other features of chronic liver disease.
- Breath (e.g. revealing hepatic fetor, alcohol, diabetic ketoacidosis).
- Respiratory pattern (e.g. Cheyne–Stokes respiration, Kussmaul's respirations of diabetes mellitus or uraemia).
- Cyanosis (e.g. due to hypoxia).

Exclude hypoglycaemia or hyperglycaemia early in the assessment of an unconscious patient by performing a BM stick analysis.

Multiple sclerosis

Multiple sclerosis causes neurological lesions that are disseminated in time and place. It can be diagnosed with reasonable confidence from the history of relapses and remissions and thorough examination if it follows a typical course. Areas of demyelination

small/pin-point pupils	opiates, pontine lesion (haemorrhage/ischaemia/compression)
large fixed pupils	tricyclic antidepressant or sedative overdose, eyedrops, atropine and death
unilateral dilated fixed pupils	supratentorial mass lesion
mid-position fixed pupils	midbrain lesion
conjugate gaze to one side	cerebral lesion on that side* or contralateral pontine lesion**
dysconjugate eye movement	drug overdose, brainstem lesion
abnormal doll's eye movement direction of turn normal abnormal	the eyes move 'with the head' with a brainstem lesion†

Fig. 17.24 Examination of the pupils in an unconscious patient. Note the size and reaction to light. In addition, note the position of gaze fixation. (*Looking towards the lesion; **looking away from the lesion; †normally if the head is held and turned quickly from side to side the eyes swivel in the opposite direction to the head.)

Differential diagnosis of optic atrophy	
Site of lesion	Causes
retina	central retinal occlusion; toxic (e.g. quinine, methylated spirits)
optic nerve	optic and retrobulbar neuritis, (e.g. multiple sclerosis); chronic glaucoma; any cause of papilloedema; toxin (e.g. alcohol, tobacco, ethambutol); tumour (e.g. meningioma, optic glioma)
optic chiasm	pituitary tumour; craniopharyngioma; meningioma

Fig. 17.25 Differential diagnosis of optic atrophy.

may occur anywhere in the central nervous system, but certain patterns are more common.

Sites of involvement
The more common sites of involvement are:
- Optic nerve (optic neuritis).
- Brainstem.
- Cerebellum.
- Cervical cord.
- Periventricular region.

Eyes
Certain patterns of disease should be distinguished:
- Retrobulbar neuritis – relative afferent pupillary defect, central scotoma.
- Optic neuritis – also note swelling of the optic disc acutely, and temporal pallor following recovery.

- Optic atrophy – this is a common finding in long-standing multiple sclerosis, but should be distinguished from other pathologies (Fig. 17.25).
- Nystagmus – often jerking or ataxic; pronounced in late disease.
- Internuclear ophthalmoplegia – diplopia on lateral gaze due to failure of adducting eye to cross midline and demyelination of medial longitudinal bundle.

Brainstem
Multiple brainstem or cerebellar signs may be present, especially nystagmus, diplopia, intention tremor, scanning speech.

Spinal cord
Spastic paraparesis is common in late disease. Other signs can include bladder dysfunction, decreased limb sensation, and loss of posture sensibility, which is often marked.

Mental
Both euphoria and depression or irritability are common.

Always attempt to make a functional assessment of how multiple sclerosis might affect daily activities.

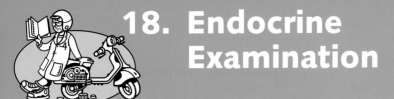
Diabetes mellitus

Inspection

Note weight and height. Calculate the patient's body mass index (BMI); diabetic control may improve with a normal BMI.

Macrovascular complications
Ischaemic heart disease and cerebrovascular disease

Diabetics have a much increased risk of stroke and ischaemic heart disease. It is important to modify any reversible risk factors. Assess these other risk factors, especially:

- Obesity – obesity is not only a risk factor for macrovascular disease, but predisposes to poor glycaemic control.
- Blood pressure control.
- Smoking – nicotine staining of fingers and hair.
- Xanthoma, arcus senilis – hyperlipaemia.

Peripheral vascular disease

Examine the peripheral pulses (femoral, popliteal, dorsalis pedis and posterior tibial arteries). Consider measuring the ratio of ankle: brachial artery pressure. Listen for bruits, especially over the abdomen and carotid and femoral arteries, which indicate turbulent flow and are suggestive of stenosis.

Look for evidence of ulcers, including between the toes. Ulcers may be painless and large without patients knowing that they have got one.

Microvascular complications
Eyes

Examination of the eyes is important in diabetic patients as they are at risk of many diseases. Diabetic patients should have a detailed fundoscopic assessment with dilated pupils at least once a year. Note the following:

- Cataracts – these are more common in diabetics.
- Evidence of background retinopathy ('dot and blot' haemorrhages, exudates).
- Proliferative retinopathy (neovascularization, vitreous haemorrhage).
- Macular oedema.

Assess eye movements (especially in long-standing diabetes mellitus) for a third nerve palsy due to mononeuritis multiplex.

Check visual acuity, which is often reduced due to maculopathy.

Peripheral neuropathy

Test for evidence of a 'stocking and glove' sensory loss. Loss of vibration and joint position sense are often the first modalities to be affected, especially in the legs. A defined peripheral nerve (e.g. median nerve) lesion (mononeuritis multiplex) may also be present.

Diabetic nephropathy

Nephropathy is particularly common in the presence of retinopathy and neuropathy. It is also a marker for an increased risk of ischaemic heart disease. Look for proteinuria. At every assessment, a urinalysis should be performed.

Urinalysis is an essential component of examination of the diabetic patient!

Feet

The feet of diabetic patients should be examined at every examination. Look at general foot care such as the presence of ulcers and the state of the nails. Test the temperature, pulses, and shape of the foot to determine vascular and neuropathic causes. The presence of abnormally sited callosities on the sole may indicate uneven weight distribution.

Assess diabetic control

Different patients use different methods for recording glucose control.

Urinalysis

Look for glycosuria, but be aware of the different renal thresholds for glycosuria. If a patient consistently has negative glycosuria, it may be worthwhile checking a blood HbA1c level.

169

BM sticks

Look at the patient's own record of BM stick assessments. This is most informative in type I diabetes mellitus. You may wish to ask patients to perform an estimate in front of you so that you can assess their technique.

Evidence of skin infections (e.g. boils, abscesses, candidiasis) may suggest chronically poor control.

Assess injection sites

Look for complications such as scarring, abscesses, and lipodystrophy, which result from not rotating injection sites frequently enough. Note any amyotrophy (painful wasting of a muscle group, e.g. quadriceps.)

Diabetic coma

A young patient may present with diabetes and diabetic ketoacidosis. Any treated patient may have hypoglycaemia complicating therapy.

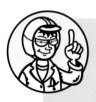 If there is any doubt about the cause of a coma in a diabetic patient and the glucose level is not known, treat with intravenous glucose first.

Diabetic ketoacidosis (DKA)

This typically occurs in a younger person. In particular:

- Note the respiratory pattern – Kussmaul's respiration suggests acidosis ('air hunger').
- Note the mental state – may be alert, but usually confused or stuporose.
- Smell the breath – ketones may be detectable.
- Consider fluid status – the patient is invariably dehydrated with dry skin and mucous membranes, decreased (or undetectable) jugular venous pressure (JVP), and hypotension.
- Consider the underlying cause.
- Fever is often absent before therapy even in the presence of infection, but sources of infection should be carefully sought.
- Do arterial blood gases. Patients can be extremely acidotic and this needs to be monitored.

Most centres now have DKA protocols. Know where to find yours and have a look at it before you start working there.

Hyperosmolar non-ketotic coma

Hyperosmolar non-ketotic coma usually presents in a similar fashion as diabetic ketoacidosis, but in elderly and middle-aged subjects. Many of the clinical signs are the same, as are the basic management strategies as follows:

- Rehydrate.
- Optimize acid–base balance.
- Replace insulin deficiency.
- Look for and treat the underlying cause.
- Provide general supportive care.

The management differs only in the fine tuning.

Hyperthyroidism

Like hypothyroidism (see below), many systems may show signs of hyperthyroidism, and although marked hyperthyroidism due to Graves' disease is unmistakable, the signs are often non-specific, and hyperthyroidism occurs in the differential diagnosis of many symptoms and signs.

Inspection

General inspection often provides clues that are easily overlooked (Fig. 18.1). In particular, note:

- General demeanour – patients are typically agitated, restless, irritable, and have poor concentration.
- Facies, e.g. exophthalmos.
- Goitre – associated with Graves' disease, toxic multinodular goitre.

Cardiovascular system

Cardiovascular abnormalities are common in thyroid disease and may provide a sensitive measure of assessing thyroid status in a treated patient. Look for the presence of:

- Tachycardia – very common.
- Atrial fibrillation – although this is a common arrhythmia, its presence should always raise a suspicion of hyperthyroidism – this is important as hyperthyroidism is an easily treatable cause of this arrhythmia.
- Warm vasodilated peripheries with a bounding arterial pulse.
- Hypertension – occasionally a feature.

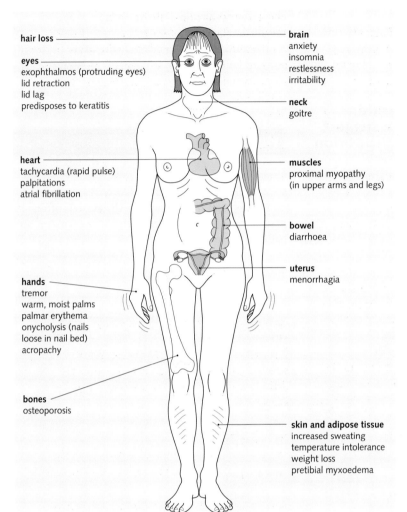

Fig. 18.1 Symptoms and signs of hyperthyroidism.

hair loss

eyes
exophthalmos (protruding eyes)
lid retraction
lid lag
predisposes to keratitis

heart
tachycardia (rapid pulse)
palpitations
atrial fibrillation

hands
tremor
warm, moist palms
palmar erythema
onycholysis (nails
loose in nail bed)
acropachy

bones
osteoporosis

brain
anxiety
insomnia
restlessness
irritability

neck
goitre

muscles
proximal myopathy
(in upper arms and legs)

bowel
diarrhoea

uterus
menorrhagia

skin and adipose tissue
increased sweating
temperature intolerance
weight loss
pretibial myxoedema

The presence of atrial fibrillation in any patient should provoke a search for the underlying cause.

- Ischaemic heart disease.
- Hyperthyroidism.
- Mitral valve disease (especially mitral stenosis).

Neurological system

A brief examination often reveals discriminatory signs, for example:

- Fine resting tremor.

- Agitated, restless, hyperactive, shaky, irritable mental state. The patient may have a frank psychosis.
- Proximal myopathy, which may be profound.

Features to suggest Graves' disease
Eye signs

Graves' disease is particularly associated with eye signs, and this can be used to differentiate it from other causes of hyperthyroidism. Note the presence of:

- Lid lag – upper eyelid does not keep pace with the eyeball as it traces a finger moving downwards from above.
- Exophthalmos.
- Chemosis.

- Ophthalmoplegia – extraocular muscles become swollen and develop secondary fibrotic changes.
- Proptosis – most common cause of unilateral and bilateral proptosis.

Pretibial myxoedema, thyroid acropachy, and features to suggest general autoimmune predisposition

Deposition of mucopolysaccharides in the subcutaneous tissues of the legs produces a non-tender infiltration on the front of the shins. Occasionally, it can present acutely.

Thyroid acropachy is a syndrome resembling clubbing with new bone formation in the fingers. It is classically associated with exophthalmos and pretibial myxoedema.

Thyroid disease is associated with other autoimmune processes. In particular, look for alopecia and vitiligo.

Hypothyroidism

Hypothyroidism often develops insidiously and non-specifically, especially in the elderly. A keen level of awareness is important, and the diagnosis is often made by an observant doctor who has never seen the patient previously.

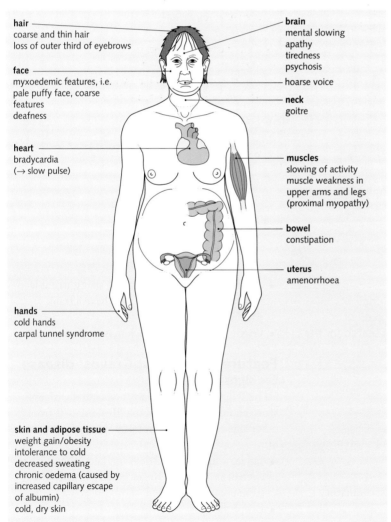

hair
coarse and thin hair
loss of outer third of eyebrows

face
myxoedemic features, i.e. pale puffy face, coarse features
deafness

heart
bradycardia
($\rightarrow$ slow pulse)

hands
cold hands
carpal tunnel syndrome

skin and adipose tissue
weight gain/obesity
intolerance to cold
decreased sweating
chronic oedema (caused by increased capillary escape of albumin)
cold, dry skin

brain
mental slowing
apathy
tiredness
psychosis

hoarse voice

neck
goitre

muscles
slowing of activity
muscle weakness in upper arms and legs (proximal myopathy)

bowel
constipation

uterus
amenorrhoea

Fig. 18.2 Symptoms and signs of hypothyroidism.

Cardiovascular system

Discriminatory features may include:

- Cold peripheries.
- Bradycardia – a useful sign, especially if it is out of context with the patient's condition.
- Hypothermia.
- Pericardial effusion (i.e. difficult to locate apex beat, quiet heart sounds), heart failure.

It is very easy to overlook a diagnosis of hypothyroidism. Always maintain a high index of suspicion, especially if the patient is seen on a regular basis, as it is easy to miss.

Slow-relaxing reflexes are a particularly useful sign for confirming a clinical suspicion of hypothyroidism.

Inspection

It is easy to overlook hypothyroidism, so always consider the diagnosis, especially for patients presenting with chronic fatigue, dementia, slow thought, or non-specific difficulty coping with previously simple tasks (Fig. 18.2). Note the:

- Facies.
- Body shape – obesity, which is usually mild.
- Presence of a goitre – for example if due to Hashimoto's thyroiditis, iodine deficiency.
- Non-pitting oedema.
- Dry scaly skin.

Neurological system

It is common to find neurological signs, for example:

- Slow-relaxing deep tendon reflexes (classically at the ankle joint)
- Proximal myopathy.
- Carpal tunnel syndrome.
- Deep, hoarse voice.
- Mental slowing, which may present with dementia, stupor, or even coma.

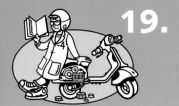

19. Reticuloendothelial Examination

Examination of lymph node groups is important in many disease states. It is important to know the anatomical drainage pattern of the major organs as regional lymphadenopathy may be the first manifestation of local disease.

Normally, lymph nodes are not palpable, except in some thin people. If a single lymph node is found to be enlarged, it is important to adopt a systematic approach.

Examination routine

How to examine any lump

You need to expose the area in question and then:

Inspect

Look at shape of the lump and its position. Is there any associated colour change or change in the skin overlying the lump? Now, remember to ask if the lump is painful before:

Palpation

Ask yourself is there any difference in temperature between the lump and the surrounding temperature. Feel and measure the shape, size (it is a three-dimensional structure so length, breadth and depth) and surface.

- Determine the edge of the lump, is it well or poorly demarcated? What is the consistency of the lump?
- Is it pulsatile? If so, is it expansile or is it a transmitted pulse?
- Is the lump compressible or even reducible? e.g. a form of hernia. Is there a cough impulse present?
- Is there a fluid thrill present in the lump or is it fluctuant?
- Now try moving the lump. What is it fixed to? Is it in the skin or is it fixed to muscle?

Auscultate

You should listen over the lump for both bowel sounds and bruits. And lastly, try to transilluminate the lump to see if it is fluid filled. You may need to switch off the light to get a clear idea of this.

Now that you've finished with the lump examine the surrounding tissue. Is there any change in power or sensation?

Examine all lymph node groups

Examine all the lymph node groups systematically to define the anatomical distribution of the enlarged lymph nodes (Fig. 19.1). It is important to examine the liver and spleen as well as these are also reticuloendothelial organs and may be enlarged in the presence of generalized lymphadenopathy.

Define the characteristics of the enlarged lymph node(s)

Define the texture, size, mobility, and fixation to superficial and other tissues of the enlarged lymph node(s) (as with the examination of any lump). Certain characteristics are suggestive of different disease processes. For example:

- Rubbery texture is suggestive of lymphoma.
- Hard, matted, fixed lymph nodes suggest malignancy.
- Tender lymph nodes suggest infection or other inflammatory state.

Explore the region drained by the enlarged lymph node group

If a single lymph node group is enlarged, try to identify the cause. The broad causes of lymphadenopathy are:

- Infection.
- Metastatic tumour.
- Lymphoproliferative disorder.
- Sarcoidosis.

In cases of cellulitis or other bacterial infection, it is sometimes possible to see lymphangitis. It is visible as thin red streaks following the line of the lymphatics in the skin.

Perform a systemic examination

Consider the pathological cause by performing a systemic examination, concentrating on inflammatory or malignant conditions draining into that lymph node group. Consider the more common causes of localized and systemic lymphadenopathy (Fig. 19.2).

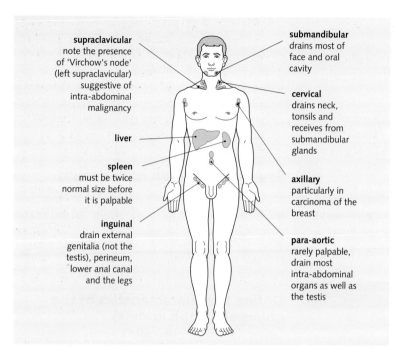

Fig. 19.1 Position of the major lymph node groups and lymphoid organs.

supraclavicular
note the presence of 'Virchow's node' (left supraclavicular) suggestive of intra-abdominal malignancy

submandibular
drains most of face and oral cavity

cervical
drains neck, tonsils and receives from submandibular glands

liver

spleen
must be twice normal size before it is palpable

axillary
particularly in carcinoma of the breast

inguinal
drain external genitalia (not the testis), perineum, lower anal canal and the legs

para-aortic
rarely palpable, drain most intra-abdominal organs as well as the testis

Usually the cause of lymphadenopathy is apparent from a detailed history and systemic examination, but if further investigation is needed, the most useful tests include:

- Full blood count and film – for infection, leukaemia.
- Erythrocyte sedimentation rate (ESR) and C-reactive protein (CRP) – for malignancy, systemic inflammatory disease, systemic lupus erythematosus (SLE) – these are markers of an acute inflammatory response, and a differential rise in ESR or CRP is occasionally discriminatory.
- Biochemical profile, especially liver function.
- Chest radiography – for example for sarcoid, malignancy, chest infection.

Fig. 19.2 Differential diagnosis of localized and generalized lymphadenopathy. SLE, systemic lupus erythematosus.

Differential diagnosis of localized and generalized lymphadenopathy

	Lymphadenopathy	Features and examples
localized	infection (bacterial, viral, fungal)	pharyngitis, dental (cervical); lymphogranuloma venereum (inguinal)
	lymphoma (Hodgkin's; non-Hodgkin's)	can present anywhere, but cervical group is the most common
	malignancy	Virchow's node (left supraclavicular lymphadenopathy due to intra-abdominal or thoracic disease); breast cancer (axillary or supraclavicular)
generalized	infection	infectious mononucleosis; syphilis; tuberculosis; toxoplasmosis; HIV
	malignancy	lymphoma; leukaemia (especially CLL); carcinoma (unusual)
	autoimmune disease	SLE, rheumatoid arthritis, sarcoidosis, other connective tissue diseases
	drugs	
	hyperthyroidism	

- Viral screens, autoantibody profiles, blood culture.
- Lymph node biopsy – often provides diagnostic information if sinister pathology is suspected.

If a single lymph node is enlarged, explore the region drained by that lymph node in detail.
Regional lymphadenopathy is common, but usually transient. Persistent lymphadenopathy always warrants investigation.

Skin examination

The definition of a dermatologist: someone who tells you in Latin what you just told them in English!

The skin is the single largest organ in the body and yet is often overlooked. Rashes are common things to be asked about and you need to be able to describe the lesion even if you cannot make a precise diagnosis so you can communicate with others about it. Differing institutions have differing expectations about which terms they expect students to be familiar with (Fig. 19.3). During your dermatology attachment(s) they should provide you with a dictionary of what they expect. Try to assimilate some of it!

When examining a rash you will need to expose the patient in a well-lit room. The patient may well be shy about their lesion and feel it is unsightly, so be sensitive. Have a chaperone present. Firstly consider the distribution of the rash, so take a step back and look. Is it only on areas exposed to sunlight, is it dermatomal in distribution (e.g. herpes zoster), is it related to jewellery or buttons? Is the rash generalized or localized, bilateral or unilateral? Are there any areas that are spared?

Next, what is the morphology of the lesion? You need your dictionary to help with this. Try and determine the shape, size, colour and the margins of any lesions you can see. If you can't remember the special phrase just describe exactly what you see in plain English.

Fig. 19.3 Some dermatological terms.

Some dermatological terms	
alopecia	absence of hair where it normally grows
bulla	a circumscribed elevation of skin greater than 5 mm containing fluid
crusting	scale composed of either dried fluid or blood
erythema	a flushing of the skin due to the dilation of the capillaries
excoriation	an erosion or ulcer secondary to scratching
lichenification	thickening of the epidermis of the skin with exaggeration of the normal creases
macule	small flat area of altered skin colour or texture
nodule	a solid mass in the skin greater than 5 mm
papule	a small solid elevation of skin less than 5 mm
petechia	pinhead sized flat collection of blood in the skin
plaque	elevation area of skin greater than 20 mm without depth
purpura	a large flat or raised collection of blood in the skin
pustule	visible accumulation of pus in the skin
ulcer	a loss in the continuity of an epithelially lined surface
vesicle	circumscribed elevation of skin less than 5 mm, containing fluid

20. Breast Examination

Examination routine

Breast examination forms an integral part of a full medical clerking. However, a more detailed breast examination is always necessary if the presenting symptoms:

- Are breast symptoms (e.g. lump, pain, nipple discharge, change in appearance).
- Arouse suspicion of disseminated malignancy with an undiagnosed primary (e.g. presentation with pleural effusion, hepatomegaly, bony tenderness).
- Include fever of unknown cause.

As with any system, a methodical approach is needed. Anticipate what information might be obtained from each part of the examination and how each elicited sign is placed into context with the presenting illness.

Patient exposure and position

Clearly great sensitivity is essential. Very often the patient feels uncomfortable or embarrassed, especially if the doctor is male. Remember that many patients will be terrified, not only of the examination, but of the potential underlying diagnosis. It is not uncommon for women to 'ignore' a breast mass for several months or even years.

Explain clearly why the examination is being performed and the useful information that is likely to be gained. Ensure complete privacy. It is clearly unacceptable for a secretary or another doctor to burst through the door or screens revealing a semi-clad patient to the waiting room or ward! The room should be warm, and a blanket should always be provided so that the patient can remain covered until the examination is performed.

Explain clearly what the examination will entail before asking the patient to undress. Ask the patient to remove all clothing (including bra) from the waist upwards, and to sit on the side of the examination couch. You must always have a female chaperone with you at all time.

The examination follows the usual sequence of:

- Inspection.
- Palpation.
- Systemic examination.

Inspection

Remember to look at the whole patient. Make a mental note of:

- Age. Breast carcinoma is more common in older women, but can occur in any age group from the third decade onwards. Fibroadenoma is more common in premenopausal women. Abscess is much more common in women of childbearing age.
- Sex. Men also get breast disease!
- General health.

Breast substance

Ask patients to sit still facing you with arms by their side (Fig. 20.1) and with their arms raised above their head – a mass tethered to the skin may then become apparent, and the undersurface of the breasts can be seen. Note:

- Symmetry. It is not uncommon for one breast to be slightly larger than the other, but underlying masses, infections, or nipple disease can also cause asymmetry of size, shape, or nipples.
- Any obvious mass.
- Skin discoloration. Infections and occasionally malignancy may cause a red discoloration.
- Skin puckering or 'peau d'orange' (Fig. 20.2). Peau d'orange is caused by infiltration of the skin lymphatic system, and as the name implies, its appearance resembles the peel of an orange.

Nipples

Inspect the nipples carefully, especially noting the following:

- Symmetry.
- Retraction or deviation. If one or both nipples are retracted, ask the patient if this is a new phenomenon. This is an ominous sign. As well as carcinoma, it is associated with chronic abscess and fat necrosis.
- Discharge. If present note whether it appears milky (galactorrhoea), bloody, or pustular.
- Skin colour. Particularly note the presence of an eczematous rash suggestive of Paget's disease of the nipple.

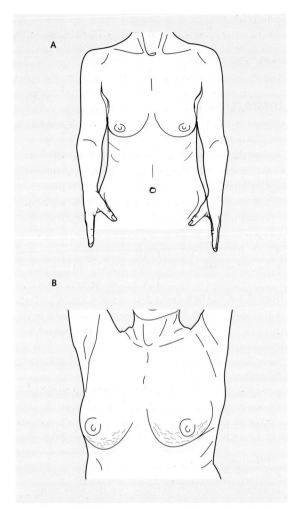

Palpation

The normal consistency of a breast varies considerably. It is recommended to start the examination with palpation of the normal breast. Palpate with the palmar surface of the fingers. It is helpful to divide the breast into quadrants (Fig. 20.3). Palpate each quadrant in turn noting:

- Consistency and texture of the breast.
- Tenderness.
- Presence of any mass.

Examine the breast with symptoms. Before palpating, ask patients to point to the area of tenderness or to any lump that they may have felt. Once again, examine each quadrant in turn. If a mass is felt, it should be systematically examined as described below.

Breast mass

If any lump or mass is identified on systemic examination, the essential features should be described. This is well illustrated with a breast mass. The following characteristics should be noted.

Position

It is usual to describe a breast mass in relation to the quadrant it is located in. A breast carcinoma is more common in the upper outer quadrant. Remember to palpate the axillary tail as this also contains breast tissue.

Size

Describe the size of the mass in three dimensions. Ideally measure the mass objectively with a tape measure or calipers to decrease interobserver error.

Fig. 20.1 (A) Ask the patient to sit facing you with hands on hips. (B) Then ask the patient to lift her arms in the air. Skin tethering may become apparent, and abnormalities on the undersurface of the breast will become visible.

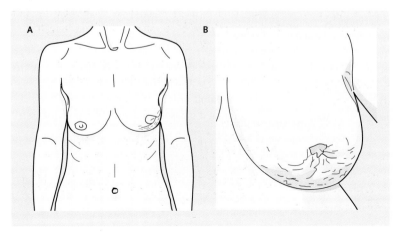

Fig. 20.2 Inspection often reveals obvious asymmetry. (A) A retracted nipple and skin tethering on the left breast. (B) Peau d'orange in association with a retracted nipple.

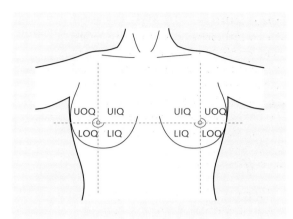

Fig. 20.3 Quadrants of the breast. Upper outer quadrant (UOQ), upper inner quadrant (UIQ), lower outer quadrant (LOQ), lower inner quadrant (LIQ).

This is essential when assessing the progression or regression of a lesion (e.g. judging the response of breast carcinoma to chemotherapy).

Consistency
Note the consistency of any mass. In practice, it is easiest to use terms such as:
- 'Craggy' – literally like a rock.
- 'Hard' – like pressing on your forehead.
- 'Rubbery' – like pressing on the tip of your nose.
- 'Soft' – like pressing on your lips.

Relation to the skin
Note the presence of tethering or fixation to the skin. Fixation suggests an infiltrating carcinoma; tethering occurs in carcinoma, abscess, or fat necrosis.

Relation to underlying tissue
Note the mobility of any lump. A mass fixed to deeper tissue is much more likely to be a carcinoma.

Fibroadenomas are typically described as highly mobile, and may be difficult to palpate. Trapping a fibroadenoma between finger and thumb can be tricky, and has been likened to chasing a mouse, hence the term 'breast mouse'.

Tenderness
Breast carcinoma is rarely tender on presentation. A tender mass is much more likely to be an abscess, cyst, or fat necrosis.

Skin discoloration
Note any change in the appearance of the skin overlying the mass. Erythema is common in association with infections. Paget's disease of the nipple presents with an eczematous rash, a carcinoma occasionally has a red or blue hue.

Temperature
Inflammatory lesions often produce palpable warmth.

Associated lesions
It is essential to examine the rest of the breast for the presence of a second mass. It is not rare for breast carcinoma to present with bilateral disease. Fibroadenosis often presents with multiple lumps.

If breast carcinoma is suspected, a full systemic examination is essential. Look for evidence of metastatic spread. In particular, check for the presence of:
- Hepatomegaly – liver metastases result in a grim prognosis; note the presence of jaundice.
- Pleural effusion – the lung is a common site of metastatic spread.
- Bony tenderness – bony metastases are the most common site of secondary breast malignancy after axillary lymph nodes and the axial skeleton is often involved; disease may be present for several years.
- Ascites – peritoneal deposits often present with ascites.

Lymphatic drainage
Palpation of the axillary lymph nodes forms part of the routine breast examination (see below).

An example of a recording of the presence of a breast mass in the medical notes is illustrated in Fig. 20.4.

Axillary examination
Breast examination is incomplete without examination of the axilla as these are the natural site of lymphatic drainage of breast tissue. Inspect the axilla for any obvious lumps.

Axillary lymphadenopathy can only be palpated if the muscles forming the walls of the axilla are relaxed. Stand on the patient's right-hand side, support the patient's right upper arm with your right hand, and encourage the patient to allow you to take the weight of the arm (Fig. 20.5). Palpate the axilla with your left hand flat against the lateral chest wall, reaching high up into the axilla with your fingertips, sweeping around all of the walls. The left axilla is examined in a similar manner, but with the opposite hand.

The key to successful examination of the axilla is to ensure that the arm is totally relaxed and supported by your hand.

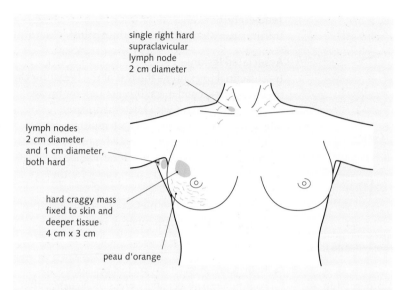

single right hard
supraclavicular
lymph node
2 cm diameter

lymph nodes
2 cm diameter
and 1 cm diameter,
both hard

hard craggy mass
fixed to skin and
deeper tissue
4 cm x 3 cm

peau d'orange

Fig. 20.4 Example of a recording of the presence of a breast mass in the medical notes. A simple diagram provides unambiguous objective information.

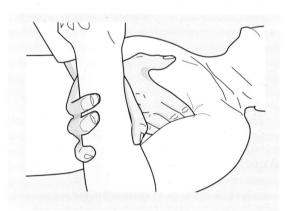

Fig. 20.5 Examination of the axilla for lymphadenopathy. It is important to support the patient's arm to relax the muscles of the axillary folds.

If any mass is detected in the breast or axilla, the supraclavicular and cervical lymph nodes should also be examined.

Finally, note the size of the patient's arms. Lymphoedema can result from tumour invasion of the lymphatics, axillary dissection, or radiotherapy.

Breast mass

Presentation with a breast mass is common. Clearly, the most important diagnosis to exclude is carcinoma of the breast. The most common causes are listed below.

Carcinoma of the breast

In the presence of a breast mass, features to suggest carcinoma include:

- A hard, craggy mass.
- Fixation of the mass to skin or deeper tissues.
- Nipple deviation or retraction.
- Skin changes (peau d'orange, tethering, ulceration).
- Axillary lymphadenopathy.
- Signs of systemic disease.

Fibroadenoma

A fibroadenoma is typically a well-demarcated, highly mobile, non-tender mass in a young or middle-aged woman.

Fibroadenosis (cystic hyperplasia, fibrocystic disease)

The features of fibroadenosis are highly variable and depend upon the degree of cystic change, fibrosis, and masses. Often there is a diffuse change in texture in the breasts and there are multiple masses, which are poorly defined. Mild tenderness is common

Abscess

Abscesses usually present in lactating women and are easily distinguished by the presence of:

- Tenderness.
- Erythema.
- Poor definition.
- Axillary lymphadenopathy.
- Systemic features of infection (e.g. fever, tachycardia).

Fat necrosis

Fat necrosis is much more common in large breasts following a history of trauma. The lump is usually hard and may be tethered to the skin. It may be distinguishable from a breast carcinoma by the lack of axillary lymphadenopathy or peau d'orange.

Breast pain

The more common causes of breast pain are:
- Fibroadenosis.
- Premenstrual tension.
- Mastitis.
- Abscess.

The cause is usually apparent from the history and physical examination. Breast carcinoma rarely presents with pain.

Gynaecomastia

Gynaecomastia results from an increase in breast tissue. It may be unilateral or bilateral, and is confirmed by palpation. The most common causes are:
- Puberty. Normal finding (very common) including in boys.
- Old age.
- Liver failure (look for stigmata of chronic liver disease).
- Carcinoma of the lung.
- Testicular tumours.
- Adrenal tumours.
- Drugs (e.g. spironolactone, cimetidine, digoxin).
- Testicular feminization (very rare).
- Pituitary tumours.

Investigations

The cause of many breast lesions is often apparent from a careful history and physical examination.

However, in many circumstances it is important to exclude breast carcinoma. The most reliable procedure for such exclusion is to perform an excision biopsy, but it is clearly desirable for this to be avoided for benign lesions.

Mammography is performed as a screening procedure in the UK for women over 50 years of age. In the presence of a lump, mammography provides a useful adjunct by detecting areas of calcification, which are indicative of an underlying carcinoma. In addition, a second suspicious area may also be revealed, which should also be investigated clinically.

Ultrasound can be used to identify the composition (i.e. solid versus cystic) of a mass. Cystic lesions can be aspirated as a diagnostic or therapeutic procedure. Ultrasound is often requested to localize masses before surgery. In addition, ultrasound can be used to identify masses for fine needle aspiration (FNA). FNA may provide adequate cytological information to increase or decrease the clinical index of suspicion of malignancy, and so determine the urgency of treatment.

Within every region women should have access to triple assessment clinics via their GP. At the clinic the women will be able to have a clinical examination of her breast by an experienced clinician. This will be complimented with FNA of the lump (with reporting facilities) and mammography with experienced reporting available. This ensures a one-stop visit where the women can have full investigation of any lump and get the results that day. There must also be counselling services on site if bad news is going to be given.

One last thought, men also get breast cancer although it is rare. It also carries a worse prognosis as often the lump will already be adherent to the chest wall at presentation.

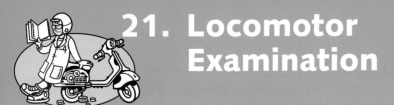
Examination routine

Locomotor assessment is fundamental to even the shortest medical clerking as information on the patient's functional ability is assessed and integrated with other physical signs. Clearly, if a patient describes decreased mobility, weakness, or joint pain a more detailed general assessment is necessary. Equally, if a focal abnormality is detected, this should be fully examined.

This chapter is not intended to provide a detailed description of examination of every joint and muscle group, but illustrates a methodical and functional approach to examining the system.

Patient exposure and position

When examining muscle groups or mobility it is important to ensure that patients are properly exposed. They should be provided with a blanket and asked to strip to their underwear in a warm, well-lit room. The initial formal assessment is usually performed on the examination couch. The approach to examining a joint should follow the scheme of 'Look, Feel, Move'.

The most important part of the locomotor examination is inspection.

Inspection
General inspection

Remember that the examination begins as soon as the patient walks into the examination room! It is often possible to form an impression of functional ability by observing how easily the patient gets out of the chair, walks to the examination room, and climbs onto the examination couch. Note the following.

Always try to relate pathological signs to a functional disability such as difficulty in performing routine daily activities (e.g. getting out of bed, writing, walking, picking up a knife and fork).

Age and sex

Different disease processes are more likely to occur at different ages, for example:

- Osteoarthritis and polymyalgia rheumatica are more common in the elderly.
- Osteoporosis is primarily a disease of postmenopausal women.
- Ankylosing spondylitis usually presents in young men.
- Many inflammatory arthritides first present in young women.

Racial origin

Many forms of arthritis or diseases presenting with impaired mobility have a strong genetic predisposition and are more common in certain racial groups. Others have a predominantly environmental cause that varies geographically, for example:

- Systemic lupus erythematosus (SLE) is much more common in Afro-Caribbean women.
- Paget's disease is more common in Caucasians.
- Multiple sclerosis is more common in patients from temperate climates.

General health and appearance

Note whether the patient appears well or is cachexic. Obesity predisposes to osteoarthritis of the back and weight bearing joints. Cachexia may indicate chronic systemic disease or carcinoma. Note whether the patient appears to be in pain at rest or on walking. An obvious focal weakness may be apparent. These visual clues may contrast with the information obtained from the history or when the patient knows that a formal examination is being performed.

Facial appearance

Note the appearance of facial asymmetry or obvious weakness. In addition, note the general appearance (e.g. myopathic facies of muscular dystrophy with unlined expressionless facies and wasting of the facial muscles).

How easily does the patient get out of a chair?

Proximal muscle weakness (e.g. due to polymyalgia rheumatica, steroid myopathy, hyperthyroidism) will have a profound effect on getting up from a seated position. The significance of a patient wincing with pain when they rise from the chair is unclear.

Does the patient require any aids for walking?

Observe whether the patient walks unaided into the examination room or walks with the aid of a walking stick or zimmer frame, or holding on to another person for support. The patient will hold a walking stick in the hand opposite the weakest leg.

If the patient has a zimmer frame, observe how he or she uses it. It is not infrequent for a nervous but mobile patient to become reliant upon a frame, and on observation they will be seen to carry the frame in front of themselves, rather than rely upon it for support.

Gait

If the patient walks unaided, make a quick assessment of gait. A more formal assessment should be made later in the detailed examination.

How easily does the patient climb onto the examination couch?

A certain amount of agility is needed for elderly patients to climb onto the examination couch. It may be instructive to observe the patient during this process.

Detailed inspection

Once the patient is properly exposed and positioned a detailed inspection should be performed. This process forms the key to a successful examination.

A detailed examination of the locomotor system is time consuming and tiring for the patient. With the benefit of the history, a focused examination is possible after detailed inspection. The more important features to note are outlined below.

Skin rash

Skin rashes may suggest an underlying inflammatory:
- Infection.
- Malignancy.
- Pain (erythema ab igne from a hot-water bottle).

Muscle bulk

Note the general muscle bulk and the distribution of any atrophy, for example:
- Disuse atrophy in a hemiplegic limb.
- Atrophy of the quadriceps in the presence of a proximal myopathy.
- Atrophy of the distal muscles of the lower limbs (Charcot–Marie–Tooth disease).
- Old polio.

Deformity or swelling

Observe any obvious deformity that may be the result of bone, joint, or muscle disease, for example:

- Scoliosis.
- Varus or valgus deformity. This is common in the knees in osteoarthritis.
- Rigid back with loss of lumbar lordosis and fixed posture in ankylosing spondylitis.
- Obvious joint swelling. The distribution of swollen (or inflamed) joints should be mapped out as the distribution is often characteristic of the underlying disease and variations can be correlated with changes in disease activity (Fig. 21.1).

Gait

A formal assessment of the gait should be part of the routine examination, especially in an elderly patient. Apart from highlighting a possible aetiological factor for impaired mobility, it provides a direct functional assessment and an impression of the problems with daily living.

Ask the patient to walk in a straight line, turn around, and then walk back to you. Balance and

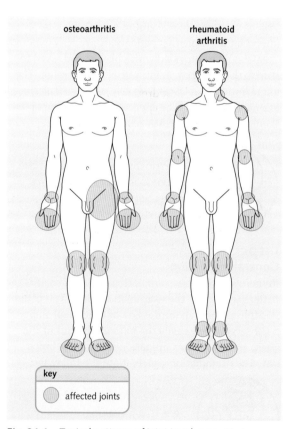

Fig. 21.1 Typical patterns of joint involvement in two different forms of polyarthritis. In rheumatoid arthritis there is usually a symmetrical polyarthropathy. Osteoarthritis is less likely to be symmetrical, but often is symmetrical in its widespread form.

ataxia may be additionally tested by asking the patient to walk 'heel-to-toe'. Characteristic gaits may be noted as follows.

Ataxic gait
An ataxic gait is characteristically wide-based. The arms are often held out wide to aid balance. Marked clumsiness is obvious on walking heel-to-toe. The patient often staggers to the left or right. This is associated with cerebellar pathology.

Spastic gait
If the patient has spastic paraplegia, the gait is stiff and described as a 'scissor gait'. The appearance may resemble someone wading through water. If the patient has a hemiplegia, the affected leg is extended and the leg is swung around the hip joint.

Sensory ataxia
Peripheral neuropathy with sensory ataxia results in a high-stepping gait with the appearance that the feet are being 'thrown'. The feet tend to be 'slapped' on the floor and the patient walks on a wide base. Romberg's test is positive (see Chapter 17). Patients often appear to be concentrating hard on where their feet are being placed.

High-stepping gait
In the presence of foot drop the affected foot is lifted high off the ground to avoid scraping the toes on the floor. Such patients are unable to stand on their heels.

Parkinsonian gait
The patient has a characteristic stooped appearance. The gait is shuffling and hesitant with short steps and a lack of associated arm movement. The arms do not usually swing during walking. The gait is described as 'festinant' – having the appearance that the patient is always chasing his or her own sense of gravity. The patient often has great difficulty when asked to stop and turn around and there are usually other features of Parkinson's disease.

Osteogenic gait
Patients with legs of unequal length may walk normally in shoes with appropriate shoelifts, but the abnormality should be obvious when they walk barefoot.

Waddling gait
A proximal myopathy is associated with a waddling gait. The patient walks on a wide base with the trunk moving from side to side on each step and the pelvis drooping as the leg leaves the ground.

Observe whether the patient has any pain on walking, and if so which movements appear to provoke the pain.

Regional examination

The history from the patient will point you to the region of the body that needs to be examined. Specific regional examination can now begin. As with other systems of the body, it is important to follow a strict routine. When examining any region of the body or joint, use the following routine.

Inspection
Note the bones, alignment, joint swelling, redness, deformity, local swelling, and the presence of any scars.

Palpation
Palpate the area concerned paying particular attention to:
- Skin temperature. In particular, note any areas of increased warmth. Compare the two sides.
- Tenderness. Map out any areas of tenderness and try to relate it to the affected structure.
- Deformity. Note the bony contours and any fixed flexion deformity.
- Soft tissues. Note the presence of any abnormal swellings (e.g. fluid in the joint, cysts, bursae, tumours). Palpate the muscles for bulk, etc.

Assessment of joint movement
Assess the range of active and passive movement, muscular power, and whether movement is accompanied by pain. It is important to have an appreciation of the range of normal movement around each joint. It is often helpful to test the unaffected side first so that any deviation can be more easily appreciated.

Sensation
Test the sensory modalities (see Chapter 17). Light touch, pin prick and vibration are the most discriminatory.

Function
The most useful part of the examination is to assess the function of the relevant body part. Try to relate your assessment to daily activities, for example:
- In the lower limb test the ability to walk, jump, hop, run.

- In the hand test the ability to hold a pen and grip strength.

General examination

It is very important to perform a systemic examination. The localized joint symptoms may form part of a systemic disease or be referred from another site. Furthermore, it is only possible to place the disability into context when the patient is considered as a whole.

Hands

Most systemic examinations start with examination of the hands as stigmata of systemic disease are often manifest in the hands. This is also true for a patient presenting with impaired mobility. Furthermore, many patients specifically complain of symptoms directly related to their hands (e.g. paraesthesiae, weakness, joint pain). A methodical approach to examination of the hands is therefore useful.

Inspection

Remember to look at the face of the patient first for any clues to the underlying disease or treatment (e.g. scleroderma, Cushingoid facies). Look at both hands. Ask the patient to place his or her hands flat on the table, palmar surface downwards. Look at:

- The general shape of the hands and note any deformity (e.g. ulnar deviation in rheumatoid arthritis).
- The colour of the skin (e.g. pigmentation, icterus, erythema, rash).
- The nails. Look for signs of psoriasis (e.g. pitting, onycholysis), clubbing, splinter haemorrhages, nailfold infarcts.
- Soft tissue. Note any swellings (e.g. Heberden's nodes in osteoarthritis on the proximal and distal interphalangeal joints, gouty tophi).
- Joints. Look for any swelling or redness suggestive of an active arthritis.

Ask the patient to turn his or her hands over so that the palmar aspect can be inspected. Repeat the same process of inspection. In particular, note the presence of palmar erythema, and pay close attention to the muscle bulk of the thenar eminence (atrophy in carpal tunnel syndrome) and hypothenar eminence (atrophy in T1 root lesion or in the presence of severe rheumatoid arthritis). Note the presence of any scars (e.g. carpal tunnel decompression).

Palpation

Palpate over the joints of the hand and wrist gently, noting any tenderness of the joints. Record the distribution of any tender joints (Fig. 21.2). Many forms of polyarthritis have a characteristic distribution of joint involvement. In addition, palpate for the presence of any swellings or palmar thickening (e.g. Dupuytren's contracture, trigger finger).

Movement of the joints

Assess the movement of the joints of the hand. Try to relate this to functional activity. First, test passive movement and then active movement. If the primary problem is joint disease, useful tests might include:
- Grip strength.
- Pincer grip (ask the patient to pick up a pen and write his or her name).

Assess whether movement is limited by deformity, pain, or muscular weakness. Some of the signs of rheumatoid arthritis are illustrated in Fig. 21.3.

Neurological assessment

Symptoms in the hand may result from a nerve lesion. Test sensation on the middle finger (median nerve), little finger (ulnar nerve) and the anatomical snuff box (radial nerve). The most common pathologies are:

- Peripheral nerve/Radial nerve injury, most commonly at the spiral groove of the humerus, leads to wrist drop and a weak grip. The ulnar nerve is most commonly injured at the elbow and this leads to claw hand with wasting of the muscles between the metacarpals. The medial nerve is also commonly injured at the wrist (as in carpal tunnel syndrome) and this leads to wasting of the thenar eminence.
- Nerve root or brachial plexus lesion (e.g. Pancoast's tumour).
- Sensory neuropathy.

When examining motor and sensory function, consider the implication of each elicited physical sign and whether the underlying problem is likely to be nerve root, peripheral nerve, muscular, or joint pathology.

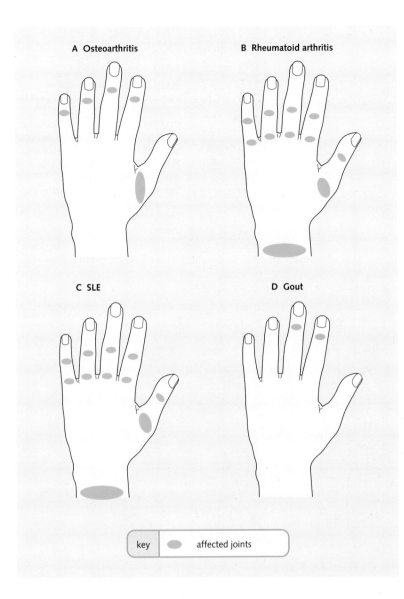

Fig. 21.2 Patterns of joint involvement in some systemic polyarthropathies. (A) Osteoarthritis (OA). Joint swelling of the first carpometacarpal joints is characteristic. Joint involvement is usually symmetrical in the hands and typically affects the distal interphalangeal joints. (B) Rheumatoid arthritis (RA). Active synovitis is detected by joint warmth, swelling, redness, and tenderness. During a flare, arthritis is usually symmetrical, affecting the wrists and metacarpophalangeal and proximal interphalangeal joints. The distal interphalangeal joints are usually spared. (C) Systemic lupus erythematosus (SLE). The distribution of joint involvement is similar to that of rheumatoid arthritis in the hands, but the signs are usually less marked and pain is often out of proportion to the signs of synovitis. (D) Gout. Initial attacks of gout usually present in the lower limb, especially the first metatarsophalangeal joint. However, it may present in the hands. It is often monoarticular. The distal interphalangeal joints are more prone to attacks.

Motor function tests

The tests of motor function are illustrated in Fig. 21.4. If the problem is unilateral, it is very helpful to directly compare strength in the two hands, testing the normal hand first.

Sensory function tests

Test sensory function in the hand including the different modalities (pinprick, light touch, vibration, and joint position). The distribution of sensory loss is illustrated for the three peripheral nerves as well as the dermatomes in Fig. 21.5. Remember that the areas of skin providing sensory fibres for the peripheral nerves or nerve roots often overlap, so it is important to test in the more discriminating areas.

Clues from the systemic examination

It should be apparent from the history and assessment of the hands whether the lesion is articular, vascular, neurological, etc. There are often clues to be obtained from a systemic survey. For example:

- Look at the elbows for rheumatoid nodules or a psoriatic rash.
- Note the presence of gouty tophi on the ear lobes.
- If the patient has an arthritis, it is essential to examine each joint so that the distribution of joint involvement can be mapped out.

Shoulder examination

The shoulder is a difficult joint to examine as it moves in so many different ways! Expose the patient.

189

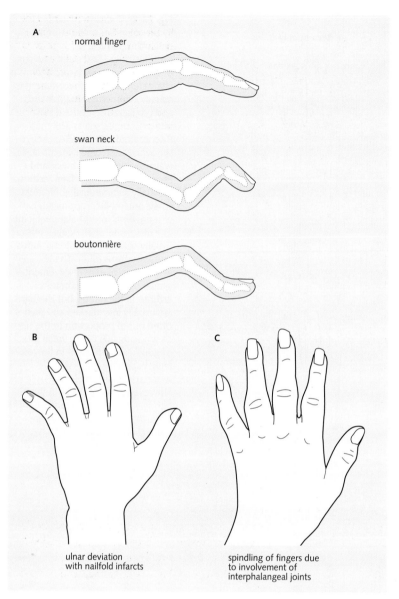

Fig. 21.3 Signs of rheumatoid arthritis in the hands. (A) Deformities of the fingers result from tendon rupture and joint laxity. Characteristic patterns include swan neck and boutonnière deformities. The thumb may develop a Z deformity. (B) Ulnar deviation results from subluxation at the metacarpophalangeal joints. Nailfold infarcts are one of the manifestations of vasculitis. (C) Spindling of the fingers is an early sign due to involvement and swelling of the interphalangeal joints.

Ask them to strip to the waist and sit on the end of the bed.

Look
Inspect the patient for any signs of skin erythema or scars. Note any asymmetry between the two shoulders. Look for evidence of wasting of the deltoid muscles and effusions or joint swelling. Observe the position of the shoulders.

Feel
Palpate over all the joints that encompass the shoulder: the sternoclavicular joints, the acromioclavicular joints and the glenohumeral joints. Pay attention to any joint line tenderness or swelling.

Move
First, ask the patient to do the moving (active movement). Ask them to move their shoulder through abduction, flexion, extension, and internal and external rotation. See Fig 21.6. A good way to do this is to ask them to place their hand behind their neck and slide their hand down between their shoulders.

Second, you should move the shoulder through a full range of movement (passive movement) and see how far you can move the shoulder before the patient

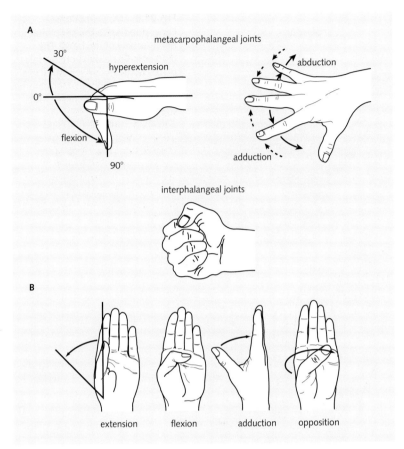

Fig. 21.4 Movements of (A) the fingers and (B) the thumb. Finger abduction and adduction (e.g. 'Grip a piece of paper between your fingers!') rely on the ulnar nerve. Thumb extension relies on the radial nerve; opposition, flexion, and abduction rely on the median nerve.

experiences pain. You should have a hand over the joint feeling for crepitus or restrictions to movement.

Then test the power of the patient shoulder against resistance.

Examining the glenohumeral joint

Immobilize the scapula by placing a hand on it to restrain it. Ask the patient to abduct their arm (which must start down by their side). If they can not initiate this movement there is probably a rotator cuff tear. If abduction is restricted and further passive movement causes more pain this is classed as 'impingement pain', and the patient is likely to have painful arc syndrome.

The rotator cuff comprises the supraspinatus, subscapularis and infraspinatus tendons. An incomplete tear leads to painful arc syndrome (pain on movement from 45–140°). A complete tear results in the patient being unable to initiate abduction. If you abduct the patient's arm to greater than 45°, then the patient should be able to continue the abduction to 180°.

Elbow
Look

Expose the patient to the waist and inspect both elbows from behind with the arms in extension. Look for any obvious deformity, or is there an effusion filling out the hollow at the head of the radius?

Feel

Palpate the bony contours of the elbow. Palpate over the epicondyles and radial head. Feel for any signs of inflammation or bursae.

Move

The elbow should move freely from 0 to 150° (normal people also get a little extension). While doing this palpate over the elbow joint and the head of the radius feeling for crepitus.

Now fix the elbow at the patient's side and flex the arm to 90°. Now test pronation and supination. With the elbow fully extended, test the integrity of the collateral ligaments.

191

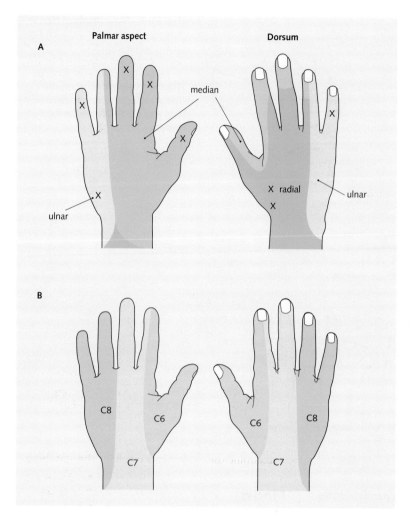

Fig. 21.5 (A) Dermatomes corresponding to the peripheral nerve supply of the hand. The crosses indicate the more useful places for assessing sensation in a quick examination. (B) Dermatomes corresponding to the nerve root supply.

To test for tennis elbow (lateral epicondylitis) ask the patient to fully extend their elbow and then to squeeze your hand. Then ask them to slightly flex their elbow and squeeze your hand. If the patient has tennis elbow the second manoeuvre should be less painful. Figure 21.7 shows how to test for golfer's elbow (medial epicondylitis). They will also be tender over the respective epicondyles.

Back

Back pain is a very common presentation, both to general practitioners and hospital doctors. It is necessary to develop a systematic approach when examining patients with back pain so that potentially serious disease can be recognized early and investigated, while appropriate advice offered to the vast majority with less serious but none the less disabling problems.

In the context of back pain, neurological examination of the legs is important. Spinal cord compression warrants urgent investigation.

Inspection

A brief survey of the patient often provides invaluable clues. In particular, note:
- General health (e.g. cachexia suggestive of underlying malignancy).
- Posture and deformity (e.g. kyphosis, scoliosis, loss of lumbar lordosis).
- Scars (e.g. previous surgery to the back).
- Pain. Note if the patient appears to be in pain and is lying very still for fear of provoking worse pain,

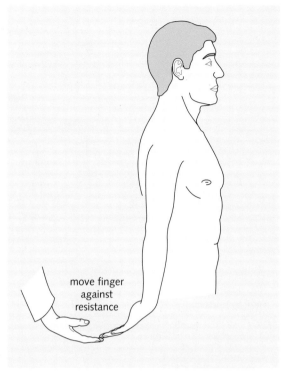

Fig 21.7 Golfer's elbow. If moving the fingers against resistance causes pain then the patient has golfer's elbow.

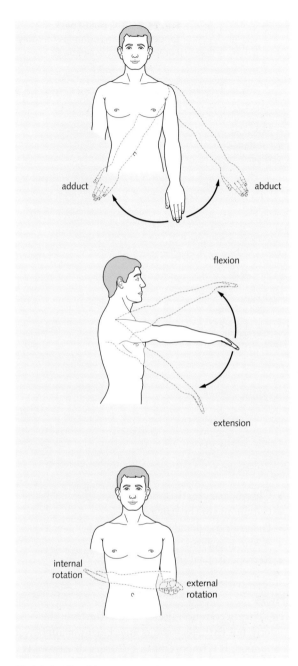

Fig 21.6 Shoulder movements.

comfortable at rest and whether or not they are pain free on moving around.

Examination of the back

Palpate the back for local tenderness suggestive of an inflammatory process. Record in the notes, the site of elicited tenderness. This may indicate the underlying disease (Fig. 21.8).

Examine the movements involving the vertebrae (flexion, extension, lateral flexion, rotation) and record both the range of movement and any pain elicited (Fig. 21.9). If ankylosing spondylitis is suspected, the sacroiliac joints must be assessed as these are often the first site of inflammation. Lateral compression of the pelvis may elicit pain in the presence of sacroiliitis.

Peripheral joints and systemic examination for arthritis

A full survey of other joints may reveal a more widespread arthropathy (e.g. ankylosing spondylitis, psoriatic arthropathy). Note the distribution of joint involvement and the presence of active synovitis.

In addition, there may also be non-articular clues to the presence of a systemic arthritis, for example:

- Psoriatic arthropathy is associated with a classic rash and nail changes.
- Ankylosing spondylitis is associated with decreased chest expansion, upper lobe fibrosis, iritis, and aortic regurgitation.

193

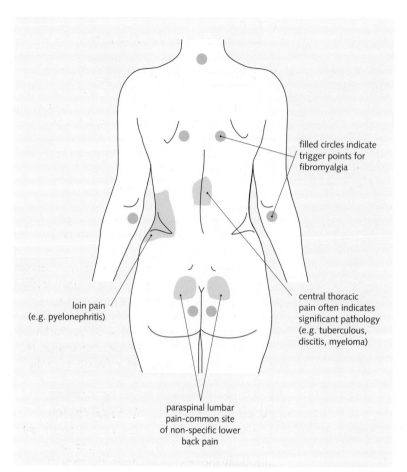

Fig. 21.8 The site of back tenderness is important as this may correspond to the aetiology.

filled circles indicate trigger points for fibromyalgia

central thoracic pain often indicates significant pathology (e.g. tuberculous, discitis, myeloma)

loin pain (e.g. pyelonephritis)

paraspinal lumbar pain-common site of non-specific lower back pain

Test for evidence of nerve root entrapment

Acute or chronic back pain may be due to a prolapsed intervertebral disc which may be associated with sciatic nerve root entrapment. The presence of nerve root entrapment and its localization may be elicited by testing:

- Straight leg raising.
- Femoral stretch test (Fig. 21.10).

Neurological examination of the legs

It is important to exclude nerve root pressure or spinal cord compression. A description of the neurological assessment of the legs is given in Chapter 17.

Detailed systemic examination

A detailed systemic examination should always be performed in a patient presenting with new-onset or progressive back pain. The back pain may be a manifestation of a systemic disease (e.g. metastatic carcinoma) or be referred from a source in the abdomen or pelvis, for example:

- Chronic pancreatitis.
- Carcinoma of the pancreas.
- Posterior duodenal ulcer.
- Aortic aneurysm.
- Retroperitoneal fibrosis.

Hips

The hip is a common site of osteoarthritis in the elderly, but pathology sometimes begins in infancy or childhood. It is important to recognize disease early in its natural history so that appropriate treatment can be instituted.

The initial part of the examination is performed with the patient lying flat and properly exposed. Later posture and gait can be formally assessed.

Position

Start by ensuring that the pelvis is set square so that leg length and deformity can be assessed accurately (Fig. 21.11). Attempt to position the line joining the anterior superior iliac spines perpendicular to the

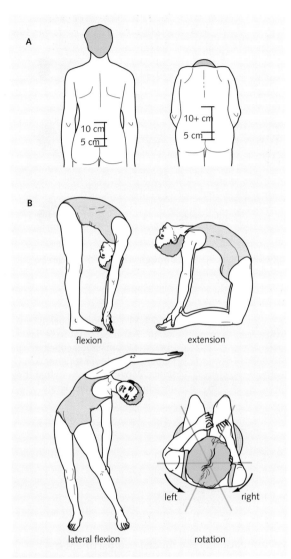

Fig. 21.9 Assessing movements of the (A) lumbar and (B) thoracic spine. Flexion of the lumbar spine can be objectively measured. Ask patients to touch their toes keeping their knees straight. Mark the spine at the lumbosacral junction 5 cm and 10 cm above this point. The distance between the upper two points should move approximately 5 cm on full flexion. This movement is impaired in ankylosing spondylitis.

legs. If this is not possible, there is a fixed abduction or adduction deformity.

Inspection

Note the presence of any scars (e.g. previous hip replacement), abnormal bony or soft tissue contours, and any abnormalities of the skin (e.g. erythema, sinuses).

Palpation

Palpate for any tenderness or warmth.

Measurement of leg length

If the pelvis is square, it is easy to estimate relative leg length by inspection. However, if there is any doubt, the leg can be measured from the anterior superior iliac spine to the medial malleolus (Fig. 21.12). An apparent discrepancy can be excluded by measuring the distance from the xiphisternum to the medial malleolus.

Examination for fixed deformity

Long-standing arthritis commonly results in a contracture of the joint capsule or muscles and subsequent fixed flexion deformity. Often, patients compensate by increasing their lumbar lordosis (Fig. 21.13). This may be assessed by placing a hand behind the lumbar spine to detect a lordosis and then asking patients to fully flex their good leg. Push the leg further into flexion to obliterate the lordosis and observe the angle of fixed flexion deformity in the affected hip.

Assessment of movements about the hip

It is important to assess movement about the hip and to eliminate movement of the pelvis that may compensate for deficiencies. Assess the range of movement for passive and active movements. The normal range of movement is illustrated in Fig. 21.14.

Active movement should also be tested to assess power using the Medical Research Council (MRC) grading of strength (see Fig. 17.11).

Gait and posture

Ask the patient to stand up. The Trendelenburg test should be performed to assess the postural stability of the hip joint (particularly the gluteal muscles). Normally, if one leg is lifted off the ground, the abductors will stabilize the leg and the pelvis will tilt up on the side of the lifted leg. If the abductors are ineffective, the body weight is too much for the adductors and the hip will tilt downwards (Fig. 21.15).

The causes of a positive Trendelenburg test are:

- Paralysis of the abductor muscles (e.g. polio).
- Absence of stability (e.g. ununited fracture of the femoral neck).

Finally assess the gait.

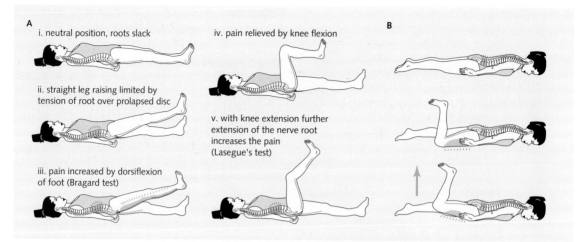

Fig. 21.10 Stretch tests. (A) Straight leg raising. Record the angle (normally 80–90°) through which each leg can be raised. (B) Femoral stretch test.

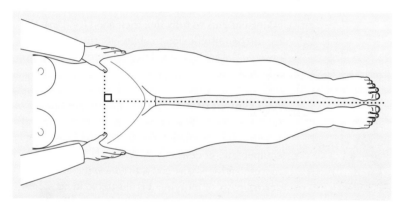

Fig. 21.11 Setting the pelvis square. Ask the patient to lie flat upon the examination couch. Palpate the anterior superior iliac spines. Move the pelvis so that they are square to the lower limbs.

Systemic survey

Remember to perform a systemic survey for other causes of hip symptoms.

Knee
Inspection

With the patient properly exposed and supine on a couch, inspect the knee, thigh, and lower leg, noting:

- Muscle bulk and evidence of wasting.
- Bony deformity (e.g. genu varum, genu valgum, Fig. 21.16).
- Evidence of soft tissue swelling or effusion.

Palpation

Palpate the bony contours of the knee joint noting any areas of tenderness or warmth. Specifically examine for an effusion. A small effusion may only be detectable by massaging fluid into the suprapatellar pouch and observing accumulation in the medial compartment by pressure over the superior and lateral aspects of the joint. A larger effusion is detectable by the patellar tap.

Movements

Assess for the presence of a fixed flexion deformity, the range of passive movement, and strength of active movement.

Tests of stability

The four major ligaments should be tested in turn as follows:

- Medial and lateral ligaments (Fig. 21.17). Support the knee in a position close to full extension and ask patients to relax their muscles. Apply an abduction and adduction force in turn to test the integrity of the medial and lateral ligaments respectively.

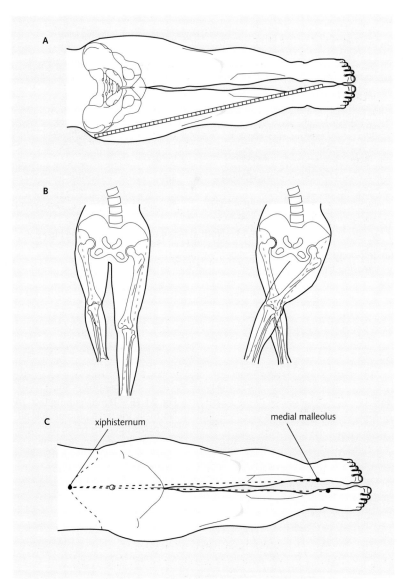

Fig. 21.12 Assessing relative leg length. (A) Measure from the anterior superior iliac spine to just below the medial malleolus on each side. (B) If the pelvis is tilted, the leg length may appear discrepant. (C) Apparent shortening may be detected measuring the distance from the xiphisternum to the medial malleolus.

xiphisternum

medial malleolus

- Anterior and posterior cruciate ligaments (Fig. 21.17). The anterior cruciate ligament prevents anterior displacement of the tibia on the femur. The posterior cruciate prevents posterior displacement. Flex the knee and fix the foot firmly on the couch by sitting lightly on it. Clasp the knee joint with both hands, holding your fingers behind the joint and thumbs laterally so that the tips are resting on each femoral condyle. Alternately push and pull the tibia to assess anteroposterior stability.

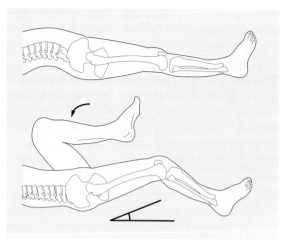

Fig. 21.13 Examination for fixed flexion deformity of the hip. A fixed deformity may be hidden by increasing the lumbar lordosis. This should be eliminated.

Normal range of movement at the hip joint	
Movement	**Range (degrees)**
flexion	0–120
extension	0 (extension occurs by rotating the pelvis)
abduction	0–30
adduction	0–30
lateral rotation	40
medial rotation	40

Fig. 21.14 Normal range of movement at the hip joint.

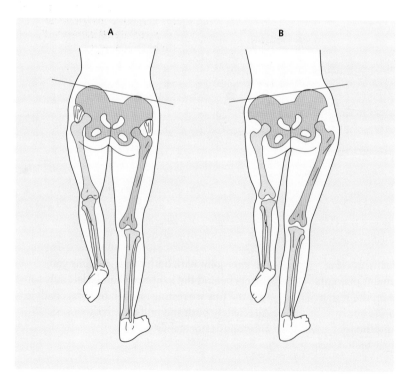

Fig. 21.15 Trendelenburg test. (A) Normally the hip abductors will tilt the pelvis upwards when the leg is lifted off the ground. (B) If the abductors cannot sustain the weight, the pelvis will droop.

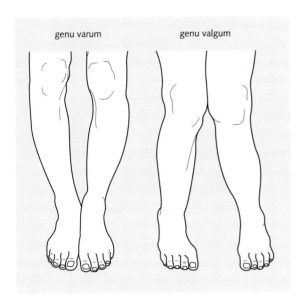

Fig. 21.16 Genu varum and genu valgum.

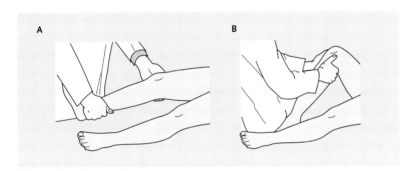

Fig. 21.17 Testing for stability of the knee joint. (A) Medial and lateral collateral ligaments. (B) Cruciate ligaments.

22. Ophthalmic Examination

Ophthalmic examination is essential in any detailed assessment of a patient. Not only may the cause of visual symptoms be determined, but the retina is the only place where the small blood vessels of the body can be directly visualized, providing clues to a host of systemic diseases.

Examination routine

Inspection

Before fundoscopy, look at the eyes for:

- Red eye (e.g. conjunctivitis, iritis, acute glaucoma, scleritis).
- Pupil size, symmetry, and irregularity.
- Pupil reflexes.
- Arcus senilis (significant in young adults).
- Squint.
- Ptosis.

Visual acuity

Test near and distant vision. Visual acuity should be tested in any complete physical examination. Test each eye individually with patients wearing their own spectacles or contact lenses to correct any refractive error. This need take only a few seconds, and can be adapted to different circumstances. For example:

- Read a newspaper headline from the other side of the room.
- Count fingers from the end of the bed.
- Identify light from dark, perceive hand movements.

If time permits, perform a formal assessment with a Snellen chart (Fig. 22.1). The patient should be placed 6 metres from a standard chart and asked to read the letters or a mini Snellen chart (used at 3 metres). The last line that can be clearly distinguished by the patient should be recorded for each eye. For example if the patient can read the line with '12' written under it, but not the next line, acuity in that eye is recorded as 6/12. Accepted normal vision is 6/6. The numerator refers to the distance from the chart that the patient is seated and the denominator is the last line that can be read.

Near vision can be formally tested with special books with text of a defined font and pitch size.

Eye movements and nystagmus

These are discussed in Chapter 17. Squint may be assessed by the cover test. If the eye fixating an object is covered, the squinting eye will move to take up fixation.

Fundoscopy

Examine in a darkened room to maximize pupil size. Ophthalmologists and diabetologists will dilate the pupil if there is no contraindication. The patient should look straight ahead and focus on the far wall. First set the ophthalmoscope so that you can see through it in an undistorted manner (especially if you normally wear glasses). Familiarize yourself with the way a fundoscope works so that, if asked in an exam, you can at least demonstrate you have lifted one up before!

 Practice fundoscopy on as many normal people as possible. It will become easier to recognize any pathological signs.

Red reflex

Start by shining the light from about 30 cm on the pupil to look for a red reflex. Loss of red reflex is usually due to vitreous haemorrhage or a dense cataract. Bring the ophthalmoscope closer to the eye and focus on the retina, looking systematically at the following.

Anterior chamber

Using a +10 lens, focus on the iris and examine for rubeosis, hypopyon, etc. Then by decreasing the power of the ophthalmoscope focus through the anterior chamber, lens, and posterior chamber. Small cataracts appear black and well-demarcated using this technique.

Optic disc

Note the size of the disc and colour. The most important pathologies to note are:

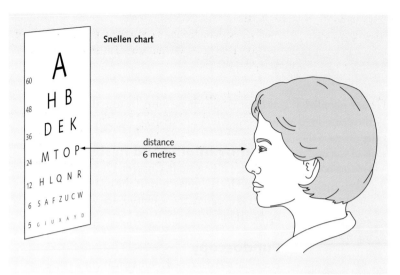

Snellen chart

60 A
48 H B
36 D E K
24 M T O P
12 H L Q N R
6 S A F Z U C W
5 G J U X A Y D

distance
6 metres

Fig. 22.1 Use of Snellen chart to test visual acuity.

- Optic atrophy (Fig. 22.2) may be due to multiple sclerosis, compression of the optic nerve (e.g. by pituitary tumour, aneurysm).
- Papilloedema (Fig. 22.3) may be due to accelerated hypertension, a space-occupying lesion, hydrocephalus, benign intracranial hypertension (especially in obese women), cavernous sinus thrombosis, central retinal vein thrombosis.
- Glaucoma – pathological cupping of the disc due to gradual loss of nerve fibres and supporting glial cells, resulting in a pale disc with an enlarged cup.
- Myelinated nerve fibres.

Retina

Note the retinal vessels. Trace the vessels away from the optic disc towards each quadrant of the retina in turn. The veins are darker and appear wider than the arteries. The main features to observe about the retinal vessels are:

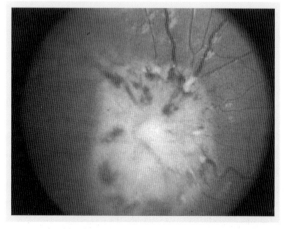

Fig. 22.3 Papilloedema (swelling of the optic disc) caused by acute lymphoflastic leukaemia. (Courtesy of Myron Yanoff.)

- Engorgement of the veins, which imply slow flow (e.g. retinal venous occlusion, polycythaemia).
- Attenuation of the arterioles (e.g. due to retinal artery occlusion, widespread retinal atrophy).
- Arteriovenous (AV) nipping in hypertension.

Note the retinal background in each quadrant. In particular, look for:
- Haemorrhages. The most common haemorrhages are flame-shaped haemorrhages, which are superficial and occur in severe hypertension. 'Dot haemorrhages' are not true bleeding areas, but represent microaneurysms, which are prone to rupture, forming 'blot' haemorrhages.
- Hard exudates (true retinal exudates). These are usually small, sharply defined, and intensely white.

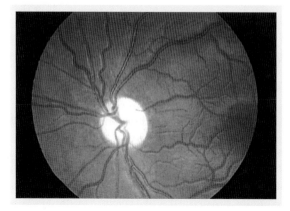

Fig. 22.2 Optic atrophy. (Courtesy of Myron Yanoff.)

- Soft exudates (areas of infarction). These have a fluffy appearance resembling cotton wool. They usually have an ill-defined edge.
- Neovascularization. New blood vessel formation is an important sign of diabetic retinopathy. These new blood vessels are fragile and appear as a tuft of delicate vessels on the surface of the retina.
- Photocoagulation scars.
- Pigmentation (retinitis pigmentosa).

Some of the more important fundal abnormalities are illustrated in Figs 22.4 and 22.5.

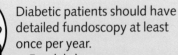

Diabetic patients should have detailed fundoscopy at least once per year.
 Fundal changes are sensitive markers of end-organ damage in diabetes mellitus and hypertension.

Macula

Ask the patient to look briefly directly at the light of the ophthalmoscope. Macular disease is common in the elderly.

Visual fields

The examination routine for testing by confrontation is discussed in Chapter 17 (p. 147) . More formal visual field testing can be performed by assessing the visual threshold in different regions, but this relies upon special equipment and skilled interpretation.

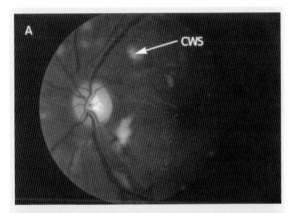

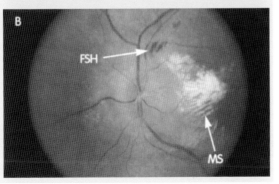

C	Features of hypertensive retinopathy
Grade I	silver wiring of arterioles
Grade II	AV nipping
Grade III	soft exudates (due to small infarcts) flame-shaped haemorrhages
Grade IV	papilloedema

Fig. 22.4 (A, B) Grade III hypertension. CWS, cotton wool spot; FSH, flame-shaped haemorrhage; MS, macular star. (C) Features of hypertensive retinopathy. Grades III and IV indicate accelerated hypertension. (Courtesy of Myron Yanoff.)

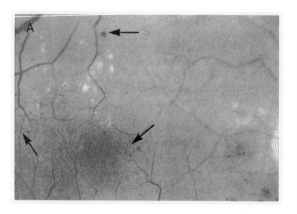

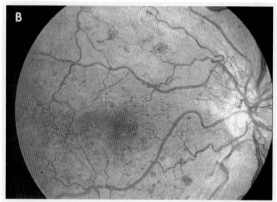

C   Features of diabetic retinopathy

background diabetic retinopathy
dot haemorrhages (micro-aneurysms)
blot haemorrhages (discrete bleed)
hard exudates

proliferative retinopathy
neovascularization
(laser coagulation scars)

Fig. 22.5 Diabetic retinopathy. (A) Background changes. Arrows indicate haemorrhages. (B) Neovascularization at the optic disc. (C) Features of diabetic retinopathy. (A, B courtesy of Myron Yanoff.)

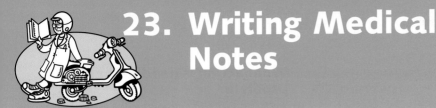

23. Writing Medical Notes

General points

When writing up the medical notes, it is extremely important to adopt a systematic and objective style. Your notes form a permanent record of your impression of the patient at that moment in time. It should be possible for another health care professional to read your notes and to understand them and your conclusions. Although the following points appear to be obvious, it is alarming how often simple good clinical practice is ignored. Always ensure that:

- Each piece of paper has the patient's name at its head – notes have an uncanny knack of falling apart!
- Each entry is dated, and ideally a time recorded.
- Each entry is followed by a legible signature, your name, grade (printed), speciality and your bleep number. Scrawled initials are inadequate. Someone else has to read your notes and be able to identify who has written them.
- Your handwriting is legible. This point sounds ludicrously obvious, but unfortunately anyone who has looked through a set of notes will testify that it is often forgotten.
- Each statement is objective. It is no longer acceptable to write value judgements in the notes if they cannot be justified. Avoid the use of meaningless phrases such as the commonly written NFN (Normal For Norfolk) or NLM (Nice Looking Mum). These are not acceptable. You could end up in world of hurt in court if a lawyer got hold of these.

Your handwriting must be clear and legible. It is potentially dangerous to write in hieroglyphics!

- You write in the notes every time you see the patient. You do not have to write an essay – a short statement of the patient's progress is an important record. Even noting a lack of any change since your last consultation is important.
- You avoid the use of abbreviations as much as possible. If they have to be used, use only accepted terms such as MI (myocardial infarction), LVF (left ventricular failure).
- You use diagrams where appropriate as they are often much more descriptive than long paragraphs.
- You keep your record as concise as possible.

Remember that patients (or their lawyers) may gain access to the notes. Avoid the use of statements that you cannot justify.

Often the history given by the patient is recounted in an unconventional manner. When writing your notes, it is usual practice to record the history in the order described in Part I of this book. This helps to structure your own thoughts as well as those of anyone who subsequently reads the notes. There is an example of this in the chapter. Clearly the history is a dynamic process, and there are infinite variations and exceptions to this general aim.

Finally, it is important to make a note of what information has been given to the patient. Poor communication between the doctor and patient is responsible for the vast majority of instances of patient dissatisfaction, complaints and litigation. It is helpful, not only to yourself, but also for other doctors to be aware of exactly what information the patient has when starting the next consultation.

Structuring your thoughts

When you first start to take medical histories, it is a struggle to remember the traditional order of questions to ask and the normal examination routine. However, your job has only just begun! Remember that the aim of a clerking is to:

- Identify any problems.
- Formulate a differential diagnosis of these problems.
- Consider a plan of initial investigations to elucidate the underlying cause, severity, and prognosis of each problem.
- Initiate treatment and advice for the patient.

Once your examination has been completed, it is helpful to go through a routine and ask yourself the following questions.

In an examination setting, it is important to spend time reflecting on the significant points of the history and examination. Always allow enough time to gather your thoughts before presenting your findings.

What is the patient's presenting complaint?

Never forget the initial reason for the patient seeking medical attention. Although you may have identified more significant medical problems during your history and examination, you must show patients that you are addressing their primary concern.

What problems have I identified?

Problems can take many forms and be physical, social, or psychological. Before trying to dissect the differential diagnosis, it may be helpful to write down a list of each problem. A problem may be:

- A proven diagnosis (e.g. diabetes).
- A pathological state (e.g. renal failure).
- An abnormal symptom (e.g. coughing up blood – haemoptysis).
- An abnormal sign (e.g. pulmonary consolidation, tachypnoea, pitting oedema).
- An abnormal investigation result (e.g. raised plasma creatinine concentration, increased carbon monoxide transfer coefficient, a raised C-reactive protein, haematuria and red cell casts in the urine).
- A past medical history (e.g. pneumonia).
- A social or psychological problem (e.g. unemployed, homelessness, intravenous drug abuser).
- Significant risk factor for illness (e.g. smoking).

It is only by identifying these individual problems and considering them as a group that their relative importance and relationship to each other can be systematically assessed.

What action is needed for each problem?

Try to prioritize the importance of each problem and decide upon the urgency of treatment and investigation of each.

What is the differential diagnosis of each problem?

By assessing each problem in turn it may become apparent that a unifying diagnosis could explain a number of features. Equally, some diagnoses may be excluded by the presence of certain features. When you see a patient always remember that unusual presentations of common problems are still more frequently encountered than the common presentations of rare diseases.

What is the most likely underlying diagnosis?

Once a differential diagnosis has been formulated, it is important to make a mental note of the order of probability of each diagnosis. This is important, as immediate treatment and investigations are aimed at the diagnoses at the top of your list and those that require urgent therapy.

What investigations should be requested?

In the examination setting, as in real life, it is important to consider which investigations are appropriate, and their urgency. When requesting investigations it is essential to consider how the result of a particular test is going to help refine your management of the patient. It is no longer acceptable to adopt the mentality of 'I always request chest radiography, an electrocardiogram, full blood count and biochemical profile for all medical patients!' Consider each problem in turn and assess which investigations are appropriate. It is by this systematic approach that potentially important and useful investigations are not omitted.

Start by considering the simple and non-invasive tests, and then consider the value of more discriminatory but invasive investigations. Weigh up the potential usefulness of the result against the potential morbidity, cost, (and mortality) of each test. For example:

- Many simple blood tests are cheap and non-invasive so a low threshold is needed.
- A positron emission tomograph is expensive, but in limited situations offers very specific

information that cannot be reliably obtained from other sources.

- Coronary angiography is the gold standard for diagnosing structural causes of angina, but does have a defined mortality.

Ideally you should have an idea about the sensitivity (ability to detect something when its there), specificity (ability to recognize when something isn't there) and the predictive values of the test in the population of the patients you are involved with.

Presenting your findings

It is important to get as much practice as possible in presenting your findings to your colleagues. The easiest part of a consultation is taking a history and performing an examination. Most students struggle when trying to collate the vast amount of information obtained from a clerking and reformat it in a digestible form.

Remember how dull it can be listening to inexperienced students presenting their findings. It is essential to be as concise as possible so that important information is not lost among masses of irrelevant detail. Further, examination formats such as structured long cases and OSCEs, which are increasingly common, require students to give focused case presentations.

When presenting a clerking, put yourself in the audience's position and consider what information you would like to hear.

Start with a pithy introductory phrase describing the patient and his or her reason for presenting for medical attention. This is important as it provides a frame for the subsequent information. Your audience will already have started the process of differential diagnosis and be anticipating certain specific facts.

Describe the detailed history, using the patient's words where possible, and avoid placing value

judgements at this stage. You will have asked the patient many specific questions. Your listeners are interested in a limited number of these. Using your judgement, introduce important negative responses, but do not overburden your audience with irrelevant detail. For example, if your patient presents with exertional chest pain your audience needs to know about risk factors for ischaemic heart disease and other cardiac symptoms even if there are none, but introducing information about myopia or the patient's stool habit will only cloud the important issues. The rest of the history should be presented in a similarly edited form. Unrelated symptoms described by the patient can be mentioned at the end of the history.

When presenting your examination findings:
- Start by describing the vital signs.
- Then concentrate on the system primarily affected. Discuss your findings in this system at length.
- For the other systems of the body, describe any positive findings and any important negative signs that may affect interpretation of the main findings.

It is important to sound confident. It is very difficult when you first begin, but you must commit yourself. Good problem presentation has been shown in itself to aid the process of clinical reasoning. Many students start by making excuses for having difficulty in eliciting a sign. This does not impress examiners and is not helpful – in the real world, your interpretation of physical signs affects your management of the patient.

At the end of your examination findings, provide:
- A short summary encompassing the main features of the history and examination.
- Your interpretation and analysis of the problems with a brief differential diagnosis with a note of features in favour of or against each differential diagnosis.

Sample clerking

A sample medical clerking is shown in Fig. 23.1 and illustrates some of the points discussed at the start of this chapter.

Hospital No: X349182

BLOGGS, Joe

29/4/40

20/6/05 19:30   65 yr old man   Referred by GP

PC   Productive cough ↑ SOB
            Background of COPD 15 years.

> 1. Presenting complaint should be brief, but it is helpful to mention relevant background information.

HPC   1/52 cough and green sputum. No haemoptysis. ↑ SOB over last 3/7.
            + Wheezy. + Feverish and sweaty.
            Reduced ex. Tolerance – now < 20 yds. Normally > 200 yds.
            Using home nebs – only minimal relief.
            + Aching, dull chest pain. Worse on inspiration.
                    - no radiation
                    - onset 3/7 ago, gradual
                    - not getting worse.
            No weight loss.

> 2. Mention only the relevant negatives. In this case it is important to mention the absence of haemoptysis and weight-loss because of the history of cancer. It is always wise to document whether or not there is chest pain.

PMH   COPD Dx 1989 – on home nebs. Not on home O2.
            Hypertension Dx 1995
            Ca sigmoid colon 2001 – resected. Has colostomy.
            Appendicectomy as child.
            °DM/IHD/CVA/Ep/Renal/J/An

> 3. A useful way of recording important negatives on one line. This stands for: No history of diabetes, ischaemic heart disease, stroke, epilepsy, renal disease, jaundice or anaemia.

DH   Beclomethasone MDI 100mcg 2 puffs tds
            Atrovent MDI 20mcg bd
            Salbutamol 100mcg MDI or 2.5mg nebulas prn
            Lisinopril 20mg od
            Aspirin 75mg od

> 4. Always record the dose and frequency of any drugs – remember you'll be writing the drug chart later! Always document that you have asked about drug allergies.

Allergies NKDA   Smoking – stopped 15 yrs ago
                              - 30 pach-years total

                       Alcohol – occasional. < 20 units/week.

Fam Hx   Nil of note   Social Hx   Lives with wife – currently well
                                          Retired factory worker
                                          No social package.

Fig. 23.1   Sample medical clerking.

O/E   Thin man. Breathless at rest.
       Looks distressed. Short sentences only.

       Afebrile 37.0   156/80   Sats 96% on air

       °J/A/Cy/Cl/O/L   HR 100 reg
                                         HS I + II + 0
                                         JVP →
                                         Apex = Ⓝ

       Widespread wheeze
       Good air entry
       Coarse creps Ⓛ base
       PNR
       RR = 36   PEFR = 150

sigmoid colectomy
2001

Appendix

       Abdo soft now tender
       °Masses
       BS = N

       CNS   Grossly intact. GCS 15 PERLA
              Alert and responsive.

       Imp   Infective exacerbation of COPD
                       Cardiac event
                ⌂⌂ PE
                       Note prev Hx Ca colon – consider risk of secondaries.

       Plan   Admit
              28% O2 by mask
              ECG ✓
              IV access ✓
              Bloods ✓ CXR ✓ ABG ✓
              salbutamol nebs 5mg – 1 hourly
              Atrovent 500 mcg nebs – 1 hourly
              IV co-amoxiclav 1.2g tds
              Prednisolone 40mg orally
              Review progress. Await results

                       HORTON-SZAR   437

5. Record your initial observations –
   they are important. 'Alert & chatty' or
   'Distressed & looks unwell' tell you a lot
   about the patient.

6. Always use diagrams to clarify
   your examination findings.

7. If there is no abnormality of the
   CNS, simply include a one-line summary.

8. Always include a management plan –
   even when you are still a student. It might
   not be right but you need to start training
   yourself to think like a doctor.

9. Sign your notes,
   including printed surname
   and bleep number.

Fig. 23.1, cont'd

24. Further Investigations

Once the history and examination have been performed, it is necessary to assess your differential diagnosis and to plan a management strategy for the patient. Part of this process includes arranging further investigations in order to refine the differential diagnosis. The tests may be performed to:

- Exclude serious conditions.
- Confirm the presence of a suspected pathology.
- Obtain a baseline against which further progress may be assessed.
- Assess the severity of the current illness.
- Assess the response to therapy.
- Predict prognosis.

Before requesting any investigations think how the patient will benefit from the result.

Remember that it is easy to request investigations, but the results may require great skill in interpretation. Furthermore, each test has a cost and produces a defined morbidity (however small) to the patient. It is essential to anticipate how the results of the investigation may alter your management at the time of the request. If you cannot see how the results of an investigation will alter your management, there is absolutely no point requesting that test. For each test, be prepared to justify:

- Why it is being requested.
- How the result will affect management.
- That the potential benefit of the information outweighs the cost and morbidity incurred.
- The urgency of a request.

The lists given below are not intended to be comprehensive, and certainly do not imply that every test should be requested for each system. The tests requested need to be tailored to the clinical scenario. For each system, consider:

- Urine.
- Blood.
- Radiological imaging.
- Electrical recording.
- Special investigations.

Cardiovascular system

The diagnosis of acute MI is made on the basis of two of the following three factors being present: chest pain, ECG changes consistent with MI and an increase in cardiac enzymes.

Blood tests

The following blood tests may help in the diagnosis of cardiac pathologies:

- Full blood count. Anaemia may be the cause of, or exacerbate heart failure or angina.
- Erythrocyte sedimentation rate (ESR). Inflammatory conditions (e.g. endocarditis) are associated with a raised ESR. The C-reactive protein (CRP) is an acute phase protein and is often more sensitive in changing inflammatory states (e.g. monitoring the response of infective endocarditis to antibiotic therapy).
- Cardiac enzymes. Tropinin T is released by cardiac muscle breakdown. It should be measured 12 hours post chest pain or a change in rhythm.
- Biochemical profile. Exclude electrolyte disturbance as a cause of arrhythmia.
- Thyroid function tests. Hyperthyroidism is a common cause of atrial fibrillation. Hypothyroidism may present as a pleural effusion or heart failure.
- Blood cultures. Essential if endocarditis is suspected.

If infective endocarditis is suspected obtain at least six sets of blood cultures.

Urinalysis

Look for microscopic haematuria if infective endocarditis is suspected.

Imaging
Chest radiography

A chest radiograph is usually requested for a patient who presents with cardiological symptoms. Note the presence of:

- Cardiac enlargement – cardiothoracic ratio should be less than 50% (posteroanterior film).
- Signs of increased left atrial filling pressure – upper lobe blood diversion, septal lines, pulmonary oedema, pleural effusion (Fig. 24.1).
- Signs of left atrial enlargement – prominence of atrial appendage (straight left heart border), double contour of right heart border, splaying of the carina.
- Left ventricular aneurysm – post-myocardial infarction.
- Abnormal calcification – valvular calcification in rheumatic heart disease, tuberculous pericardial disease (Fig. 24.2).

Echocardiography

Echocardiography may be transthoracic (non-invasive) or transoesophageal, which provides better images of the left atrium and aorta. It is useful for assessing chamber size, valvular pathology, pericardial disease, and contractility of the heart. Echocardiography is usually requested to:

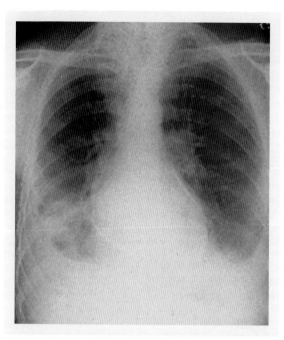

Fig. 24.2 Radiograph of pericardial calcification. Note the associated pleural effusions.

- Comply with the ruling that the National Service Framework now says all cases of heart failure should have an echo to investigate the cause of heart failure.
- Investigate heart murmurs.
- Look for vegetations in suspected infective endocarditis.
- Investigate pericardial effusions and tamponade.
- Assess the severity of cor pulmonale.
- Investigate aortic aneurysms.

Modifications of echocardiography such as stress echo and contrast echo may also be used to investigate angina and septal defects, respectively. The two most common views are illustrated in Figs 24.3 and 24.4.

Nuclear imaging

Nuclear imaging (e.g. thallium scan) can be used to investigate suspected angina in a patient who cannot perform an exercise test.

Electrocardiography (ECG)
12-lead ECG

ECGs are very widely performed. They can be used to assess rhythm disturbances, ischaemia or infarction, left ventricular hypertrophy, right ventricular hypertrophy; a useful ECG resource can be found at *medstat.med.utah.edu/kw/ecg*.

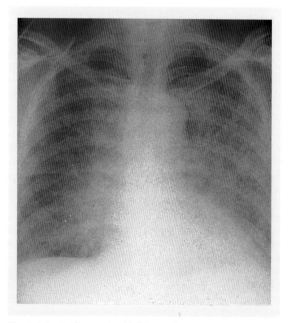

Fig. 24.1 Radiograph of left heart failure. Note the cardiomegaly, bilateral alveolar shadowing in a perihilar distribution, and the presence of fluid in the horizontal fissure.

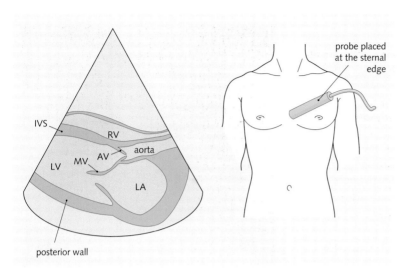

Fig. 24.3 Diagrammatic representation of an echocardiogram of a normal long-axis view of the left ventricle. The probe is placed in the left parasternal region. This provides a good view for assessing chamber size, left ventricular wall motion, and ejection fraction as well as mitral and aortic valve regurgitation using colour Doppler. AV, aortic valve; IVS, interventricular septum; LA, left atrium; LV, left ventricle; MV, mitral valve; RV, right ventricle.

24-hour tape (Holter monitor)

A 24-hour tape is used to investigate paroxysmal cardiac arrhythmias that may be associated with symptoms. Patients should be instructed to indicate when they have palpitations or other symptoms such as lightheadedness so that their symptoms can be correlated with electrical disturbances.

Event recorder (cardiac memo)

If the palpitation lasts long enough, it is desirable to record the ECG at the time of the arrhythmia. Symptoms can then be directly related to the electrical activity of the heart.

Exercise ECG

The exercise ECG is used as a screening test in the investigation of ischaemia. Many cardiologists do not refer patients for angiography if the exercise test is normal. In addition, exercise testing provides collateral information on exercise tolerance. Remember that it is a waste of time requesting an exercise test for a wheelchair-bound 90-year-old!

Coronary angiography

This invasive investigation is used:

- To assess the coronary arteries.
- To measure pressures in the heart chambers in the assessment of valve pathology or cor pulmonale.

Respiratory system

Blood tests

Patients with respiratory disease often have infections or unexplained dyspnoea. The more common blood tests requested include:

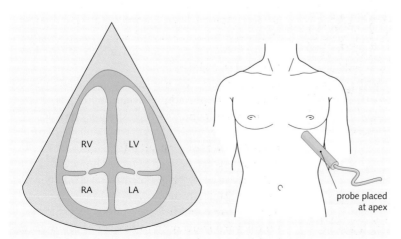

Fig. 24.4 Diagrammatic echocardiogram representing of a four-chamber view. The probe is placed at the apex. This view allows assessment of the left ventricular apex and quantification of the severity of aortic and tricuspid valve pathology. LA, left atrium; LV, left ventricle; RA, right atrium; RV, right ventricle.

- Full blood count. A raised white cell count suggests infection. A raised eosinophil count may occur in rare conditions.
- You can check the C-reactive protein as a non-specific marker of inflammation. As the disease state resolves the level should drop.
- Blood cultures – important in the diagnosis of pneumonia.
- Arterial blood gases – essential in the assessment of severe asthma attacks and for providing baseline function for patients with chronic obstructive pulmonary disease (COPD).

Sputum assessment

Sputum culture is part of the routine assessment of a patient with a chest infection. When investigating pneumonia, especially in sick patients, liaison with the laboratory is important for diagnosing some of the less common infections (e.g. *Pneumocystis*, mycobacteria, *Nocardia*).

Sputum cytology is used in the investigation of malignancy and certain pneumonias.

Imaging
Chest radiography

In the context of respiratory disease, the important features to note are:

- Area of consolidation – for example lobar or widespread.
- Evidence of COPD – paucity of lung vascular markings, hyperinflation, flat diaphragms, narrow mediastinum, bullae.
- Pneumothorax or areas of collapse in asthmatic patients.
- Hilar masses – lung carcinoma may underlie many respiratory disorders (Fig. 24.5); bilateral lymphadenopathy occurs in sarcoidosis.
- Pleural effusions.
- Fibrosis.

Computerized tomography (CT) scan

Occasionally CT scanning is needed to clarify features on the radiograph, for example:

- Investigation of direct or metastatic spread of suspected lung cancer.
- Investigation of bronchiectasis.
- Investigation of pulmonary fibrosis.

Lung function tests

Assessment of gas exchange and airway function may be performed by the following methods.

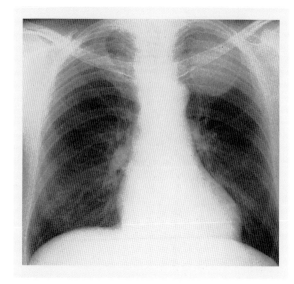

Fig. 24.5 Radiograph of a Pancoast tumour with destruction of the first left rib.

Peak expiratory flow rate

This should be considered as part of the routine examination of the asthmatic patient.

Arterial blood gases

These are useful for assessing gas exchange in acute pulmonary disease. In addition they provide a baseline assessment for patients with COPD when they are stable (e.g. 3 months after any infective exacerbation).

Spirometry

The most simple assessments of forced expiratory volume in 1 second (FEV_1) and forced vital capacity (FVC) can provide invaluable information in respiratory disease. The ratio of FEV_1/FVC and absolute values will help in the diagnosis of:

- Obstructive disease – low ratio ($<70\%$) and low absolute values.
- Restrictive disease – normal or high ratio, reduced FVC (Fig. 24.6).

In addition, the absolute value of FEV_1 is often used to assess patients with respiratory muscle weakness (e.g. myasthenia gravis, Guillain–Barré syndrome).

Variations can be used to record bronchial reactivity to allergens or potential reversibility with bronchodilators.

The transfer coefficient of carbon monoxide (K_{co}) provides a measure of the efficiency of gas exchange and permeability of the alveolar membrane:

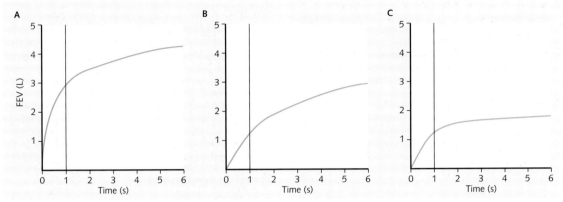

Fig. 24.6 Examples of spirometry. (A) Normal patient – FEV_1/FVC = 3.0/4.0 (75%). (B) COPD – FEV_1/FVC = 1.5/3.0 (50%). (C) Fibrosis – FEV_1/FVC = 1.5/1.8 (83%).

- Diseases resulting in impaired ventilation or perfusion reduce K_{CO}.
- Diseases such as pulmonary haemorrhage increase K_{CO}.

Bronchoscopy

Bronchoscopy allows direct visualization of the upper airways and abnormal areas can be biopsied. In addition, bronchoalveolar lavage can be performed to collect specimens for culture and cytology and to assess the differential cell types in the alveoli.

Abdominal system

Blood tests

Blood tests are required for a wide range of abdominal presentations including the investigation of anaemia, jaundice, palpable masses, abdominal pain, and bowel disturbance.

The more commonly requested investigations include:

- Full blood count. This may reveal anaemia. The mean cell volume (MCV) provides a starting point for further investigation. A raised white count suggests an inflammatory process.
- ESR. Raises the suspicion of inflammatory lesions.
- Biochemical profile. Assesses liver function, renal function, and calcium. Electrolyte levels may fluctuate during diarrhoeal illnesses or fluid replacement.
- Vitamin B_{12}, iron studies, red cell folate levels. These are initial investigations in anaemia.
- Amylase. Exclude pancreatitis as a cause of abdominal pain.

Urinalysis

Urinalysis is part of the routine assessment during a detailed examination. Note the presence of:

- Glycosuria – diabetes mellitus.
- Haematuria – for example due to glomerulonephritis, renal stone, bladder lesion.
- Proteinuria.
- Ketonuria – diabetic ketoacidosis.
- Nitrites or leucocytes – indicate infection.

Imaging
Chest radiography

An erect chest radiograph is often requested for patients presenting with acute abdominal pain. The important features to note are:

- The presence of free air under the diaphragm – suggests perforated viscus (Fig. 24.7).
- Lower lobe consolidation – pneumonia masquerading as acute abdominal pain.

Abdominal radiography

The main features to note are:

- Distended loops of bowel – suggestive of bowel obstruction.
- Double contour to the bowel – perforation with free air in the abdomen (Wriggler's sign).
- Radio-opaque gallstones – unusual (only 10%).
- Radio-opaque renal calculi – common (i.e. 90%).

Abdominal ultrasound and CT scan

These are performed to localize and identify any abnormal masses, detect free fluid in the abdomen, and assess the size and parenchyma of intra-abdominal organs.

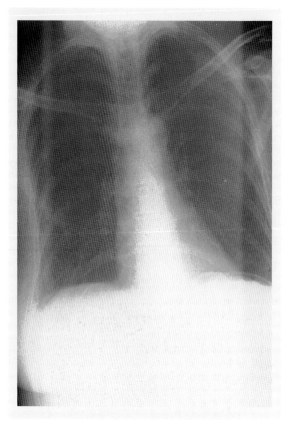

Fig. 24.7 Air under the diaphragm. This suggests the presence of a perforated abdominal viscus.

Ultrasound is particularly useful in the assessment of jaundice as biliary tree dilatation and gallstones are readily identified.

Following trauma, CT or ultrasound may be used to diagnose damage to the liver, kidney, or spleen.

Barium studies
Barium studies are used to assess abnormalities of the mucosa or motility disorders. The four main studies are:
- Barium swallow – to assess the oesophagus (e.g. for dysphagia, heartburn).
- Barium meal – to assess mucosal abnormalities of the stomach and duodenum (e.g. for dyspepsia, iron deficiency anaemia).
- Small-bowel meal or enema – to assess the small bowel, in particular the terminal ileum (e.g. for malabsorption, suspected Crohn's disease).
- Barium enema – to investigate the colon (e.g. for anaemia, change in bowel habit, rectal bleeding).

Endoscopy
Endoscopy is performed to visualize the mucosa of the bowel directly and to biopsy any abnormal area. Upper gastrointestinal (GI) endoscopy will assess as far as the duodenum. A good colonoscopy will reveal the whole of the large bowel.

Endoscopic retrograde cholangiopancreatography (ERCP) can be performed to image the pancreatic or hepatic and bile ducts and to treat any strictures or remove stones.

Stool assessment
Stool assessment may involve:
- Culture – for diarrhoeal illnesses.
- Microscopy – for ova cysts and parasites.
- Faecal fat estimation.

Neurological system

Imaging
CT scans and magnetic resonance imaging (MRI) of the brain or spinal cord are often requested to investigate acute and chronic neurological symptoms. CT is the modality of choice in the investigation of acute trauma or subarachnoid haemorrhage.

Electroencephalography (EEG)
The EEG relates to the brain in the same way that the ECG relates to the heart. However, correlation between the traces and physiological function is less understood. The main uses of the EEG are in:
- Diagnosis of epilepsy.
- Diagnosis of encephalitis.

Lumbar puncture
Lumbar puncture provides essential information in the assessment of patients with neurological disease, especially those with suspected meningitis. The main indications are:
- Investigation of meningitis.
- Pyrexia of unknown origin.
- Subarachnoid haemorrhage.
- Inflammatory central nervous system (CNS) disease (e.g. multiple sclerosis, vasculitis).

 In the presence of decreased level of consciousness or focal neurological sign, obtain a CT scan of the brain before performing a lumbar puncture.

Lumbar puncture is contraindicated in the presence of:

- Suppuration of the skin overlying the spinal canal.
- Undiagnosed papilloedema.

Electromyography (EMG)

EMG is used in the assessment of the peripheral nervous system. It is particularly useful if the patient reports:

- Weakness or wasting.
- Undue fatiguability.
- Sensory impairment or paraesthesia.

EMG will establish a diagnosis of a neuropathy and identify the pathological process as a demyelination or axonal neuropathy. In addition, diagnostic information may be provided for some myopathies.

Evoked potentials

Visual evoked potentials are sometimes used in the assessment of a patient with suspected multiple sclerosis.

Locomotor system

X-rays are the usual investigation in the diagnosis of muscular and joint problems. Figures 24.8 and 24.9 show the changes associated with osteoarthritis in the knee and hip, respectively.

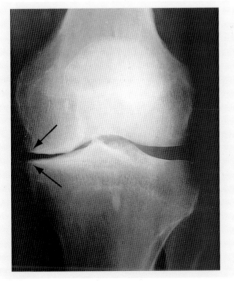

Fig. 24.8 X-ray of knee showing osteoarthritic changes. Note the loss of joint space, bone sclerosis, osteophytes and subchondral cysts.

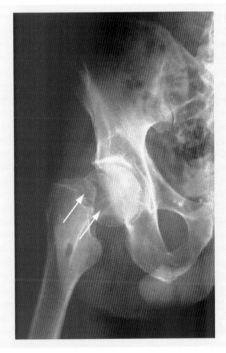

Fig. 24.9 X-ray showing a fractured neck of femur.

217

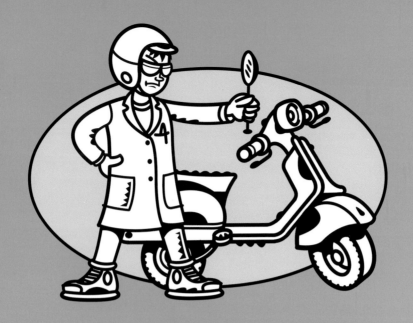

SELF-ASSESSMENT

Exam Technique

By the time you read this book you will probably have passed lots of exams at medical school. The aim of this short section is to share with you some of the tips my friends and I found useful.

Study groups are useful; a minimum of three people is really needed and everyone needs to prepare for them. I found that groups worked best for refining physical examination technique. The group first brainstormed all the things we thought we could be asked to examine. I have included the list here:

- CVS
- RS
- GI
- Cranial nerves
- Eye function
- Upper limbs
- Lower limbs
- Cerebellar screen
- Speech language
- Higher functions
- Hands
- Elbow
- Shoulder
- Back
- Knee
- Hip
- Neck
- Thyroid screen/goitre
- Describe the lump/mass
- Varicose veins
- Peripheral vascular system
- Skin lesion
- Lump in groin/scrotum
- Developmental assessment
- Baby check
- Examination of legs
- Examination of ears nose/throat
- Breast examination
- CPR
- Fluid balance charts
- Prescription kardexes
- Warfarin/insulin presciptions
- Death certificates

This list is not exhaustive so add to it if you wish. Remember, examiners get more devious all the time!

Then we pulled our resources to try to come up with the best answers. We all brought with us some good ideas, so will you. We set it up as follows. One person would be the patient, one the medical student and one the examiner.

Once we had all the questions and answers, we wrote the OSCE questions onto slips of paper and placed them all in a bag. The session then went as follows. The 'examiner' put his hand into the bag and pulled out a question. The 'student' then had to examine the 'patient'. The 'examiner' timed and marked the 'student'. At first we were hopeless but we all got there in the end and 'passed'. This has the advantage that it mimics the surprise of walking into an OSCE and it means you do not concentrate on one area to the detriment of the others.

If you want to practise alone, then your old teddy bear makes a good patient. One of my friends made a life-size paper man and took it to her attachments throughout the region so she had something to practise on!

The groups should be sociable and are also a good way of helping share the stress of examinations.

Spin the bottle has always been popular. Try it with a bottle of wine. Get a group of friends together. Everybody should bring some sample questions and put them in a bag. Have some food, drink the wine, then sit in a circle and spin the bottle. Whoever the bottle ends up pointing to has to answer a question pulled from the bag. This worked best for Friday night revision sessions.

When you are revising allow yourself time off. Say 'I'm not doing anything on Sunday evening. I'll see friends or go to the cinema but I'm not going to feel guilty about not revising'. There comes a point with revision when all you are doing is appeasing your conscience.

The aim of revising at this stage is not to have a detailed knowledge of everything; this is impossible. It is also why, in the postgraduate world, people specialize. The aim is rather for broad strokes. Know a little about as much as you can. Study guides and/or learning outcomes should detail which conditions your examiners feel important. Let that guide your learning.

On the day there are some points to remember. Read the questions and do what you are asked to do. It sounds simple but *every* year people do not. If you mess up a question put it behind you and move on. There will not usually be 'killer stations' that you must pass, so accept that you have failed a question and move on.

There are two key facts that are the absolute bottom line when it comes to exams:

1. The world will still turn.
2. Mummy and Daddy still love you.

Everyone will tell you that the examiners are actually out to pass you by the time you come to Finals. (After all if they don't who is going to be their house officer in 2 months' time?). It does not matter how many times you are told this, you will not believe it until you have sat Finals, and only then will you understand what people meant.

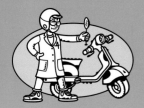

Multiple-choice Questions (MCQs)

In the following indicate whether each answer is True or False.

1. In the fetal circulation:

(a) The placental blood flow is perfusion dependent
(b) Venous blood flow is deflected from the right atrium to the left atrium via the ductus arteriosa
(c) There is no blood flow through the fetal lungs
(d) Systemic venous return is a mixture of oxygenated and de-oxygenated blood
(e) At birth the first breath increases pulmonary arterial pressure.

2. In matters pertaining to contraception:

(a) Eisenmenger's syndrome is an indication for early female sterilization
(b) Focal migraine is not a contraindication to the CoC
(c) A condom is as efficacious as a diaphragm at preventing the spread of sexually transmitted diseases
(d) The return of normal menstruation may be delayed after progesterone-only contraceptives
(e) Male sterilization is associated with less morbidity than female sterilisation.

3. Features associated with aortic stenosis include:

(a) A systolic murmur which radiates to the neck
(b) Left ventricular hypertrophy on ECG
(c) Right axis deviation on ECG
(d) Fainting on exertion
(e) A collapsing pulse

4. Regarding acute myocardial infarction:

(a) A diagnosis can be made solely on elevated troponin levels
(b) ST elevation of >2 mm in 2 or more chest leads associated with chest pain is diagnostic
(c) ST elevation in II, III and aVR would be consistent with an inferior lesion
(d) The ST segment can be usefully interpreted in people with left bundle branch block
(e) VF is a common arrhythmia following MI

5. Causes of dyspnoea on exertion include:

(a) Anaemia
(b) Pulmonary embolism
(c) Pulmonary hypertension
(d) Hypothyroidism
(e) Constrictive pericarditis

6. A collapsing radial pulse may be associated with:

(a) Hypertrophic cardiomyopathy
(b) Aortic reflux
(c) AV fistula
(d) Persistent ductus arteriosus
(e) Hypovolaemic states

7. Risk factors of a pulmonary embolus include:

(a) Long bone fracture
(b) First trimester abortion
(c) Malignancy
(d) Atrial fibrillation
(e) Thrombocytopenia

8. In patients with GI bleeding:

(a) A PR is mandatory to confirm or deny the presence of melena
(b) A drop in haemoglobin is a marker of blood loss
(c) One blue venflon is sufficient for effective fluid resuscitation
(d) A normal BP in the presence of tachycardia is not a cause for concern
(e) Those with cirrhosis and oesophageal varices have a good prognosis

9. Gastrointestinal causes of clubbing include:

(a) Crohn's disease
(b) Cirrhosis
(c) Rectal cancer
(d) Irritable bowel syndrome
(e) Chronic pancreatitis

10. During the examination of the abdomen:

(a) Start at the site of the pain
(b) Palpate from the LIF when examining the liver
(c) Palpate from the RIF when examining the spleen
(d) Look for spider naevi
(e) Ascites can be detected by shifting dullness.

11. Regarding oesophageal cancer:

(a) There is a higher incidence in Japan compared to the UK
(b) 5 year survival is around 65%
(c) Patients present with difficulty swallowing solids more than liquids
(d) 20% of patients will have lymph node involvement at presentation
(e) Heavy smoking is a risk factor

12. Patients with peptic ulcers are at an increased risk of:

(a) Perforation
(b) Haemorrhage

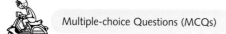

(c) Short bowel syndrome
(d) Pancreatitis
(e) Peripheral vascular disease

13. In patients with COPD:

(a) Their activities of daily living are a useful guide in assessing their pre-morbid state in acute exacerbations
(b) Home oxygen should be used for at least 16 hours a day
(c) Home oxygen is prescribed to help with the symptomatic relief of shortness of breath
(d) An FEV_1 of <1litre when well would be grounds for an admission to ITU for artificial ventilation
(e) An arterial blood gas measurement prior to discharge is a useful prognostic indicator

14. Physical features of hypercapnia include:

(a) Peripheral vasodilation
(b) A resting tremor
(c) A low volume pulse
(d) Confusion progressing to drowsiness
(e) A raised ALT

15. Causes of haemoptysis include:

(a) Pulmonary oedema
(b) Pulmonary TB
(c) Infective exacerbation of COPD
(d) Oesophageal cancer
(e) Thrombophilia

16. Regarding aspiration of a foreign body:

(a) It is treated in babies by placing them head down on your arm and firmly patting them on the back
(b) The Heimlich manoeuvre is now no longer considered safe
(c) It can lead to lung abscess
(d) They typically go down the left main bronchus
(e) The sensation of something stuck in the throat warrants laryngoscopy

17. In the management of asthma:

(a) Serial peak flows are a guide to treatment
(b) Volumatics are as efficacious as nebulisers
(c) You can be reassured by a normal arterial $PaCO_2$ in someone having an asthma attack
(d) The inability to complete a sentence is a concerning feature.
(e) The incidence of asthma is falling in developed nations

18. Risk factors for the successful completion of suicide include:

(a) Traumatic means
(b) Young and female
(c) Schizophrenia
(d) Alcoholism
(e) Having children

19. Common features of a significant depressive episode include:

(a) A persistently low mood of 1 week's duration
(b) Anhedonia
(c) Flight of ideas
(d) Increased libido
(e) Early morning wakening

20. Neurological causes of difficulty in walking include:

(a) Tourette's syndrome
(b) Epilepsy
(c) Parkinson's disease
(d) Proximal weakness
(e) Cerebellar ataxia

21. Common causes of headache:

(a) Temperomandibular joint dysfunction
(b) Alcohol excess
(c) Increased intracerebral pressure
(d) Migraine
(e) Middle ear infection

22. When performing a lumbar puncture:

(a) A CT scan excluding increased intracerebral pressure must be avaliable
(b) Clotting abnormalities should be excluded
(c) The pressure of the CSF should be measured
(d) Oligoclonal bands are normally present in the CSF
(e) Cellulitis of the overlying skin is not a contra-indication

23. In patients with peripheral vascular disease:

(a) Medical management is the first line treatment
(b) Patients should be encouraged to exercise within their claudication distance
(c) Ankle/brachial pressure indices should be measured pre and post angioplasty
(d) As a PRHO you should take consent for angioplasty
(e) Diabetes is a risk factor for peripheral vascular disease

24. Definitions:

(a) A hernia is the protrusion of a viscus or tissue out of the body cavity which contains it
(b) A fistula is a normal communication between two epithelial surfaces
(c) An ulcer is a break in the continuity of an epithelial surface
(d) A sinus is a blind-ending tract communicating with an epithelially lined surface
(e) An aneurysm is the abnormal dilation of a vein

25. In patients presenting with a fractured neck of femur:

(a) Clinically they will have a shortened leg
(b) The affected leg will be internally rotated
(c) A positive family history is likely

(d) They are at high risk of a DVT
(e) Minor trauma is a common cause

26. Diffuse alopecia:

(a) Is associated with pernicious anaemia
(b) Can be caused by iron deficiency
(c) Can be caused by zinc deficiency
(d) Can be caused by IV heparin administration
(e) Is genetically determined in women

27. Acute tonsillitis:

(a) An elevated anti-streptolysin titre suggests bacterial infection
(b) Does not occur following tonsillectomy
(c) The most common lymph glands affected are the pre-auricular glands
(d) Is associated with a leucocytosis
(e) Can cause referred pain to the ear

28. Deep vein thrombosis after hip replacement:

(a) Is commoner in patients with an increased BMI
(b) Usually leads to pulmonary embolism
(c) Is easy to clinically diagnose
(d) Can be prevented by the use of SC heparin prophylactically
(e) Happens in more than 20% of cases

29. Urinary tract infections in children:

(a) Are more common in boys than girls at six years of age
(b) Are commoner in boys than girls in the newborn period
(c) Can present as febrile convusions
(d) Can present as failure to thrive
(e) May be diagnosed on microscopy

30. A small for dates baby is liable to suffer from:

(a) Significant weight loss in the neonatal period
(b) Meconium aspiration
(c) Intrauterine hypoxia
(d) Hypoglycaemia
(e) Hyaline membrane disease

31. Breath-holding attacks:

(a) Can be precipitated by frustration
(b) Are a risk factor for the development of epilepsy
(c) Rarely present in infants over the age of one
(d) Can be associated with unconsciousness
(e) Can be prevented with phenobarbitone

32. The following are contained within the broad ligament:

(a) The ovary
(b) The ureter
(c) The uterine artery
(d) The fallopian tube
(e) The ovarian artery

33. The management of bronchiolitis in infants includes:

(a) A reducing course of hydrocortisone
(b) Clarithromycin
(c) IV aminophylline
(d) Humidified oxygen
(e) Tube feeding

34. Stress incontinence of urine:

(a) Should be investigated by cystoscopy before surgery
(b) Can be a transient difficulty post-delivery
(c) Is commoner in multiparous women
(d) Can be distinguished from urge incontinence by a cystogram
(e) Can coexist with detrusor instability

35. Difficulty with swallowing can occur as a result of:

(a) A cerebrovascular accident
(b) Recurrent larygneal nerve trauma
(c) Carcinoma of the stomach
(d) Dementia
(e) Motor neurone disease

36. Absent ankle jerk reflexes can be caused by:

(a) Syphilis
(b) Diabetes mellitus
(c) Gonorrhea
(d) Parkinson's disease
(e) Motor neurone disease

37. In alcoholic liver disease:

(a) The sensitivity to sedative drugs is increased
(b) Prothrombin time is increased
(c) Synthetic liver function is best assessed by clotting studies
(d) The pattern of alcohol excess determines the development of liver disease
(e) Liver damage is mainly due to dietary insufficiencies

38. The normal metabolic response to trauma includes:

(a) The release of antidiuretic hormone
(b) Potassium loss
(c) A negative nitrogen balance
(d) Glycolysis
(e) A decrease in the lean body mass

39. In Colles' fracture, the distal radial fragment:

(a) Is usually impacted
(b) Is associated with median nerve damage
(c) Is deviated to the radial side
(d) Is ventrally angulated on the proximal radius
(e) Is usually torn from the intra-articular triangular disc

40. Regarding multiple pregnancies:

(a) They commoner in younger women
(b) They are associated with a shorter pregnancy
(c) There is an increased risk of postpartum haemorrhage
(d) They are usually monozygotic following IVF
(e) Twin pregnancies occur in roughly 1:50 pregnancies

41. The following confirm ovulation:

(a) In a 28 day cycle, blood progesterone level on day 21
(b) In a 28 day cycle, blood oestrogen level on day 14
(c) A basal body temperature drop of at least 0.5°C on the day 12
(d) 'Spinbarkeit' in cervical mucus
(e) Histological examination of a premenstrual endometrial biopsy

42. With regard to termination of pregnancy:

(a) Must be approved by 3 different medical professionals
(b) Can be performed with prostaglandins
(c) Can be legally performed at any point in pregnancy
(d) Can be safely performed by suction termination of pregancy before 14 weeks' gestation
(e) Can be carried out with mifepristone (RU 486) up to 12 weeks' gestation

43. Following a medial nerve injury the patient will demonstrate:

(a) The inability to abduct the thumb
(b) The inability to oppose the thumb and little finger
(c) Have altered sensation of the forearm
(d) Pain in the upper arm
(e) Sensory loss over the medial fingers

44. Regarding developmental milestones in childhood:

(a) A 10 month old will demonstrate opposition
(b) A 12 month old will release objects on request
(c) A 3 month old can roll from back to front
(d) An 18 month old can put 3 words together
(e) A 4 month old can localize sound

45. Successful suicide is:

(a) Rare in young men
(b) At a similar rate in all developed countries
(c) An event which commonly occurs without warning
(d) Associated with unemployment
(e) Increased in mental illness

46. Schizophrenia:

(a) Carries a 1 in 10 risk of lifetime suicide
(b) Is strongly associated with violence to others
(c) Is a lifelong diagnosis
(d) Is influenced by the patient's emotional environment
(e) If chronic is associated with marked cognitive defects

47. A swelling just below the angle of the mandible in a 25-year-old male may be:

(a) Ectopic thyroid tissue
(b) A thyroglossal cyst
(c) An enlarged lymph node
(d) A pharyngeal pouch
(e) A carotid body tumour

48. The following are associated with hyperthyroidism:

(a) Weight loss
(b) Atrial fibrillation
(c) Lid lag
(d) Onycholysis
(e) Feeling tired all the time

49. Dementia:

(a) Is invariably progressive
(b) If onset occurs before 75, is termed pre-senile
(c) The sleep–wake cycle is preserved
(d) May be caused by a head injury
(e) Can be diagnosed with a mini-mental test score of 8 or less

50. In Parkinson's disease:

(a) Urinary incontinence is an early symptom
(b) The gait is typically shuffling
(c) The onset of symptoms is typically before the age of 50
(d) There is typically cog-wheel rigidity
(e) Tremor is most noticeable on sustained movement

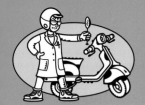

Short-answer Questions (SAQs)

It is important to only answer the question set, especially in short-answer questions. Examiners are looking for specific points and will not give marks for superfluous information. For example the first question only asks for features of severe aortic stenosis, so do not waste time discussing the auscultatory signs of aortic stenosis.
Only list three causes in any answer as only the first three will score marks.

1. What features from the history and examination would suggest the presence of severe aortic stenosis in the presence of an ejection systolic murmur?

2. An elderly patient presents with cough and dyspnoea. What features on physical examination would favour a diagnosis of heart failure?

3. What features on the examination would alert you to a severe attack of asthma?

4. List three of the more common causes of a median nerve palsy at the wrist and describe the physical signs.

5. Describe the features of Parkinson's disease on physical examination.

6. A patient complains of acute lower back pain radiating down the legs. What signs on physical examination would raise the suspicion of an acute disc prolapse of L5–S1?

7. List three causes of massive splenomegaly. Describe the features of a palpable spleen on physical examination.

8. List seven features that may be found on examination of the upper limbs of a patient with long-standing rheumatoid arthritis.

9. List three major causes of papilloedema, and a suggestive feature for each on physical examination.

10. A patient has a breast lump. Describe features on examination that would make you concerned that she has a carcinoma.

11. What mode of transmission is illustrated in Figs 1 and 2? Give two examples of each.

12. Give an example of opportunistic infections that may cause disease in the following.
   (a) Eye.
   (b) Lungs.
   (c) Central nervous system.
   (d) Gastrointestinal tract.

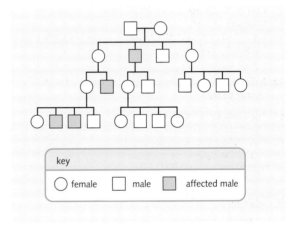

key		
⭘ female	☐ male	▦ affected male

Fig. 1

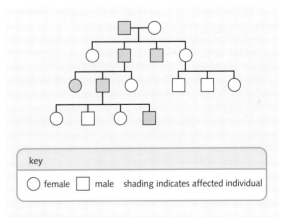

key	
⭘ female ☐ male	shading indicates affected individual

Fig. 2

Give two other groups of patients who may be susceptible to opportunistic infections.

13. A patient presents with anaemia. Give some examples of food that may provide a good dietary source of iron, folate, and vitamin B_{12} to the patient. Give two other examples of causes for each type of anaemia.

14. How may a patient present with hypercalcaemia? Give four causes.

15. A nulliparous woman who is 30 week' pregnant complains of swollen ankles. What are the three most likely causes? What features on clinical examination would help the differential diagnosis? Which investigations may exclude the more serious causes?

16. List five skin rashes that may be associated with an occult malignancy.

17. Indicate two features in the history and three findings on physical examination that may help to differentiate a hypoglycaemic coma from diabetic ketoacidosis in a diabetic patient.

18. What four questions might you ask a patient with suspected hypothyroidism? Indicate three discriminatory signs that may be present.

19. List four classes of drug that might cause hyperkalaemia and indicate the mechanism.

20. List four risk factors for human immunodeficiency virus (HIV) infection.

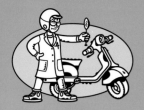
1. Theme: Limp (musculoskeletal)

(a) Chondromalacia patellae
(b) Compartment syndrome
(c) Congenital dislocation of the hip
(d) Fractured neck of femur
(e) Gout
(f) Osteoarthritis of hip
(g) Osteoarthritis of knee
(h) Perthe's disease
(i) Slipped femoral epiphysis
(j) Trochanteric bursitis

Instruction: *For each scenario described below, choose the SINGLE most likely diagnosis from the above list of options. Each option may be used once, more than once or not at all.*

1   On a GP visit to a nursing home you are asked to see an 85-year-old woman with dementia and recurrent falls. She can only walk with assistance. On examination when lying supine she has a shortened externally rotated left leg.

2   A 65-year-old man with high blood pressure and ischaemic heart disease presents with a hot erythematous knee joint. His regular medications include a thiazide diuretic.

3   A 13-year-old boy presents with niggly pain in the hip which is much worse after being tackled at football.

4   A 25-year-old man presents in A&E with a limp and excruciating pain in the lateral aspect of his lower leg following training for a marathon.

5   A 58-year-old man who presents to his GP with pain in his left knee of several months' duration. On examination he has a restricted range of movement in his left hip.

2. Theme: Gastrointestinal bleeding

(a) Anal fissure
(b) Colonic carcinoma
(c) Crohn's disease
(d) Diverticular disease
(e) Duodenal ulcer
(f) Gastric carcinoma
(g) Haemorrhoids
(h) Laryngeal carcinoma
(i) Mallory–Weiss tear
(j) Oesophageal varices

Instruction: *For each scenario described below, choose the SINGLE most likely diagnosis from the above list of options. Each option may be used once, more than once or not at all.*

1   A 60-year-old man presents with altered bowel habit, crampy abdominal pain and blood mixed in with his stools.

2   A 40-year-old woman presents with a long history of indigestion, worse recently, black tarry stools and feeling light-headed.

3   A 32-year-old woman presents to her GP following childbirth, worried about the fresh, painless red blood on the toilet paper.

4   A 22-year-old medical student presents to A&E with haematemesis and chest pain following celebrations on passing his Finals.

5   A 17-year-old woman with cystic fibrosis presents to A&E vomiting profuse volumes of fresh blood.

3. Theme: Liver problems

(a) Alcoholic liver disease
(b) Biliary atresia
(c) Gallstones
(d) Hepatitis A
(e) Hepatitis B
(f) Hepatitis C
(g) Metastatic liver disease
(h) Physiological jaundice
(i) Primary biliary cirrhosis
(j) Wilson's disease

Instruction: *For each scenario described below, choose the SINGLE most likely cause from the above list of options. Each option may be used once, more than once or not at all.*

1   An obese 60-year-old man presents to the medical admissions unit following haematemesis with unsteadiness, a flapping tremor and erythematous palms.

2   2 years after major abdominal surgery a 75-year-old woman presents to her GP with weight loss and jaundice. On examination she has an enlarged knobbly liver.

3   A 4-week-old baby girl is taken to see the GP by a concerned breast-feeding mother from a professional family. The baby is deeply jaundiced.

4   A 20-year-old soldier returning from the Gulf has abdominal pain, vomiting and pale stools with jaundice. His liver edge is just palpable, smooth and slightly tender.

5   An overweight, 45-year-old woman presents with right upper quadrant pain associated with meals. On examination she is slightly tender in the right upper quadrant on deep inspiration.

4. Theme: Cardiac murmurs and added sounds

(a) Aortic regurgitation
(b) Aortic stenosis
(c) Bicuspid aortic valve
(d) Mitral regurgitation
(e) Mitral stenosis
(f) Patent ductus arteriosus
(g) Transposition of the great vessels
(h) Tricuspid regurgitation
(i) Ventricular septal defect

Instruction: *For each scenario described below, choose the SINGLE most appropriate cardiac lesion from the above list of options. Each option may be used once, more than once or not at all.*

1   A 60-year-old man presents with heart failure. On examination he has a collapsing pulse, an early diastolic murmur, and a displaced apex beat.

2   A 56-year-old man gives a history of rheumatic fever. He has flushed cheeks, an irregularly irregular pulse and a mid-diastolic murmur.

3   A 75-year-old woman presents to A&E following a drop attack. Her ECG shows left ventricular hypertrophy. On examination a harsh systolic murmur is heard over both carotid arteries.

4   Three days following his myocardial infarction Mr Thompson has a sudden deterioration, developing left ventricular failure. He has a new pansystolic murmur radiating from the apex to the axilla.

5   A baby who is cyanotic at birth with a loud long systolic murmur in whom Fallot's tetralogy is suspected.

5. Theme: Finger clubbing

(a) Alcoholic liver disease
(b) Crohn's disease
(c) Emphysema
(d) Familial clubbing
(e) Fibrosing alveolitis
(f) Infective endocarditis
(g) Pulmonary abcess
(h) Scleroderma
(i) Squamous cell carcinoma

Instruction: *For each scenario described below, choose the SINGLE most likely cause of finger clubbing from the above list of options. Each option may be used once, more than once or not at all.*

1   A 40-year-old man with right sided chest pain with weight loss of 3 months duration and a grumbling pyrexia.

2   A 20-year-old man with intermittent lower abdominal pain on defaecation associated with blood and mucus.

3   A 48-year-old woman presents with dyspnoea. On examination she has bilateral, fine, late inspiratory crackles.

4   An 18-year-old i.v. drug abuser who presents with fever and weight loss who is short of breath.

5   A 15-year-old boy who presents to his GP surgery with asthma.

6. Theme: The painful joint

(a) Ankylosing spondylitis
(b) Fibromyalgia
(c) Gout
(d) Osteoarthritis
(e) Pseudogout
(f) Psoriatic arthritis
(g) Reiter's syndrome
(h) Rheumatoid arthritis
(i) Septic arthritis
(j) Systemic lupus erythematosus

Instruction: *For each scenario described below, choose the SINGLE most likely cause of pain from the above list of options. Each option may be used once, more than once or not at all.*

1   A 27-year-old man with low back pain and morning stiffness. He had an episode of iritis a year previously.

2   A 40-year-old woman with symmetrically painful fingers and wrists. There is little evidence of synovitis. Her ESR is raised and she has an erythematous rash over her nose and cheeks.

3   A 37-year-old man with gonococcal urethritis presents with pain in the hip and a limp.

4   An 82-year-old woman presents with a painful right hip and knee, worse on exercise. On examination she has a positive Trendelenburg test and walks with a limp.

5   A 75-year-old man with a painful great toe, 1 week after starting therapy for mild heart failure.

7. Theme: Trauma

(a) Airway obstruction
(b) Cardiac tamponade
(c) Flail chest
(d) Haemothorax
(e) Myocardial infarction
(f) Open pneumothorax
(g) Pulmonary contusion
(h) Ruptured diaphragm
(i) Ruptured oesophagus
(j) Ruptured spleen
(k) Tension pneumothorax
(l) Traumatic aortic rupture

Instruction: *For each scenario described below, choose the SINGLE most likely diagnosis from the above list of options. Each option may be used once, more than once or not at all.*

1. An unconscious 30-year-old male with weak pulse who previously complained of left sided pleuritic chest pain. Examination reveals the left chest to be hyperresonant to percussion with decreased breath sounds.

2. A 20-year-old girl is brought in with a stab wound to the right side of her chest. She is in respiratory distress and air can be heard moving through the defect in the chest wall.

3. A 60-year-old man is hit by a lorry while out walking his dog. He has injured his chest and is in obvious respiratory distress. Initial observations show he has a pulse of 120, BP 120/60 and respiratory rate of 45. Examination reveals paradoxical chest wall movement.

4. A 3-year-old girl who has been eating peanuts and who now has a cough and stridor.

5. A 38-year-old man is brought into A&E after a high speed RTA. He has chest pain and a BP of 70/50 and a widened mediastinum on his CXR.

8. Theme: Heavy periods (or menstrual problems)

(a) Adenomyosis
(b) Break-through bleeding
(c) Endometrial polyp
(d) Fibroids
(e) Hypothyroidism
(f) Hyperthyroidism
(g) Pelvic inflammatory disease
(h) Physiological bleeding
(i) Salpingitis
(j) Thrombocytopenia
(k) von Willebrand's disease

Instruction: *For each scenario described below, choose the SINGLE most likely diagnosis from the above list of options. Each option may be used once, more than once or not at all.*

1. A 34-year-old woman who presents with a 15-month history of worsening painless menorrhagia. The bleeding is so heavy she is having to take time off work. On examination she has a bulky uterus and is anaemic.

2. A 36-year-old woman who complains of feeling tired all the time. She has been gaining weight and losing her hair. She now has heavy irregular periods.

3. A 20-year-old woman present to her GP 4 months after stopping the combined oral contraceptive pill. She has developed prolonged and heavy periods. Investigations and blood tests are all normal.

4. A 25-year-old woman complains of lower abdominal pain and menorrhagia. Her smear shows *Chlamydia trachomatis*.

5. A 17-year-old A-level student presents to her GP with fatigue and heavy periods. She is anaemic with a prolonged bleeding time.

9. Theme: The diabetic eye

(a) Arc light damage
(b) Background retinopathy
(c) Central retinal artery occlusion
(d) Central retinal vein occlusion
(e) Cortical blindness
(f) Maculopathy
(g) Optic atrophy
(h) Pre-proliferative changes
(i) Prololiferative retinopathy
(j) Snowflake cataracts
(k) Snow blindness
(l) Vitreous haemorrhage

Instruction: *For each scenario described below, choose the SINGLE most likely diagnosis from the above list of options. Each option may be used once, more than once or not at all.*

1 Fundoscopy in a 75-year-old woman with NIDDM demonstrates widespread microaneurysms, blot haemorrhages and hard exudates with macular sparing.

2 A 50-year-old man with long-standing IDDM presents to A&E with acute onset, complete loss of vision in a left eye. Fundoscopy reveals loss of the red reflex with grey haze obscuring the retina.

3 Fundoscopy in a 29-year-old man with poorly controlled IDDM reveals microaneurysms and blot haemorrhages with hard exudates, cotton wool spots and neovascularization.

4 A 68-year-old man presents to his GP with sudden loss of vision in his left eye. Examination reveals that acuity in the left eye is diminished to the perception of light only. The fundus is pale with a cherry red spot at the macula.

5 A 57-year-old man with NIDDM present with sudden loss of vision in his left eye. Fundoscopy reveals a swollen optic disc with cotton-wool spots and haemorrhages across the retina.

10. Theme: Delirium

(a) Concussion
(b) Diabetic ketoacidosis (DKA)
(c) Encephalitis
(d) Hepatic encephalopathy
(e) Hypercalcaemia
(f) Hypercapnia
(g) Hyperosmolar, non-ketotic state
(h) Hyponatraemia
(i) Opiate analgesia
(j) Subarachnoid haemorrhage
(k) Subdural haematoma

Instruction: *For each scenario described below, choose the SINGLE most likely cause of delirium from the above list of options. Each option may be used once, more than once or not at all.*

1 A previously fit and well 13-year-old boy presents to A&E with a 24-hour history of increasing confusion. On examination he is unwell, smells of ketones and is dehydrated.

2 A 70-year-old lifelong smoker who is attending the oncologists diagnosis presents to the medical admission unit with a 48-hour history of increasing confusion and vomiting. His blood gases are normal but he is dehydrated.

3 A 60-year-old smoker with a 75-pack year history presents with a productive cough and feeling short of breath. He is drowsy but rousable. He has a bounding pulse and a flapping tremor.

4 An 82-year-old lady with a history of dementia and falls presents with increasing confusion and more frequent falls. She is drowsy with a mental test score of 2/10. She has a right-sided weakness and up-going plantars.

5 A previously fit 25-year-old man presents to A&E with a severe headache and increasing confusion. Whilst you are examining him he starts to fit. While applying the oxygen mask you notice a cold sore.

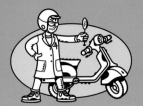

Objective Structured Clinical Examination (OSCE)

The following OSCE stations are designed to both help and direct your learning. They are intended to be used as part of group revision and involve role play.

Suggestion for using the OSCE scenarios

- Obviously someone may need to volunteer as simulated patient, someone as candidate, and one (or more) as examiner/observer.
- Time the station to simulate exam pressure – anything between 5 and 10 minutes, depending on how experienced and/or confident you're feeling, and what the norm is in your medical school.
- Grade each element as 'Achieved', 'Partially achieved' or 'Not achieved/not attempted'.
- Get into the habits (a) of talking through what you're doing as you do it and (b) summarizing your findings at the end. Some medical schools run OSCE stations where this is expected. You will usually be told this in the instructions, but it is good practice in any case, both for exams and for 'real life'!
- The volunteer undertaking a role play should spend a few minutes thinking themselves into the role, being guided by the content of the OSCE checklist as to what to emphasize (or conceal!) in the history. The story should be believable and the details consistent, and although a little bit of embellishment may add spice to the role, remember that the focus is on the candidate's clinical skills, not on the role player's thespian talents!

1. The newborn baby check

Equipment/resources required
You could use a doll or mannequin

Instructions to candidate
This baby was born yesterday and is now due a newborn baby check. Please carry this out, checking for any problem or abnormality. Describe what you are doing, and why, as you proceed.

Station-specific tasks
- Washes hands (or indicates intention to wash hands)
- Checks birth weight and estimates gestational age
- Tests general tone and observes skin colour, including jaundice
- Establishes history of labour and pregnancy
- Checks anterior fontanelle
- Checks for
  - dysmorphic features
  - red eye reflex
  - integrity of palate (looking for cleft palate)
- Measures head circumference
- Feels for apex beat and listens to heart
- Palpates for abdominal masses
- Asks if baby passed meconium
- Checks femoral pulses
- Checks hips using Ortolani and/or Barlow tests
- If male, checks
  - both testes have descended
  - whether hypospadias present
- Checks spine for
  - dimples
  - spina bifida
- Checks feet and hands
  - fingers and toes?
  - talipes?
- Washes hands at end (or indicates intention)

Generic skills
- Introduces self and explains what they're doing
- Establishes identity of baby and mother
- Elicits mother's concerns
- Is gentle with baby
- Fluent approach to examination

2. Examination of a neck lump

Equipment/resources required
A volunteer

Instruction to candidate
Please examine this patient's neck.

Station-specific tasks
- Washes hands (or indicates intention to wash hands)
- Exposes the neck with the patient sitting up
- Observes the patient from the front and both sides
- (If asked indicates that they are looking for scars, goitre, distended veins)
- Asks the patient to swallow a sip of water
- (Ideally this should be a two-stage command: first take water into mouth, then swallow when asked. It avoids the patient drinking the water before you are positioned to observe!)
- Asks the patient to stick out their tongue
- (Does the mass move? If yes, a thyroglossal cyst would be likely)

For goitre

- Asks if the mass is painful
- Stands behind the patient
- Explains to the patient what they are about to do
- Palpates the mass
- Feels for
  - tenderness
  - degree of swelling
  - single/multiple nodules
  - texture
  - surface features
  - size

asks patient to swallow

- Checks for associated lymphadenopathy
- Looks over top of patient's head checking for exophthalmos
- Assesses the position of the trachea
- Percusses out lower border of thyroid
- Listens over the mass for a bruit
- Looks at eyes for
  - lid retraction
  - lid lag
  - ophthalmoplegia
- Checks the conjunctivae
- Goes on to examine for other signs of hyper- or hypothyroidism
  - Facial appearance
  - Skin texture
  - Build
  - Dress
  - Behaviour
  - Feels pulse for presence of atrial fibrillation
  - Tremor
  - Increased sweating
  - Palmar erythema
- Asks patient to get out of chair without using hands (proximal myopathy)
- Checks for slow relaxing reflexes (especially ankle reflex)
- Washes hands at end (or indicates intention)

Generic skills

- Introduces self
- Explains what they're doing
- Is gentle throughout
- Gives clear instructions
- Systematic and fluent exam technique
- Correct technique

3. Examination of knee joint

Equipment/resources required

A volunteer, ideally in shorts

Instructions to candidate

Please examine this patient's knee.

Station-specific tasks

- Washes hands (or indicates intention to wash hands)
- Asks the patient about any pain
- Asks the patient about range of movement
- Lies the patient supine
- Adequately exposes both legs

Looks

- Comments on any joint deformity, muscle wasting, swellings
- Compares one side with the other
- Measures both quadriceps at same point above tibial tuberosity

Feels

- Checks skin temperature of both knees
- Checks for effusions
  - patellar tap test
  - cross fluctuation
- Flexes the knee and palpates the joint line in a methodical manner
- Palpates popliteal fossa
- Comments on
  - tenderness
  - synovitis
  - bony swelling
  - masses

Moves

- Checks firstly active flexion and extension, then passive range
- On passive flexion and extension comments on any crepitus
- Assesses stability
  - medial collateral ligament
  - lateral collateral ligament
  - anterior cruciate ligament
  - posterior cruciate ligament

Extra tests

- Asks patient to stand
- Looks for varus/valgus deformity
- Looks for popliteal swelling
- Asks the patient to walk and observes gait
- Washes hands at end (or indicates intention)

Generic skills

- Introduces self
- Explains what they're doing
- Is gentle throughout
- Gives clear instructions
- Systematic and fluent exam technique
- Correct technique

4. Neurovascular examination of legs

Equipment/resources required
A volunteer, ideally in shorts

Instructions to candidate
Please examine circulation and peripheral nervous system in this patient's legs.

Station-specific tasks
- Washes hands (or indicates intention to wash hands)
- Exposes both patient's legs
- (With a real patient any dressings should already have been taken off)

Inspection
- Inspects posterior and anterior aspects of legs
- Comments on any scars
- Pays close attention to feet and pressure point
- Comments on
  - nutrition of skin
  - wasting of muscles
  - obvious ulcers

Palpation
- Feels for pulses
  - femoral
  - popliteal
  - dorsalis pedis
  - posterior tibia
  - checks capillary return
- Compares right with left side
- Comments on character of pulses
- Auscultates for bruits over femoral pulses
- Tests *tone*
- Tests *sensation*
  - dermatomes
  - glove-and-stocking distribution
- Tests in *a systematic manner* (comparing right with left)
- Tests *power*
  - hip flexion (L1/2)
  - hip extension (S1)
  - knee flexion (L5/S1)
  - knee extension (L3/4)
  - ankle dorsiflexion (L4/5)
  - ankle plantar flexion (S1)
- Reflexes
  - knee (L3/4)
  - ankle (S1)
  - plantar
- Tests for *clonus*
- Tests for *coordination*
  - heel-to-shin
- Asks patient to walk
  - notes any difficulty in getting up
  - observes gait

- Calculates ankle/brachial pressure index
- Comments on significance
- Washes hands at end (or indicates intention)

Generic skills
- Introduces self
- Explains what they're doing
- Is gentle throughout
- Gives clear instructions
- Systematic and fluent exam technique
- Correct technique

5. Change in bowel habit

Equipment/resources required
A volunteer to role play

Instructions to candidate
Please take a history from this patient who has presented with an alteration of bowel habit.

Instruction to role-player
You have presented with a change of bowel habit. Make up plausible answers to the following questions consistent with an alteration in bowel habit.

Station-specific tasks
- Ascertains name and age of patient
- Occupation
- Elicits presenting complaint
- Defines duration, severity and the nature of the change

Associated features
- Asks about pain
  - nature
  - location and any radiation
  - relieving and exacerbating factors
- Enquires about any PR bleeding
  - nature of bleeding
  - any mucus being passed
- Asks about general health
- Appetite
- Weight loss
- Malaise
- 'Tired all the time'
- Short of breath

Generic skills
- Introduces self
- Active listening (eye contact, appropriate body language)
- Appropriate question style (clarity of question, balance of open and closed questions)
- Elicits ideas, concerns and expectation

237

- Accurate summary of the history given by the patient
- Empathic approach

6. History of headache

Equipment/resources required
A volunteer to role play

Instructions to candidate
Please take a history from this patient who has presented with a history of headache.

Instruction to role-player
You have presented with headache. Make up plausible answers to the following questions consistent with headache.

Station-specific tasks
- Ascertains name and age
- Occupation
- Characteristics of headache
  - duration
  - character
  - frequency
  - severity
- Site
- Radiation
- Aggravating and relieving factors
- Associated features
- Visual disturbance (e.g. blurring and photophobia)
- Nausea and vomiting
- Asks about general health
- Any stress(ors) in patient's life?
- Family history of headache

Generic skills
- Introduces self
- Active listening (eye contact, appropriate body language)
- Appropriate question style (clarity of question, open and closed question)
- Elicits ideas, concerns and expectation
- Empathic approach
- Accurate summary of the history given by the patient

7. Examination of a patient with a murmur

Equipment/resources required
A volunteer

Instruction to candidate
Please examine this patient's heart.

Station-specific tasks
- Washes hands (or expresses intention to wash hands)

Inspection
- Looks at hands for finger clubbing
- Checks mucus membranes for cyanosis
- Inspects jugular venous pulse (note correct positioning of patient)

Palpation
- Takes radial pulse
- Assesses rate, rhythm and character
- Asks to measure BP (or actually measures it)
- Feels praecordium for thrills and heaves
- Defines position of apex beat and comments upon its nature

Auscultation
- Listens in four areas
- Alters patient's position for each valve
- Asks patient to hold breath

Generic skills
- Introduces self
- Explains what they're doing
- Is gentle throughout
- Gives clear instructions
- Systematic and fluent exam technique
- Correct technique

8. Visual fields

Equipment/resources required
A volunteer

Instruction to candidate
Please examine this patient's visual fields

Instructions to volunteer
Try and simulate someone with a visual field loss, e.g. a hemianopia

Station-specific tasks
- Correctly positions patient and self
- Inspects both eyes briefly
- Asks patient to cover an eye and covers opposing eye
- Candidate brings wagging finger into view
- Checks all four quadrants
- Asks patient to identify when they see the finger.
- Tests for visual inattention
- Correctly identifies visual field defect

Generic skills
- Introduces self
- Explains what they're doing

- Is gentle throughout
- Gives clear instructions
- Systematic and fluent exam technique
- Correct technique

9. Assessment of suicide risk

Equipment/resources required
A volunteer willing to role play

Instruction to candidate
You are the on-call SHO in psychiatry. You have been called to A&E to assess a patient complaining that they feel there is no point to life.

Instructions to role player
You have been depressed for some time, and feel that there is no point to life. You have been building up a store of paracetamol over a week, and expect the quantity to kill you. You have recently amended your will.

Station-specific tasks
Planning
- Elicits the stockpiling of tablets
- Ascertains that the patient
  - is planning on not being discovered
  - expects this to be lethal
- Asks if any other methods have been considered
- Discovers any preparatory actions
- Asks if they have talked to anyone else about this
- Altruistic motive (i.e. 'They would be better off without me')
- Insight into aetiology
- Asks why they haven't made the attempt

Risk factors
- Symptoms of depression sought
- Biological features
- Family history

Generic skills
- Introduces self
- Active listening (eye contact, appropriate body language)
- Appropriate question style (clarity of question, open and closed question)
- Empathic approach
- Elicits ideas, concerns and expectation
- Accurate summary of the history given by the patient

10. History of alcohol abuse

Equipment/resources required
A volunteer willing to role play

Instruction to candidate
You are the PRHO on duty for medicine, and are asked to see a patient with blood test results compatible with alcohol abuse (raised gammaGT). Explore the possibility of alcohol abuse and the effect this has on the patient's life.

Instructions to role player
You work behind the bar in a pub, and drink at least a bottle of strong cider per day, along with extra shots of spirits in the form of 'tips'. Your wife is threatening divorce if you continue drinking.

Station-specific tasks
- Clarifies reasons for consultation
- Quantifies the patient's drinking habits
- Asks the CAGE questions:
  - Have you ever attempted to **C**ut down on your drinking?
  - Have people **A**nnoyed you when they criticized your drinking?
  - Have you ever felt **G**uilty about how much you drink?
  - Do you ever have to have a drink first thing in the morning (**E**ye opener)?
- Elicits other symptoms (e.g. hallucinations, blackouts, etc.)
- Asks about previous medical history and general health
- Asks if patient had considered quitting and/or would they like to have a go
- Explains the consequences of excess alcohol
- (Elicits what the patient already knows and gives an honest explanation including liver damage, heart disease, hypertension, stroke, brain damage, etc.)

Generic skills
- Introduces self
- Active listening (eye contact, appropriate body language)
- Appropriate question style (clarity of question, open and closed question)
- Elicits ideas, concerns and expectation
- Empathic approach
- Accurate summary of the history given by the patient

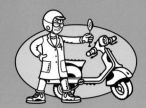

Essay Questions

1. A 62-year-old man presents with a sudden-onset weakness in his left arm and leg. Discuss how you would assess him in the casualty department and what investigations you would perform.

2. A 30-year-old man is referred to you because his general practitioner hears a systolic murmur during a routine examination. Discuss how your history and examination would guide your further management.

3. An elderly lady has been found by a neighbour lying on the floor. She appeared to be confused and was brought to the local hospital. How would you obtain a history?

4. What features in the history and physical examination would be useful in assessing the long-term control of a 16-year-old boy's asthma?

5. A 45-year-old long-distance lorry driver had been admitted to hospital six weeks earlier with an inferior myocardial infarction. What would you do at his first outpatient assessment following discharge from hospital?

6. A 45-year-old coal-miner presents with clubbing. What features on the history and physical examination might elucidate the cause?

7. A 20-year-old man presents with a dry cough, fever, and dyspnoea. What questions would you ask him?

8. An obese 45-year-old lady presents with polyuria and polydipsia. Urinalysis reveals 4+ glucose. What features are important in the history and examination?

9. A 70-year-old man presents to hospital with shortness of breath and marked swelling of his legs. What would you ask him? How would your physical examination help the assessment and what investigations would be most useful in the casualty department?

10. A 20-year-old man reports blood in his urine shortly after a sore throat? What features of the history and examination would guide your further management?

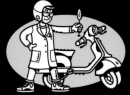

MCQ Answers

1. (a) True—The spiral arteries of the placenta are always maximally dilated so perfusion is dependent on maternal blood pressure.
    (b) False—In the fetal circulation blood flows from the right to left atrium via the foramen ovalae.
    (c) False—About 5% of the in-utero cardiac output goes through the lungs.
    (d) True—The oxygenated blood of the fetus arises from the placenta rather than the lungs.
    (e) False—5% of the cardiac outflow goes round the lungs in-utero and the first breath decreases the pulmonary arterial pressure.

2. (a) True—Since Eisenmenger's is a right-to-left shunt with pulmonary hypertension, any decrease in left sided pressure (delivery) leads to an increased shunt, which often precipitates death.
    (b) False—Focal migraine is a contraindication to the CoC due to the increased risk of CVA.
    (c) False—A condom is less efficacious than the diaphragm.
    (d) True—Progesterone-only contraceptives lead to delayed return to fertility.
    (e) True—One is an intra-abdominal procedure requiring GA, the other can be done under local anaesthetic.

3. (a) True—All aortic murmurs can radiate to the neck.
    (b) True—The increased work of forcing blood through a stenosed valve leads to hypertrophy of the left ventricle.
    (c) False—You would expect left axis deviation with aortic stenosis.
    (d) True—As the pressure gradient across the valve becomes greater, patients get syncopal symptoms.
    (e) False—A collapsing pulse is associated with aortic regurgitation.

4. (a) False—An MI can be diagnosed if two of the following three features are present – chest pain, ST changes and enzyme rises.
    (b) True—Those would be criteria for thrombolysis.
    (c) False—An inferior MI is associated with ST elevation in II, III and aVF.
    (d) False—Left bundle branch block precludes useful interpretation of the ST segments.
    (e) True—The origins of CPR/arrest team protocols in the 1960s stem from the recognition that MI patients get arrhythmias (these are particularly common in inferior MIs).

5. (a) True—Haemoglobin carries oxygen; not enough haemoglobin, not enough oxygen, so you feel short of breath.
    (b) True—Again, a significant PE will impair oxygen exchange so not enough oxygen gets into the blood.

    (c) True—People with raised pulmonary arterial pressure become short of breath.
    (d) True—Both hypo and hyper thyroid patients can become short of breath.
    (e) False—Constrictive pericarditis does not cause exertional dyspnoea.

6. (a) False—A collapsing pulse is not associated with hypertrophic cardiomyopathy.
    (b) True—Aortic reflux is a recognized cause of a collapsing pulse.
    (c) True—Depending on the site of the fistula it may be associated with a collapsing radial pulse.
    (d) True—PDAs can cause a collapsing radial pulse.
    (e) False—A collapsing pulse is not associated with hypovolaemia; the classic signs would be a weak and thready pulse.

7. (a) True—Trauma and immobility are risk factors for a PE.
    (b) True—Pregnancy at any stage is a risk factor for a PE.
    (c) True—Malignancy leads to altered coagulation states which may precipitate DVT, hence, PE.
    (d) True—People in AF get warfarinized to prevent PE/CVA.
    (e) False—Thrombocytopenia is not a risk factor for PE.

8. (a) True—If you don't put your finger in it, you'll put your foot in it!
    (b) True—That's also why you check a patient's Hb postoperatively
    (c) False—A blue venflon is small and these patients should have two large bore cannulae.
    (d) False—Tachycardia is a serious sign of shock and in itself worrying.
    (e) False—People with varices have a worse prognosis than those who don't.

9. (a) True—There are many causes of clubbing – learn them.
    (b) True—See above.
    (c) False—Rectal cancer is not a cause of clubbing.
    (d) False—Irritable bowel syndrome is not a cause of clubbing.
    (e) False—Chronic pancreatitis is not a cause of clubbing.

10. (a) False—Start palpation away from any pain to gain the patient's trust.
    (b) False—Start in the RIF for palpation of the liver.
    (c) True—Start in the RIF and work up to the left upper quadrant.
    (d) False—Spider naevi follow the distribution of the superior vena cava and are, therefore, only seen on the upper trunk.

(e) True—Fluid thrills and shifting dullness may both be used to detect ascites (an ultrasound scan is good too!).

11. (a) True—It's commoner in Japan so they screen for it.
(b) False—Oesophageal cancer has a poor 5 year survival (less than 30%).
(c) True—Difficulty swallowing solids tends to be caused by an obstructive pathology whereas difficulty swallowing liquids tends to be a neurological problem.
(d) False—50% of patients have nodal involvement at presentation.
(e) True—Smoking is a risk factor for most diseases.

12. (a) True—If you've got a partial area of weakness you more likely to breach it.
(b) True—If the area of weakness erodes a blood vessel – you bleed.
(c) False—Surgery for a peptic ulcer will not remove so much of the bowel that 'short bowel syndrome' occurs.
(d) False—Peptic ulcers are not associated with pancreatitis.
(e) False—Peptic ulcers are not associated with PVD.

13. (a) True—What people do day-to-day helps you judge not only their physical fitness but to some extent their quality of life.
(b) True—Home oxygen should be used for 16 hours a day to prevent the development of cor pulmonale.
(c) False—Home oxygen should not be used primarily to relieve breathlessness (it should be used to prevent the development of cor pulmonale) although it may do this through its effect on oxygen levels.
(d) False—An FEV_1 denoted very poor lung function and would struggle to get off a ventilator.
(e) False—ABG sample should be done 2 to 3 months post-discharge.

14. (a) True—Hypercapnia leads to vasodilation so you see warm peripheries and large veins.
(b) True—You see a tremor with hypercapnia (all tremors are easier to see if you ask the patient to close their eyes).
(c) False—Hypercapnia can cause a bounding pulse.
(d) True—Progressive hypercapnia leads to confusion and drowsiness. These are markers of severe disease process.
(e) False—Hypercapnia does not affect LFTs.

15. (a) True—The arterial/venous engorgement you see with LVF can lead to haemoptysis.
(b) True—Classically people with pulmonary TB have haemoptysis.
(c) True—Any infective process in the lungs can lead to haemoptysis.
(d) False—Oesophageal cancer will not cause someone to cough up blood.

(e) False—Haemoptysis is not associated with thrombophilia.

16. (a) True—This is basic first aid – as a doctor you will still be asked about first aid.
(b) False—However, the Heimlich manoeuvre remains in the ALS and APLS guidelines.
(c) True—If the foreign body gets lodged and isn't removed then an abscess may well develop.
(d) False—Foreign bodies typically go down the right main bronchus.
(e) True—People who feel they have something stuck very often do so – they should be referred for an ENT opinion as they may well warrant laryngoscopy.

17. (a) True—Serial peak flows should be recorded on a peak flow chart – they are an extremely useful guide to a person's asthma and how well controlled it is.
(b) True—It's true volumatics are as good as nebulizers – hospitals like nebulizers because they take less nursing time to administer!
(c) False—PCO_2 should drop due to hyperventilation. If it is normal it may suggest that the patient is getting tired.
(d) True—If someone is so short of breath that they can't talk, they are at risk of a respiratory arrest.
(e) False—The incidence of asthma is rising in the developed world.

18. (a) True—Traumatic means tend to be fatal, e.g. jumping, hanging, shooting – people with borderline personalities tend not to use such methods.
(b) False—Being young and female does not increase your risk of completing suicide.
(c) True—Schizophrenia carries a 1 in 10 lifetime risk of suicide.
(d) True—Being an alcoholic does increase your chance of completing suicide.
(e) False—Having children is a protective factor.

19. (a) False—A persistently low mood of 2 weeks' duration is suggestive of depression.
(b) True—People have less energy and don't enjoy things that they used to when they are depressed.
(c) False—Flight of ideas is a feature of mania.
(d) False—Increased libido is associated with mania.
(e) True—People with depression have a disturbance in their sleep cycle and often wake up early in the morning (NB make sure the patient isn't supposed to get up at 4 a.m., e.g. postmen).

20. (a) False—Tourette's syndrome affects people's speech.
(b) False—Epilepsy doesn't affect your gait.
(c) True—The shuffling gait is a classic feature of Parkinson's disease.
(d) True—If you have a proximal weakness it will affect how you walk.
(e) True—If you can't coordinate your movement walking will be difficult.

21. (a) True—TMJ dysfunction does lead to headaches – check the origin and radiation of the patient's pain.
(b) True—Where do you think hangovers originate?
(c) False—Whilst an ICP is associated with a headache it is not common.
(d) True—You surely know someone who suffers from migraine and complains of a headache.
(e) True—Middle ear problems (including infection) can cause headache.

22. (a) True—Have a CT report available so that you know the patient won't cone on the end of your needle.
(b) True—Causing a spinal haematoma is a 'no no'.
(c) True—You should measure the CSF opening pressure to confirm there is no ICP.
(d) False—Oligoclonal bands are associated with multiple sclerosis.
(e) False—Cellulitis over the area is a contra-indication as you do not want to cause a subarachnoid infection.

23. (a) True—Medical management is the first line management of virtually everything!
(b) True—Exercising within the claudication distance will help slow the progression of the disease.
(c) True—Do the ABPI pre and post angioplasty to document any improvement. It makes assessment of the patient in clinic in 6 months easier if they complain of their symptoms re-occurring.
(d) False—As a house officer you cannot consent patients for procedures.
(e) True—Diabetic patients develop peripheral vascular disease.

24. (a) True—That's the definition.
(b) False—A fistula is an abnormal communication between two epithelial surfaces.
(c) True—That's the definition.
(d) True—That's the definition.
(e) False—An aneurysm is an arterial pathology.

25. (a) True—A patient will have a shortened and externally rotated leg.
(b) False—A patient will have a shortened and externally rotated leg.
(c) False—A family history does not increase or decrease the likelihood of this pathology.
(d) True—All post-op or immobile patients are at an increased risk of DVT.
(e) True—A simple trip is a common cause of a fractured NoF. It is often associated with osteoporosis.

26. (a) False—Diffuse alopecia is not associated with pernicious anaemia.
(b) True—It can be caused by iron deficiency.
(c) False—Zinc deficiency is associated with the disturbance of nail growth.
(d) True—IV heparin can disturb the growth of hair.
(e) True—It is genetically determined in women.

27. (a) True—Streptococcus is a bacterium so an elevated titre suggests infection.
(b) True—If your tonsils have been removed then they cannot become infected (although tonsillectomy will not prevent an acute red throat).
(c) False—The most common glands affected are the submandibular glands.
(d) True—With infection you get an increase in the number of white blood cells.
(e) True—Tonsillitis not only causes a sore throat but the pain may be referred to the ear.

28. (a) True—If you have an elevated BMI you are likely to be less mobile and hence at increased risk.
(b) False—Most DVTs do not break off and cause PE.
(c) False—They are very difficult to diagnose clinically, hence all the ultrasound scanning that gets done.
(d) False—The use of SC heparin decreases the risk but does not remove it and they are a lot more common than you may think.
(e) True—It is alarmingly common.

29. (a) False—UTIs are more common in girls than boys at six years of age.
(b) True—Boys are more likely to get UTIs in the newborn period compared to when they are older.
(c) True—Any infection in children may present as a febrile convulsion.
(d) True—Recurrent UTIs can cause failure to thrive and it is the failure to thrive that can be picked up first.
(e) True—Look at the urine down the microscope – if you can see bacteria then there is a UTI.

30. (a) False—Small for dates babies do not suffer from significant weight loss after they are born.
(b) True—Small for dates babies are at risk of fetal distress which increases their likelihood of meconium aspiration.
(c) True—See above.
(d) True—Small for dates babies are not likely to have laid down enough glycogen stores as they have been expending all their energy on growing.
(e) False—Hyaline membrane disease is a feature of prematurity.

31. (a) True—Breath holding attacks can be precipitated by frustration in the same way tantrums are.
(b) False—Breath holding is not associated with epilepsy.
(c) False—A one year old baby is too immature to attempt to breath hold.
(d) True—Children can hold their breath to the point that they lose consciousness.
(e) False—Phenobarbitone won't help to control them. Parents need to be counselled how to cope.

32. (a) False—The broad ligament does not involve the ovary.
(b) False—The broad ligament does not involve the ureter.

(c) True—The broad ligament does involve the uterine artery.
(d) True—The broad ligament does involve the fallopian tube.
(e) True—The broad ligament does involve the ovarian artery.

33. (a) False—Hydrocortisone isn't effective in bronchiolitis.
(b) False—As viruses cause bronchiolitis antibiotics are of little use.
(c) False—An IV aminophylline infusion does not help in infancy.
(d) True—Humidified oxygen is always better tolerated as it does not lead to the drying of the upper airways.
(e) True—Feeding is a lot of work for infants (you can't eat and breath at the same time) and tube feeding decreases the amount of work.

34. (a) False—Urodynamics should be done prior to surgery and cystoscopy will add nothing in stress incontinence.
(b) True—With all the stretching of the pelvic floor during childbirth it can take some time for things to return to normal.
(c) True—The more stretching, the more problems.
(d) True—A cystogram can distinguish urge from stress incontinence.
(e) True—The two may coexist producing a management challenge.

35. (a) True—All patients who have had a CVA should have their swallowing assessed to prevent aspiration pneumonia.
(b) False—Recurrent laryeal nerve trauma will affect the vocal cords not the oesophagus.
(c) True—Carcinoma of the stomach can lead to swallowing difficulties – initially solids and then later liquids.
(d) False—Dementia does not impede a patient's swallow.
(e) True—Motor neurone disease can affect the swallow reflex.

36. (a) True—Syphilis can lead to nerve injury.
(b) True—Diabetes mellitus can affect the reflex pathways, e.g. diabetic autonomic neuropathy.
(c) False—Gonorrhea will not cause a patient to lose their ankle reflexes.
(d) False—Parkinson's disease will not cause a patient to lose their ankle reflexes.
(e) True—Motor neurone disease can alter your reflexes.

37. (a) False—As the liver is used to metabolizing large quantities of alcohol (a sedative) it is very good at clearing other sedative drugs through enzyme induction.
(b) True—The liver manufactures clotting factors – if the liver is damaged it can't make the clotting factors so you have an increased PT.

(c) True—See 37b.
(d) True—The degree of alcohol excess determines the onset of liver disease.
(e) False—While alcoholics do have many dietary insufficiencies the alcohol excess in itself damages the liver.

38. (a) True—There is a release of antidiuretic hormone to try and conserve body fluid as a response to blood loss.
(b) True—The body loses potassium after trauma.
(c) True—This because the body requires nitrogen for protein synthesis.
(d) False—The body needs sugar to deal with trauma so there is an increase in gluconeogenesis.
(e) True—The body will use lean body mass in the initial response to trauma.

39. (a) True—Colles' fractures are impacted.
(b) False—Colles' fracture is not associated with median nerve damage.
(c) True—Colles' fractures are deviated to the radial side.
(d) False—Colles' fracture will have a posterior and radial displacement, the angulation of the distal fragment will be dorsal. There may be impaction leading to the shortening of the radius compared to the ulnar. Good alignment is required to prevent the development of carpal tunnel syndrome.
(e) False—The fragment is not torn off the intra-articular triangular disc.

40. (a) False—Multiple pregnancies occur in older women.
(b) True—Twin pregnancies are shorter (there's less space).
(c) True—Multiple pregnancies are at a higher risk of most complications.
(d) False—They are usually dizygotic following IVF.
(e) False—Twins occur 1:105 and triplets 1:10,000.

41. (a) True—This does indeed confirm ovulation.
(b) False—Oestrogen does not help in confirming ovulation.
(c) False—There is a temperature rise with ovulation at mid cycle.
(d) False—Spinbarkeit cervical mucus does not confirm ovulation.
(e) True—Histological examination of an endometrial biopsy can confirm ovulation.

42. (a) False—Abortion only requires 2 medical professionals to agree.
(b) True—A medical termination involves giving the woman intravaginal prostaglandins to soften the cervix and stimulate an early labour.
(c) True—Surprising but true.
(d) True—You can't have a suction termination of pregnancy beyond 14 weeks.
(e) False—Mifepristone can be used up to 9 weeks.

43. (a) False—Median nerve injury will cause weak flexion at the wrist and loss of movement at the IP joint of the thumb.
(b) False—The motor deficit leads to loss of opposition of the thumb.
(c) True—The median nerve supplies sensation to the forearm.
(d) False—Upper arm pain is not associated with median nerve injury.
(e) False—Median nerve lesions lead to loss of sensation over the palmar aspect of the thumb, index and middle fingers.

Learn your milestones!

44. (a) True—A 10 month old will demonstrate opposition and will pull themselves to a sitting position.
(b) True—A 12 month old will release objects on request and can walk with one hand held.
(c) False—A three month old child will have a slight head lag when pulled to sit and will hold their hand loosely open.
(d) True—An 18 month old can put 3 words together and can build a tower of 3–4 blocks.
(e) False—A four month old child will hold their hand together, pull clothes over their head and laugh.

45. (a) False—Young men have an increased chance of completing suicide.
(b) False—The rates of suicide vary across the world.
(c) False—A significant proportion of people who complete suicide will have seen a doctor in the week before.
(d) True—People who are unemployed are more likely to complete suicide.
(e) True—People who have a definable mental illness are at increased risk – many psychiatrists feel that depression is almost always present in people who commit suicide.

46. (a) True—Having schizophrenia puts you at a high risk of suicide.
(b) False—Schizophrenia is not generally associated with violence to others.
(c) False—Patients may recover from it. Even if recovery is not complete, there may be remission for long periods.
(d) True—A patient's state of mind surprisingly is not influenced by things around them.
(e) True—Chronic schizophrenics often have a burned out appearance with cognitive impairment.

47. (a) False—Ectopic thyroid tissue would not be at the angle of the mandible.
(b) False—A thyroglossal cyst is a midline structure.
(c) True—There are lymph nodes around the neck which can become inflamed.
(d) False—A pharyngeal pouch is a midline structure.
(e) True—A carotid body tumour arises in the neck.

48. (a) True—Hyperthyroidism is associated with weight loss.
(b) True—Atrial fibrillation can be precipitated by hyperthyroid states.
(c) True—You get lid lag with hyperthyroidism.
(d) True—You get onycholysis with hyperthyroidism.
(e) False—Feeling tired all the time is more commonly associated with hypothyroidism.

49. (a) False—Dementia does not necessarily progress.
(b) False—Pre-senile means young or middle aged, usually defined as onset of less than 65 years.
(c) False—The sleep–wake cycle is often an early sign of dementia.
(d) True—A head injury may precipitate dementia.
(e) False—Mini-mental test scores are more useful at monitoring progression.

50. (a) False—Urinary incontinence is not an early symptom of Parkinson's.
(b) True—A shuffling gate is classic of Parkinson's disease.
(c) False—The onset of symptoms is usually after 50.
(d) True—Cog-wheel rigidity is associated with Parkinson's disease.
(e) False—Patients classically have a resting tremor, so called 'pill rolling.' It may disappear altogether on movement.

247

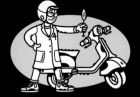

1. Features in the history include the triad of:
   - Syncope.
   - Breathlessness on exertion.
   - Angina pectoris.

   Eventually orthopnoea or paroxysmal nocturnal dyspnoea may develop.

   Features of severe aortic stenosis on examination include:
   - Narrow pulse pressure when recording the blood pressure (e.g. 90/70 mmHg).
   - A slow-rising pulse – small in volume, rises slowly to its peak, and takes a long time to pass the finger.
   - A sustained apex beat suggestive of left ventricular hypertrophy.

2. Features of heart failure include:
   - A displaced apex beat (due to left ventricular volume overload).
   - A third heart sound.
   - An elevated jugular venous pressure.
   - Peripheral oedema.

3. Features of a severe attack of asthma include:
   - Tachycardia (heart rate greater than 110/min).
   - Tachypnoea (respiratory rate greater than 30/min).
   - Pulsus paradoxus greater than 15 mmHg.
   - Peak expiratory flow rate less than 50% predicted maximum for height and weight.
   - Exhaustion.
   - Cyanosis.
   - Silent chest.
   - Bradycardia.
   - Difficulty speaking.

4. Median nerve palsy at the wrist is due to carpal tunnel syndrome. The more common causes include:
   - Pregnancy.
   - Oral contraceptive pill.
   - Hypothyroidism.
   - Rheumatoid arthritis.

   The physical signs include:
   - Wasting of the thenar eminence (if long-standing).
   - Sensory loss over the palmar aspects of the radial three and a half digits.
   - Weakness of abduction, flexion, and opposition of the thumb.
   - Tinel's sign – tingling sensation produced in the distribution of the median nerve by percussion over the carpal tunnel.
   - Phalen's sign – on flexing the wrists for 60 seconds there is an exacerbation of the paraesthesia, which is rapidly relieved when the wrist is extended.

5. The main features of Parkinson's disease are:
   - Tremor (resting, pill-rolling tremor).
   - Bradykinesia.
   - Rigidity ('cogwheel').

   Other features include an expressionless unblinking face, low-volume monotonous speech, drooling from the mouth, and micrographia. Patients have a characteristic stooping shuffling gait, holding their arms by their side.

6. The signs of an acute disc prolapse may include features of compression of the sciatic nerve roots. Straight leg raising will be impaired on one or both sides – ask the patient to lie flat and lift the leg by the ankle with the knee extended. This will reproduce pain going down the back of the leg.

   There may be:
   - Sensory loss over the back of the calf and sole of the foot.
   - Weakness of dorsiflexion of the foot.
   - A reduced ankle reflex.

7. Causes of massive splenomegaly include:
   - Chronic myeloid leukaemia.
   - Myelofibrosis.
   - Chronic malaria.

   Features of a palpable spleen on physical examination are:
   - Location in the left upper quadrant of the abdomen.
   - Movement towards the right lower quadrant on inspiration.
   - Dullness to percussion.
   - There may be a notch on the anterior surface.
   - It is not possible to get above the mass.
   - Firm consistency.
   - It cannot be felt bimanually.

8. Any of the following would be acceptable:
   - Symmetrical distribution of joint disease with redness, swelling, warmth, and tenderness.
   - Predominant inflammation in the proximal interphalangeal and metacarpophalangeal joints with relative sparing of the distal interphalangeal joints.
   - Signs of carpal tunnel syndrome.
   - Rheumatoid nodules behind the elbows.
   - Wasting of the small muscles of the hand.
   - Ulnar deviation of the fingers.
   - Deformity of the fingers (e.g. swan neck deformity, Boutonnière deformity).

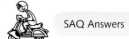

9. The three most common causes of papilloedema are:
   - Intracranial space-occupying lesion.
   - Malignant hypertension.
   - Benign intracranial hypertension.

   Features of these causes include a focal neurological deficit, very high blood pressure, and obesity.

10. Disturbing features on examination can be divided into local and systemic.

    Local features include:
    - Mass fixed to deeper tissues.
    - Mass tethered to the skin.
    - Hard and craggy mass.
    - Peau d'orange.
    - Inverted nipple.
    - Associated axillary lymphadenopathy.

    Systemic features include:
    - Hepatomegaly.
    - Pleural effusion.
    - Local bony tenderness.
    - Ascites.

11. Fig. 1 illustrates X-linked recessive inheritance. Examples include:
    - Colour blindness.
    - Haemophilia A.

    Fig. 2 illustrates autosomal dominant inheritance. Examples include:
    - Adult polycystic kidney disease.
    - Dystrophia myotonica.
    - Hereditary spherocytosis.
    - Neurofibromatosis.

12.
    (a) Cytomegalovirus.
    (b) Pneumocystis carinii, Mycobacterium avium intracellulare, cytomegalovirus.
    (c) Toxoplasma gondii, Cryptococcus neoformans.
    (d) Cryptosporidium.

    Other groups of patients who are at risk of opportunistic infection include transplant recipients who have received immunosuppression and patients receiving chemotherapy or cytotoxic drugs.

13. Iron is found in most meat. This is why vegans are susceptible to iron deficiency anaemia. Deficiency may also result from chronic blood loss (e.g. menorrhagia, hookworm) or malabsorption (e.g. gastrectomy, coeliac disease).

    Folate is found in most foodstuffs, especially liver, green vegetables, and yeast. Deficiency may also arise from malabsorption (e.g. in coeliac disease, Crohn's disease) or excess use (e.g. due to pregnancy, psoriasis).

    Vitamin B_{12} is found in foods of animal origin only such as liver, fish, and dairy produce. Deficiency may also result from pernicious anaemia, or malabsorption in the ileum (e.g. in Crohn's disease).

14. Hypercalcaemia may present non-specifically or through its effect on end-organ damage. The principal sites of presentation include:
    - Kidney – renal stones can cause renal colic, hypercalcuria can cause polyuria and consequent polydipsia.
    - Nervous system – depression, anorexia, nausea and vomiting are common.
    - Gastrointestinal tract – abdominal pain and constipation usually result from hypercalcaemia.
    - Bones – aches and pains.

    Four causes of hypercalcaemia include:
    - Hyperparathyroidism (primary or tertiary).
    - Malignant disease of the bone.
    - Vitamin D excess (e.g. sarcoidosis, iatrogenic).
    - Milk–alkali syndrome.

15. The most likely causes are:
    - Impaired venous drainage of the legs due to the enlarged uterus.
    - Pre-eclampsia.
    - Deep vein thrombosis (increased incidence in pregnancy).

    Discriminatory features on bedside examination would include blood pressure check, signs of periorbital oedema, and urinalysis for pre-eclampsia to exclude proteinuria. Features of inflammation such as redness, warmth, and tenderness would make a deep vein thrombosis more likely.

    Pre-eclampsia may be suggested by the results of a full blood count (thrombocytopenia) and urate and urea and electrolyte estimate (evidence of renal dysfunction). A Doppler ultrasound scan of the leg veins can be performed to look for a deep vein thrombosis. Venography should be avoided if possible due to the radiation exposure to the fetus.

16. The list is almost endless, but some of the more characteristic signs include:
    - Acanthosis nigricans (especially with gastrointestinal tract malignancy).
    - Dermatomyositis (heliotropic rash).
    - Herpes zoster.
    - Erythema gyratum repens (carcinoma of the breast).
    - Acquired ichthyosis (especially lymphoma).
    - Tylosis (thickening of the palms or soles associated with upper gastrointestinal malignancy).
    - Thrombophlebitis migrans (especially carcinoma of the pancreas).

17. Features in the history include:
    - A defined precipitating cause for diabetic ketoacidosis (e.g. infection, missed an insulin injection) or for hypoglycaemia (e.g. known overdosage of hypoglycaemic treatment or missing a meal).

- Time course – ketoacidosis usually develops over hours or days, hypoglycaemia is usually associated with a shorter history of illness.

Features on examination include:
- Dehydration in patients with ketosis. Patients with hypoglycaemia are usually euvolaemic.
- Kussmaul's breathing (deep sighing breathing due to acidosis) in ketosis.
- Sweating (often profound) in a patient with hypoglycaemia.

18. Some questions to ask a patient with suspected hypothyroidism include:
- 'Do you feel more comfortable in warm or cool weather?' to reveal cold intolerance.
- 'Has your weight changed over the past six months?' to reveal weight gain.
- 'Do you have more or less energy now than you used to?' to reveal tiredness, malaise.
- 'Has anyone noticed a change in your facial appearance?'

The most discriminatory signs are:
- Bradycardia.
- Slow-relaxing reflexes – easily demonstrated with the ankle reflex.
- Facial appearance (e.g. dry coarse hair, periorbital swelling, thinning of eyebrows).

19. Drugs causing hyperkalaemia include:
- Potassium supplements given in excess – due to increased gastrointestinal absorption of potassium.
- Potassium-sparing diuretics (e.g. spironolactone, amiloride) – these drugs antagonize the effect of aldosterone on the distal tubule sodium–potassium exchange pump resulting in decreased excretion of potassium into the urine.
- Angiotensin-converting enzyme (ACE) inhibitors – decreased angiotensin results in decreased aldosterone and therefore decreased urinary loss of potassium.
- Nephrotoxic drugs – for example non-steroidal anti-inflammatory drugs (NSAIDs) and aminoglycosides – may cause hyperkalaemia through impaired renal excretion of potassium.

20. Any of the following would be acceptable.
- Haemophilia.
- Blood transfusion in Africa since 1977.
- Sexual partner of a prostitute.
- Intravenous drug user.
- Anal intercourse.
- Multiple sexual partners and unprotected sexual intercourse.
- Sexual partner of an individual in any one of the above groups.

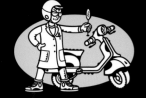

EMQ Answers

1 Theme: Limp (musculoskeletal)

1 (d) Fractured neck of femur—This is a classic presentation and must always be considered in an elderly patient who has pain or mobility problems after a fall, however trivial.
2 (e) Gout—Thiazide diuretics can also cause hyperglycaemia and hypokalaemia.
3 (i) Slipped femoral epiphysis—Avoid the pitfall of labelling such presentation as 'growing pains'.
4 (b) Compartment syndrome—Also known as 'shin splints', this is due to increased pressure in the anterior tibial compartment as a result of swelling or bleeding from a muscle tear.
5 (f) Osteoarthritis of hip—Another classic presentation with referred pain. The patient's knee would be normal on examination (unless he also had OA in that joint!).

2 Theme: Gastrointestinal bleeding

1 (b) Colonic carcinoma—The prognosis is good if detected early, so prompt referral is necessary.
2 (e) Duodenal ulcer—Altered blood almost always comes from haemorrhage in the *upper* GI tract.
3 (g) Haemorrhoids—Haemorrhoids commonly follow, or are exacerbated by childbirth but often resolve spontaneously.
4 (i) Mallory–Weiss tear—Another classic presentation due to tearing at the gastro-oesophageal junction as a result of excess vomiting.
5 (j) Oesophageal varices—Oesophageal varices are associated with portal hypertension caused, in turn, by hepatic cirrhosis.

3 Theme: Liver problems

1 (a) Alcoholic liver disease—Classic signs of hepatic failure.
2 (g) Metastatic liver disease—The patient needs an urgent ultrasound examination and possible liver biopsy; liver function tests would not be particularly helpful at this stage.
3 (b) Biliary atresia—Physiological jaundice.
4 (d) Hepatitis A—The disease is endemic in many parts of the world, and transmission is via the oro-faecal route, usually from consumption of contaminated water or food.
5 (c) Gallstones—In the classic presentation the patient might also have fat intolerance and flatulence!

4 Theme: Cardiac murmurs and added sounds

1 (a) Aortic regurgitation—The early diastolic murmur is best heard at the left sternal edge, with the patient leaning forward and the breath held in expiration.
2 (e) Mitral stenosis—Acquired mitral stenosis is usually due to rheumatic fever, now a very rare disease in the West, but still common in the developing world.

3 (b) Aortic stenosis—Patients may also present with angina even in the absence of severe coronary arterial disease, due to a combination of increased oxygen requirements and fixed flow obstruction.
4 (d) Mitral regurgitation—This often occurs because of papilliary muscle or chordea rupture.
5 (i) Ventricular septal defect—A more common presentation is an asymptomatic ejection systolic murmur detected on routine examination.

5 Theme: Finger clubbing

1 (g) Lung abcess—This is most usually a form of secondary pneumonia with aspiration a key aetological factor.
2 (b) Crohn's disease—The terminal ileum and right side of colon are the sides most frequently affected by the disease, and malabsorption is a key feature.
3 (e) Fibrosing alveolitis—This is an insidious, progressive disease, for good reasons labelled 'cryptogenic'.
4 (f) Infective endocarditis—An increasingly common presentation with a wide range of potential causative agents.
5 (d) Familial clubbing—There is no direct association between asthma and clubbing.

6 Theme: The painful joint

1 (a) Ankylosing spondylitis—The majority of affected persons carry the HLA-B27 antigen, with a male/female ratio of 4:1.
2 (j) Systemic lupus erythematosus—This is the most common multi-system connective tissue disease and is characterised by a wide variety of clinical features and a diverse spectrum of autoantibodies.
3 (g) Reiter's syndrome—There is a strong association with the HLA-B27 antigen, as there is for ankylosing spondylitis.
4 (d) Osteoarthritis—OA is by far the most common form of arthritis, shows a strong association with ageing and is a major cause of pain and disability in the elderly.
5 (c) Gout—Gout is a crystal arthropathy with a strong (over 10:1) male predominance.

7 Theme: Trauma

1 (k) Tension pneumothorax—This develops if the communication between pleura and lung is small and acts as a one way valve, allowing air to enter the pleural space during inspiration, but preventing it from escaping.
2 (f) Open pneumothorax—This occurs when the communication between lung and pleural space does not seal and allows air to transfer freely between the two.
3 (c) Flail chest—This is a clinical syndrome resulting from major trauma to the chest walls, sufficient to cause fracture of several ribs in at least two places,

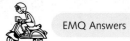

resulting in paradoxical movement of part of the chest on respiration.

4 (a) Airway obstruction—An inhaled foreign body is more likely to enter the right main bronchus.

5 (l) Traumatic aortic rupture—Similar radiological findings in association with severe chest pain radiating to the back is found in aortic dissection.

8 Theme: Heavy periods (or menstrual problems)

1 (d) Fibroids—Fibroids are the commonest uterine tumour, rarely become malignant, and are associated with nulliparity.

2 (e) Hypothyroidism—In contrast hyperthyroidism may be associated with amenorrhoea or oligomenorrhoea.

3 (h) Physiological bleeding—There is no direct association with the oral contraceptive.

4 (g) Pelvic inflammatory disease—Primary infection with Chlamydia may be asymptomic in about 80% of patients.

5 (k) von Willebrand's disease—This is a common inherited, but usually mild bleeding disorder, characterised by a reduced level of von Willebrand factor.

9 Theme: The diabetic eye

1 (b) Background retinopathy—There is no immediate threat to vision.

2 (l) Vitreous haemorrhage—Vitreous haemorrhage frequently resolves, but may be recurrent.

3 (i) Proliferative retinopathy—This requires urgent review and treatment by laser photocoagulation.

4 (c) Central retinal artery occlusion—May have prodromal episodes of transient visual loss (so-called "amaurosis fugax").

5 (d) Central retinal vein occlusion—May lead to rubeosis of the iris with neovascular glaucoma.

10 Theme: Delirium

1 (b) DKA—This is a classic first presentation of diabetes, with children more likely to complain of abdominal pain.

2 (e) Hypercalcaemia—This is a medical emergency, the mainstay of treatment being rehydration and bisphosphonates.

3 (f) Hypercapnia—Respiration in this situation is driven by hypoxia, highlighting the potential dangers of oxygen therapy.

4 (k) Subdural haematoma—A classic presentation which is often insidious in onset, and easily missed.

5 (c) Encephalitis—Herpes simplex is the commonest cause of viral encephalitis in the UK, but insect-borne causes are important in other parts of the world.

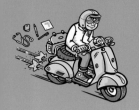

Index

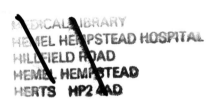